ABORTION PILLS GO GLOBAL

The publisher and the University of California Press Foundation gratefully acknowledge the generous support of Michelle C. Lerach and the Lawrence Grauman, Jr. Fund.

REPRODUCTIVE JUSTICE: A NEW VISION FOR
THE TWENTY-FIRST CENTURY

Edited by Rickie Solinger, Khiara M. Bridges, Zakiya Luna, and Ruby Tapia

"*Abortion Pills Go Global* couldn't be more timely. An important contribution to the geographies of abortion and abortion technology that speaks to how activist practice responds to—and shapes—the legal and regulatory landscapes for reproductive care. If you want to know more about how abortion technology is mobilized within and across national boundaries and how abortion services could better reach those who need them, read this book!"

Maria Fannin, Professor of Human Geography, University of Bristol

"*Abortion Pills Go Global* is excellent, incisive, exacting, and critical. Sydney Calkin's work is always of outstanding quality, and this is no different. The book offers exciting case studies that are intellectually rich and empirically grounded, offering academics and activists regional insights as well as conceptual engagements."

Kath Browne, Professor of Human Geography, University College Dublin

"I cannot think of a more timely and important book in the world right now. Calkin's *Abortion Pills Go Global* effectively situates medical abortion in wider reproductive justice and social decriminalization debates to tell us how abortion happens now and how it is changing the shape of the world we live in. It is not just a must-read for anyone interested in abortion, it is a must-read for anyone interested in geopolitics."

Sophie Harman, Professor of International Politics, Queen Mary University of London

"As well written as it is well researched, Calkin's book is an incredibly thorough and nuanced study of the activist-driven provision of medical abortion pills in Europe and the United States. A must-read for anyone who is interested in knowing, fully and completely, what is happening on the ground."

Mara Clarke, cofounder of Supporting Abortions For Everyone (S.A.F.E.)

ABORTION PILLS

GO GLOBAL

REPRODUCTIVE FREEDOM ACROSS BORDERS

Sydney Calkin

UNIVERSITY OF CALIFORNIA PRESS

University of California Press
Oakland, California

© 2023 by Sydney Calkin

Library of Congress Cataloging-in-Publication Data

Names: Calkin, Sydney, author.
Title: Abortion pills go global : reproductive freedom across
    borders / Sydney Calkin.
Description: Oakland, California : University of California
    Press, [2023] | Includes bibliographical references and index.
Identifiers: LCCN 2023002860 (print) | LCCN 2023002861
    (ebook) | ISBN 9780520391970 (hardback) | ISBN
    9780520391987 (paperback) | ISBN 9780520391994 (ebook)
Subjects: LCSH: Abortion—Political aspects. | Abortion—
    Law and legislation. | Self-management (Psychology) |
    Abortion—Moral and ethical aspects.
Classification: LCC HQ767 .C2526 2023 (print) | LCC
    HQ767 (ebook) | DDC 362.1988/8—dc23/eng/20230417
LC record available at https://lccn.loc.gov/2023002860
LC ebook record available at https://lccn.loc.gov/2023002861

Manufactured in the United States of America

32 31 30 29 28 27 26 25 24 23
10 9 8 7 6 5 4 3 2 1

CONTENTS

ILLUSTRATIONS

ACKNOWLEDGMENTS

I am grateful to all the activists, campaigners, abortion providers, and others who gave their time to be interviewed for this book.

The research for this book would not have been possible without the support of a Leverhulme Trust Early Career Fellowship from 2017 to 2021. University of Durham, University of Birmingham Institute for Advanced Studies, Maynooth University, and Queen Mary University of London School of Geography and Institute for Humanities and Social Sciences supported the research at various stages through funding, research time, and support of research activities. At the University of California Press, I want to thank Rickie Solinger and Naomi Schneider for their support. Erica Millar, Francesca Moore, and Harry Higginson generously read and commented on the full manuscript.

Many people have heard me present elements of this work at workshops and conferences across the years, and I cannot name them all individually. At Durham, where the project started, I thank my colleagues Cheryl McEwan, Louise Amoore, Lauren Martin, Noam Leshem, Kate Coddington, and Siobhan McGrath. At Queen Mary University of London, where the project finished, I am very grateful to Phillipa Williams, Tim Brown, Stephen Taylor, Regan Koch, Simon Reid-Henry, Kavita Datta, Catherine Nash, Kerry Holden, Ella Berny, and others who read chapters of the book and papers related to it. My friends and colleagues Kath Browne, Fiona de Londras, Monika Ewa Kamińska, Cordelia Freeman, Francesca Moore, Stephanie Sodero, Nishpriha Thakur, Gavin Brown, Lai Sze Tso, Sarah Hodges, and

Giulia Zanini supported this project in many different ways during the researching and writing. Olivia Engle contributed superb research and editorial assistance on many of the chapters. Pushpendra Johar, Patrycja Pinkowska, Natalia Wasinska, Paniz Nobahari, and Archanaa Seker contributed research assistance at various points. I sincerely thank them all.

At Abortion Support Network, I want to thank Mara Clarke, Rhi York-Williams, Liza Caruana-Finkel, Hannah Tipple, and the entire phone team for their friendship, support, and solidarity. It has been an honor to work with them.

My thanks and love to my family and friends who have supported me during this project. The Calkins and the Higgies, my family on both sides of the Atlantic, are so dear to me, as are my wonderful friends. I thank my partner, Harry, for our beautiful life together. Before it was on the page, so much of this book came to life through conversations with him on long walks around London.

This book is dedicated to my mother, with love.

Introduction

In summer 2022, pro-choice protesters gathered around the United States to express shock, outrage, and defiance at the Supreme Court's decision in *Dobbs v. Jackson Women's Health Organization*. The Court declared in *Dobbs* that abortion was no longer protected by the Constitution and could be banned altogether by any state that wished to do so. Some states banned abortion within hours of the decision, shuttering clinics immediately, while others committed to passing bans in the following weeks or months. As they marched, the protesters held up signs with slogans about choice, bodily autonomy, and health. They also held up signs with a familiar image of pro-choice protests: the coat hanger. In the decades before legal abortion, death from self-induced abortion with unsafe methods was so common that American coroners trained with medical textbooks that listed the dozens of ways women induced abortion: what they inserted, what they ingested, how they harmed themselves.[1] We won't go back to unsafe methods like the coat hanger, the protesters announced after *Dobbs*.

For all the political and emotional resonance of those coat hanger signs, which evoke a visceral horror at the dangers of self-induced abortion, they depict the past and not the present or future of illegal abortion. Self-managed abortion after 2022 will not be the same as it was before 1973, when the constitutional abortion right was established in *Roe v. Wade*. Abortion pills, developed in the 1980s, offer an alternative to surgical abortion and make safe abortion easier to obtain outside a clinical context. They have permanently changed the landscape of abortion care across the world, in countries with and without legal abortion. To understand the future of abortion in the United States after *Dobbs*, we must reckon with the impact of abortion pills in other countries where they have transformed the safety and availability of clandestine abortions.

———

What if abortion were as simple as ordering a small package of pills online and taking them in your home? What if your abortion could happen at the time and place of your choosing, without traveling to a clinic and without a doctor judging your reasons? What if it could happen without paying hundreds of dollars? Without legislators and courts deciding if, when, and how your abortion should proceed? Abortion would look radically different.

Governments and courts are rolling back abortion rights in the United States, Poland, El Salvador, and other countries. They are making it difficult—or impossible—to obtain a legal abortion. In spite of their efforts, the practicalities of abortion have been transformed by medication abortion, increasing the safety and availability of abortion for people who live in places with restrictive laws. It has also changed the way that restrictive abortion laws operate. Historically, laws governing abortion were written to regulate the conduct of doctors, and governments depended on doctors' cooperation to enforce those laws.[2] When people can safely self-manage abortion without medical supervision, with medication they can obtain online, they can bypass this system of oversight.[3] As a consequence, greater access to safe, self-managed abortion challenges governments' efforts to impose, enforce, and maintain restrictive abortion laws. Self-managed abortion is on the rise, but it is by no means universally available. If, how, and where a person can obtain a medication abortion depends on a complex mix of legal, political, geographic, economic, and social factors.

Abortion Pills Go Global is a book about medication abortion (MA). It follows MA across borders, asking how it changes the politics and geography of abortion when it enters countries with restrictive abortion laws. My analysis is focused on four countries in the midst of seismic shifts on abortion: the United States, Poland, Ireland, and Northern Ireland. While Ireland and Northern Ireland have recently moved from near-total abortion bans to relatively liberal abortion laws, the United States and Poland have moved in the opposite direction. Poland's already restrictive abortion law has recently been tightened. And fifty years after abortion was declared a constitutional right in the United States, this precedent has been overturned and constitutional protections on abortion have been eviscerated. Millions of Americans now live in states where they can obtain abortion only when it is necessary in order to save life, and, in practice, they might not even be able to obtain abortion in that circumstance. The United States and Poland are out of step with the global trend toward more progressive abortion laws, but they are by no means the only places in the world where clandestine abortion is a lifeline. Around the world, people have safe but illegal abortions, accompanied by community providers and lay activists who support them remotely.

Despite their differences, these four countries and their experiences with medication abortion suggest significant trends that we might expect to see in other places in the future. That being said, this book offers no predictions. It is a work of social science scholarship, drawn from abortion research in geography, politics, and law. A geography of abortion might sound puzzling at first, but understanding abortion's spatial arrangement is essential for thinking about access, care, and equality. Abortion travel—domestic and international—is a regular feature of abortion access around the world. What is unavailable at a local hospital might be available at a hospital in a neighboring city, just as what is illegal in one country might be legal across the border. Medication abortion technology challenges us to think more creatively about the geography of abortion and the kinds of mobility that are involved in obtaining it. What is illegal in one country might be easily obtained over the internet from a vendor in another country. In places where neighboring states have vastly different abortion laws, as in the United States after *Dobbs*, borders and jurisdiction will become "the central focus of the abortion battle."[4] As I illustrate in later chapters, borders are also sites of opportunity for medication abortion activists.

This book develops four key arguments. First, MA activism as a movement prioritizes practical accessibility of abortion in the short term as a means to achieve longer-term social and political change. Second, MA is able to transgress social and political boundaries because it challenges prevailing ideas about what abortion is, where it takes place, and who does it. Third, MA travels the globe in ways that make it difficult for authorities to block because it is part of globalized medicine flows that cross borders (sometimes illicitly). Fourth and finally, self-management of abortion with pills makes it very difficult for authorities to enforce restrictive anti-abortion laws because it is difficult to monitor, detect, and prevent but also because criminalizing individuals for obtaining abortions is politically unpopular. I preview each of these arguments in more detail below, after a brief discussion of some key concepts and terminology.

ABORTION IN MEDICINE AND LAW

Restrictive abortion laws do not end the need for abortion, nor do they prevent people from obtaining abortions. They do mean, however, that a greater proportion of abortions are carried out in unsafe conditions.[5] Abortion has its own geography, occurring at higher rates in places where there is greater poverty, less access to quality healthcare, and more restrictive anti-abortion laws.[6] Regardless of the law, many people have abortions. Just under half of all pregnancies worldwide are unintended; of these unintended pregnancies, 56 percent end in abortion. Every year, twenty-five million unsafe abortions occur globally. These unsafe abortions are the product of political choices: they are overwhelmingly concentrated in countries with the most restrictive laws.[7]

Advances in abortion methods have contributed to a decline in injury and death from unsafe abortion. The most important of these advances is the subject of this book: medication abortion. Abortion pills are used in hospitals and clinics around the world where abortion is legally available, but they are also widely used for self-managed abortion, in which a person "performs their own abortion without clinical supervision."[8] Safe self-managed abortion with pills has been an especially important innovation in places with very restrictive abortion laws, where it is difficult or impossible to access abortion care in a medical facility. In fact, medication abortion has transformed the safety and accessibility of abortion outside formal medical settings to the extent that new categories have been introduced to conceptualize it. Instead of seeing all self-managed abortions as unsafe, the World Health Organization (WHO) now categorizes abortions as safe, less safe, and least safe, according to whether they are done with a safe method and a trained provider. A self-managed abortion with pills is not the equivalent of the "dangerous and invasive" secret surgical abortion that many people call to mind when they imagine an illegal abortion.[9]

The legal status of abortion is also important for understanding its safety. The prevailing way of understanding illegal abortion—what scholars call the medico-legal paradigm—assumes a certain relationship between the legality and the safety of abortion. It assumes that only places with legal protections for abortion can provide safe conditions for it to take place and that abortion will almost always be unsafe in places where it is illegal.[10] However, the equation of legality with safety, and illegality with danger, has been upended by self-managed abortion with pills.[11] A safe but illegal medication abortion may not carry the physical risks we associate with earlier generations of illegal abortion, but it still presents challenges: many people lack access to accurate information about how to safely self-manage abortion, are unable to afford medication abortion or do not know where to obtain it, and risk criminalization if their abortion is discovered by state authorities.

Abortion language is always politicized, but even among proponents of medication abortion, there is some confusing terminology and blurring of concepts. For this reason, I cover a few key definitions at the outset. Medication abortion usually involves two drugs: mifepristone, followed twenty-four to forty-eight hours later by misoprostol. Mifepristone blocks the hormones that sustain a pregnancy; misoprostol induces uterine contractions that expel the pregnancy. Mifepristone and misoprostol together are the most effective, but misoprostol on its own is highly effective (and is much easier to obtain and therefore is widely used by itself). Mifepristone and misoprostol together have been shown to result in an abortion without further medical intervention in 95 percent of first trimester pregnancies, compared to 87 percent for misoprostol alone.[12] Because this book deals with medication abortion and self-managed abortion, it is primarily concerned with early abortion, that is, abortion during the first trimester. Medication abortion is also used at later stages of pregnancy, but WHO only recommends self-management of abortion with pills up to twelve weeks into a pregnancy. It is much less safe to self-manage abortion later in pregnancy, because later abortions often require greater medical intervention and clinical capacity.[13] Nonetheless, many people self-manage abortions after the first trimester in places where legal or local abortion care is lacking.

In this book, I use the term "medication abortion" or "MA" to refer to abortion by means of mifepristone and misoprostol. When I want to emphasize the material qualities of these medications, I refer to them as abortion pills, and when I want to emphasize the nonclinical context of an abortion, I use the term "self-managed abortion." Medication abortion is not the same as emergency contraception, although they are frequently confused.[14] It is also important to differentiate between the abortion methods used during the first trimester: medication abortion uses pills to make the body expel the pregnancy, whereas vacuum aspiration (commonly known as surgical abortion) uses suction to empty the uterus.[15] Although widely used, "surgical abortion" is not an accurate label as this kind of abortion involves no cutting or suturing, which is usually associated with a surgical procedure.[16] Despite these technical caveats, I speak about medication abortion and surgical abortion in the book for the sake of consistency and clarity.[17]

Self-managed abortion with pills includes a range of ways to end a pregnancy outside of clinical settings or without direct clinical supervision.[18] It is better understood as a category rather than a specific procedure. Sometimes self-managed abortion involves elements of telemedicine, meaning the provision of remote clinical services like a telephone or email consultation with a doctor. Self-managed abortion might be legal, illegal, or somewhere in between, depending on the country in which it takes place. It is best to imagine the different models of self-managed abortion on a continuum, with some points of overlap:[19]

- ✦ Traditional, in-person care: Appointments with a doctor take place in person. All consultations and tests are done in person. Medicines are prescribed and dispensed in person, and the medications might be taken in the clinic in front of the abortion provider. This model is only available in countries with legal abortion.

- ✦ Partial telemedicine: Tests are carried out in person at a nearby medical facility that is not an abortion clinic. The consultation with the abortion provider is done remotely via telephone or video. Medications are dispensed in person or by mail. This model is only available in countries with legal abortion.

- ✦ "No touch" or full telemedicine: All consultations with the abortion provider are carried out remotely, and medications are dispatched by mail directly to the person's home or somewhere safe where they can be collected later, for example, a post office box. This model is only available in countries with legal abortion. It has become much more widespread since COVID-19.

- ✦ Self-managed abortion with remote support from online feminist networks: There are no home tests, only a remote email consultation with a doctor or other support person. Medications are dispatched by mail. This model is available throughout the world, though it is illegal in many places. It is available, for example, through the organizations Women on Web and Women Help Women.

✦ Self-managed abortion without support: Some people obtain abortion pills through local networks or online pharmacy vendors. They may use these pills to self-manage an abortion without the support of a doctor, lay activist, or community health worker. People who self-manage abortion without support are especially vulnerable to criminalization.

Dividing abortion care into these categories shows the range of services available, but it provides only a rough guide because services are tailored to the geographic context where they operate. In addition, it is common for a few of these models to coexist in the same country at the same time, as in countries where it is difficult or expensive to access legal abortion care and cheaper and easier to access abortion pills through online networks or in the local informal market.

SOCIAL DECRIMINALIZATION BEFORE LEGAL DECRIMINALIZATION

There are many activist movements advocating for access to abortion across the world. They are a large and heterogeneous group, often working in domestic movements to lobby for reforms and facilitate greater local abortion access. There is also a transnational abortion activist movement of people—most of them women—who work to expand access to MA. Sometimes they do this by advocating legal change, but just as often they work outside of legal and political institutions to provide abortion medications and practical information on their safe use. MA activists are skeptical about prioritizing law as a tool to create access, instead working according to the principle that on-the-ground access leads to legal change. They engage with scientific authorities and lawmakers, but they do so by drawing on evidence generated over years of facilitating clandestine abortion.

MA activism operates according to a radical theory of change, probably most akin to what social movement scholars call "prefigurative" politics.[20] This means that rather than protest unjust institutions, activists focus on enacting change immediately, building their own institutions and embodying the changes they want to see. This is a helpful framework for understanding MA activism. It welcomes law reform—especially abortion decriminalization—but it is opposed to modes of activism that concentrate on law at the expense of the practical availability of abortion. The activist networks discussed in this book are engaged in years-long efforts to build sophisticated organizations to obtain MA, supply it, increase awareness of it, provide reliable information about how to use it, and eventually change its legal status. MA activists believe that everyday social acceptance of self-managed abortion runs ahead of legal change. As a Polish activist explained to me, "We don't believe that law creates access—we believe that access creates law."[21] MA activists argue that the informal social decriminalization of abortion pills that is generated by widespread clandestine use can contribute to formal decriminalization and abortion law reform.

Changing abortion's social status is the key goal here. Activists do this by running campaigns to break the silence surrounding abortion, sharing personal stories of abortions, and fighting stigmatizing narratives that claim abortion is traumatizing and shameful. Where abortion is legal but taboo, someone who speaks publicly about having an abortion might risk being harassed or shunned, but they do not risk imprisonment. Where abortion is illegal, speaking publicly about it is another matter entirely. Latin American feminists call this process "social decriminalization": changing abortion's social status among the public and persuading them that it is unacceptable to jail people for having abortions even while it remains criminalized by the state.[22] This strategy has several different aspects. It employs public defiance of abortion laws and facilitates access to safe self-managed abortion with pills.[23] It promotes campaigns to bring abortion into the public conversation and to persuade the public that abortion is a common procedure and a human right.[24] Campaigners counter stigma with empathetic narratives about the prevalence of abortion to persuade the public that abortion exists regardless of the law, and therefore the secrecy in which it is shrouded should end.[25] Social decriminalization combines small everyday activities with spectacular moments of protest and interventions in public institutions.[26] Public defiance of criminal abortion bans is a high-risk strategy in some places, and there are Latin American countries like El Salvador that have been willing to imprison individuals for suspected abortions.[27] Generally, however, there has been little political will among Latin American governments to enforce the criminal abortion bans that they have installed.[28]

Social decriminalization of abortion works on parallel tracks: it provides clandestine abortions regardless of abortion's legal status while mobilizing public opinion against restrictive abortion laws. It does not wait for law to

transform the status of abortion; instead it works to transform the status of abortion through "relentless illegal activism" and then campaigns for the law to catch up.[29] Latin American feminists have enjoyed hard-won successes using this strategy, with recent abortion reforms in Argentina, Mexico, Chile, and Colombia. Feminists in the Republic of Ireland and Northern Ireland have also experienced successes using this strategy, as I show in later chapters of this book. The process of social decriminalization is long and fraught, however, and by no means a linear path to abortion reform, as the chapters on Poland and the United States demonstrate.

There are a few key intellectual starting points for understanding MA activism's theory of change, emphasizing social decriminalization as a catalyst for legal decriminalization. The first is feminist legal theory, which has frequently cautioned feminists against investing too much faith in the power of law to achieve gender justice. There is a limit to what law can achieve when gender inequalities and hierarchies are so deeply entrenched across social structures. There is a further danger to imagining law is the key to unlocking gender equality: because law exercises state power, creating new laws and extending the reach of old laws can have the effect of generating new forms of surveillance and discipline. At the nexus of law, medicine, and women's bodies, Carol Smart warns, we continually see new powers to intervene in and inspect women's lives and lifestyles.[30] Abortion presents a perfect example of Smart's critique: laws that permit abortion, with the approval of a doctor, in a limited set of circumstances require abortion seekers to subject themselves to medical and/or psychological assessment and to express their request in language and behaviors that fit the available legal grounds.[31] People whose circumstances or identity characteristics do not meet expectations about what constitutes a legitimate need for abortion may find themselves refused treatment.[32]

A second key influence is the Reproductive Justice movement, which originated in the United States but whose principles have informed feminist abortion movements around the world. If feminist legal theorists come at their critique of the law from a concern about extending government power further into women's daily lives, Reproductive Justice advocates offer a critique of legal activism that emphasizes the distance between legal institutions and the lives of marginalized people. This view is also informed by the legacy of the women's health movement, which saw medical institutions and authorities as upholding an unjust hierarchy that contributed to women's subordination.[33] Reproductive Justice movement groups see law as a useful tool in some respects, but at a system level they understand law as more invested in preserving an unjust status quo than fulfilling the needs of vulnerable people. They favor grassroots organizing and movement building before engagement with law and legal institutions.[34] This is not to say that Reproductive Justice advocates disregard the law, but they do see it as a sometimes "dangerous preoccupation" of the mainstream reproductive rights movement that has not yet grappled with the limits of a legal strategy.[35] Transforming abortion at a structural level requires several simultaneous forms of feminist work, many of which do not start in the legislature or the courts.[36]

THE SOCIAL LIFE OF MEDICATION ABORTION

Reproductive technologies generate controversy when they disrupt our prevailing sense of what is "natural" in biological reproduction.[37] This is true for reproductive technologies across the spectrum, from hormonal contraception (can sex take place without the possibility of conception?) to in vitro fertilization (can conception take place without sex?). Like all technologies, reproductive technologies are never simply inert implements for human use. The social lives of reproductive technologies are shaped by the relationship between the device, the user's body, the user's geographic position, and the user's social status. The contraceptive coil IUD, for example, has been cast as a technology of both emancipation and oppression, depending on where, when, and by whom it is used. It acquired very different social and technical meanings when its users were imagined as white middle-class mothers in the United States and poor women in the global South because policy makers saw the fertility of these two groups in starkly different terms. A single technology can exist at the center of multiple "scripts" that convey different ideas about the device, its users, and its users' bodies.[38]

For reproductive technologies whose meaning is coproduced and shifts depending on the context, this ambiguity can be productive. Ambiguous reproductive technologies can travel undetected into spaces where abortion and contraception are taboo. Abortion pills are a reproductive technology that disrupts the prevailing assumptions about pregnancy and reproduction. They generate controversy around the question of what abortion is and what it means, because an abortion brought on by consuming pills blurs the lines "between pregnancy and non-pregnancy, miscarriage and abortion."[39] An abortion with pills is medically indistinguishable from a spontaneous miscarriage and sometimes resembles a heavy menstrual period.[40] This ambiguity can be useful for someone who needs to end their pregnancy but lives in a country where that is illegal as they can present at a doctor and receive aftercare without admitting to the abortion.

Misoprostol offers the best example of this productive ambiguity: it is widely accessible for abortion precisely because its effect as an abortifacient was discovered only after it had been licensed to treat stomach ulcers.[41] It is also used to manage incomplete miscarriages and stop postpartum bleeding. Activists first identified misoprostol's abortifacient properties in Brazil in the 1980s. The usage regime for self-managed abortion with misoprostol subsequently emerged through the efforts of Latin American activists and drug sellers "without legal approval and medical guidance."[42] They worked to source the medications, test their efficacy and safety, and determine the best dosage regimes, sharing this information through activist networks. Misoprostol's multiple uses are coproduced in relation to different users. The association between particular bodies and licit/illicit uses of misoprostol is deliberately manipulated by activists. In Argentina, for example, misoprostol activists recommend sending an elderly grandparent to the pharmacy to buy the medicine because their purchase will raise less suspicion about the intended purpose of the misoprostol than if a young woman were to walk into the same pharmacy and buy the same pills.[43]

While pro-choice activists capitalize on the ambiguity of misoprostol, its alternative use as an abortifacient makes the medication a target for anti-abortion forces. Misoprostol is available in many countries as an over-the-counter drug for approved gastric uses, but in the most restrictive anti-abortion countries, misoprostol's abortifacient function has prompted restrictions on its availability for any use. Countries like Brazil, Egypt, and Thailand have removed misoprostol from pharmacies and limited it to hospital physicians only.[44] Where abortion is illegal and/or highly stigmatized but self-managed abortion with pills is widespread, miscarriages can come to be regarded with suspicion, and people who present at a hospital with miscarriages may be treated as criminals.[45] Misoprostol's history of "unscripted" use for abortion makes organizations like the US foreign aid agency (USAID) reluctant to encourage its use for miscarriage management and prevention of postpartum hemorrhage, even though it is recognized as an essential medicine for maternal health.[16] Pfizer, the patent holder for misoprostol, refuses to patent misoprostol for any "reproductive uses" in order to avoid associating

the company with abortion, although it has certainly profited from the popu-
larity of misoprostol's "alternative" function.[47]

Mifepristone lacks this productive ambiguity. Its origin as a drug developed
specifically for abortion has generated a distinctive regulatory geography.[48]
In countries where all abortion is illegal or highly restricted, mifepristone is
neither licensed nor legally available. In countries where surgical abortion is
already legal but highly contested, mifepristone is usually licensed as an alternative abortion method, though it is frequently burdened by extensive
medical regulations that limit its use. The "exceptionalism" surrounding
abortion—it has many more restrictions placed on it than other medical
procedures of comparable safety—means that mifepristone is tightly controlled, even where abortion is legal.[49]

There are key differences between the pill networks that have flourished
in Latin America and those discussed in this book. Where misoprostol is easy
to obtain over the counter, sophisticated support networks to facilitate
misoprostol-only abortion have developed. Across much of Latin American,
misoprostol is approved as a prescription-only medication for the treatment
of ulcers, but in reality it is sold over the counter without a prescription.[50] As
Raquel Drovetta and other scholars show, every country in Latin America
has at least one abortion support hotline that provides information on where
to buy misoprostol, how to use it safely for an abortion, and how to avoid
detection by police.[51] Some of these groups provide in-person support (known
as "accompaniment"), but this is rarer.[52] The widespread sale of misoprostol
over the counter—or on the black market—is fundamental to pro-choice
activism because it means that abortion seekers can obtain the medications
themselves but need information and support to use it successfully. The availability of misoprostol allows Latin American abortion activists to be more
publicly visible in their information-sharing work while maintaining enough
distance to stay safe from prosecution.[53] Activists can advise people on pharmacies or clandestine vendors who will sell them misoprostol without directly
providing it themselves. In contrast, where mifepristone and misoprostol are
not available, activists have to be more directly involved in supplying the
medications. Groups that support misoprostol-only abortion remotely and
groups that facilitate medication abortion by supplying mifepristone and
misoprostol share some important features, primarily in the way they organize
themselves and share information with abortion seekers. But there are significant differences in the ways they work with the pharmaceutical products

themselves, depending on the different regulatory and legal environments in which they operate.

Medication abortion has an ambiguous legal status in some contexts.[54] Because many abortion laws were written to criminalize abortion before the introduction of MA, they concentrate on criminalizing surgical abortion by restricting abortion providers. Many of these laws did not envision a world where people could safely self-manage an abortion without a doctor present. As such, abortion laws written before medication abortion was developed are often poorly suited to regulate it. This can be a source of strength for activists such as those in Poland, discussed in chapter 5, who read their country's highly restrictive abortion law to permit self-managed abortion with pills, although it criminalizes surgical abortion by a doctor. Self-managed abortion has been used as a political tool to scramble the categories used to understand pregnancy and its termination; this is a legacy of earlier feminist abortion activism that is still essential for understanding medication abortion movements today.

Feminists' relationship to reproductive technology is complicated and ambivalent. Science and technology scholars like Donna Haraway have cautioned against the idea that women could truly transform the power relations of biomedicine and science simply by seizing the tools of medical power (e.g., the vaginal speculum).[55] This is part of a larger critique that seeks to puncture simplistic narratives about liberation through technology. Reproductive technologies are always ambiguous, particularly those that prevent or end pregnancies: a long history of feminist writing about contraceptives shows that these technologies can be emancipatory for groups who face pressure to reproduce while at the same time they can be deeply oppressive for groups who are seen as too fertile or whose reproduction is the target of state control.[56] The Reproductive Justice movement mobilized, in part, over the failure of mainstream feminist organizations to recognize that abortion rights and sterilization abuse were linked issues of equal concern for feminists.[57] This debate still resonates in discussion of abortion today.

In relation to medication abortion, feminist ambivalence stems from two main concerns. First, might this technology be coercively imposed on people who do not want to terminate pregnancies? A technology to make abortion easier might also make it easier to coerce someone into an abortion.[58] Second, since medication abortion enables a more autonomous and de-medicalized abortion, without clinical supervision, might it contribute to the rollback of health services? A technology to allow abortion without direct clinical support might harm people for whom health services are badly needed because it could be dispensed without enough caution and in the absence of quality health-care.[59] Technologies are never neutral tools. Their meanings, functions, and effects are always coproduced by their social context. The same technology can be at once empowering and exploitative, so the feminist study of technologies must always seek to hold them accountable to "freedom and justice projects."[60]

MEDICATION ABORTION ACROSS THE GLOBE

How should we understand medication abortion? We could interpret medication abortion by pairing it with surgical abortion—two ways to accomplish the morally and politically contested act of ending a pregnancy. Alternatively, we could interpret medication abortion through some of its material characteristics—as a pharmaceutical drug, a set of pills, and a manufactured product that crosses borders—in order to draw analogies between abortion pills and other biomedical technologies that are controlled or restricted but not used to end pregnancy. To that end, *Abortion Pills Go Global* explores how abortion pills are one of many pharmaceutical products that move across borders from manufacturer to consumer. It is among the first to do so; scholarship on abortion law and activism in North America and Europe has generally treated surgical and medical abortion activism as roughly equivalent methods.[61] To my knowledge, this is the first book to foreground the abortion pills themselves and follow their journeys across the world. The book argues that abortion pill flows are effectively unstoppable because they move through established pipelines that structure the global economy and move various products, including pharmaceuticals, from producer to consumer. Authorities have been unable to fully shut off these flows.

Like all pharmaceutical products, abortion pills are shaped by an intricate regulatory geography. As pharmaceuticals cross borders, they also cross conceptual boundaries, moving between legal and illegal, licit and illicit. These categories are fluid: what is legal/licit in one country might be illegal/illicit just across the border. Equally, something designated as illegal might be socially accepted or tolerated by a government, while something designated as legal might be seen as morally illicit.[62] Pharmaceuticals are able to move across borders with ease for a few reasons. First, the volume of global cargo far exceeds what state agencies can inspect. Much of the cargo that crosses borders goes uninspected.[63] Second, it is often legal to send medications between countries where they are legally produced but illegally supplied.[64] Medication abortion pills are among the medicines that are legally produced but illegally supplied, and their movement shows the fluidity of the systems used to determine the status of pharmaceutical goods. These categories can be difficult to parse as the language used to discuss pharmaceutical products frequently collapses important distinctions: labels like "falsified," "fake," "counterfeit," and "substandard" can be applied to medications depending on how they are produced, tested, packaged, stored, or traded.[65]

The complex routes that pharmaceuticals take as they move across political and regulatory borders provide opportunities for many different actors to intervene, including governments, regulators, private companies, smugglers, and activists, among others. Medications may move from the legitimate supply chain into informal markets at the behest of illicit traders, but this does not necessarily mean that they are criminal actors engaged in nefarious activities. Treatment activists known as buyer's clubs provide the best-known examples of this dynamic. A buyer's club is a community-run organization that works to improve members' access to medications through knowledge sharing and/or distribution of treatments.[66] Buyer's clubs were first identified with HIV/AIDS treatment activists who developed autonomous networks for obtaining unlicensed pharmaceuticals during the 1980s, importing drugs, making their own, and carrying out lay research on treatments.[67]

Buyer's clubs organize to obtain medications that are locally banned or prohibitively expensive. They do this by circumventing criminal laws or intellectual property restrictions on pharmaceuticals. Buyer's clubs like those for HIV/AIDS or medication abortion "organize parallel imports between countries, understanding different levels of pricing or accessibility to medicines" on a nonprofit basis.[68] To this end, buyer's clubs learn the structures of the "pharmaceutical logistics regimes" established by pharmaceutical companies, and they create corresponding "diversion logistics regimes" that make drugs accessible.[69] The anthropologist Mathieu Quet illustrates their operations with the example of Sofosbuvir, an expensive medication for hepatitis C. In 2018, a one-year supply of Sofosbuvir cost $900 in India but $84,000 in the United States. For a period of time, Sofosbuvir was not marketed at all in Australia, so an Australian buyer's club found a supplier for the medicine in India. In violation of pharmaceutical patent laws, they obtained prescriptions from Indian doctors and imported a cheaper, generic version of the branded product to Australia for users in the treatment community. Groups like the Australian Sofosbuvir network illustrate how buyer's clubs deliberately violate various laws, regulations, and social norms that limit what kinds of pharmaceutical products are available where and to whom. Medication abortion activists create their own diversion logistics regimes that play with the laws and regulations across jurisdictions where pills are manufactured, supplied, consumed, and transported.

WHAT NOT TO KNOW ABOUT ABORTION

If self-managed abortion is indeed widespread even where it is illegal, it raises an important question: Where are state authorities in this picture? If medication abortion is making illegal abortion safer, easier, and more available, then shouldn't we expect to see states increase their efforts to detect illegal abortion, criminalize abortion pill users, and intercept all medication abortion pills? I show that the answer to this question is a qualified no.

The question of how states respond to illegal abortion predates self-managed abortion with mifepristone and misoprostol. For as long as there have been restrictive abortion laws, there have been abortions that violated those laws. There have not been, with some notable exceptions,[70] large-scale efforts to identify and criminalize everyone who obtains an abortion outside of the law. Scholars who study this question—and ask, why not?—have developed a theory of abortion ignorance. They refer to it as "strategic," "choreographed," "cultivated," or "manufactured."[71] No matter the label, the meaning is similar: pretending not to know about the prevalence of illegal abortion can be useful for state authorities because it can relieve them of official responsibility to act. In pretending not to know about the reality of clandestine abortion, governments do not have to legislate for it or provide healthcare services for it, and police do not have to prosecute abortion providers or people who undergo abortion.[72] Pretending not to know about illegal abortion allows states to indulge in the comfortable myth that their abortion bans are effective. Abortions that happen in the shadows aren't necessarily invisible but concealed in strategic ways.[73]

Were authorities to decide to crack down on clandestine medication abortions, they might find it difficult for a variety of reasons. First, as discussed above, MA blurs the lines between spontaneous miscarriage and induced abortion. Medically, they are indistinguishable. A doctor could only definitively confirm the use of MA if someone admitted to using it. In practice, doctors who want to identify criminal acts of self-managed abortion distinguish between spontaneous miscarriage and induced abortion through conjecture and stereotypes.[74] Even when doctors report their patients to the police, it is difficult to prove to a legal standard that the patients self-managed an abortion. Second, laws against abortion often criminalize the abortion provider but less often criminalize the person who obtains the abortion. Laws that criminalize abortion providers sometimes require them to be caught "in the act," a designation that is more reminiscent of the backstreet clinic of the past than practices for self-managed abortion with pills today.[75] Third, many states recognize that criminalizing individual abortion seekers would provoke a public backlash. They defend restrictive abortion laws merely as deterrents, essentially admitting that ignorance of the reality of abortion will be embedded in policy. This kind of ignorance requires collective action to prevent some knowledge from being acquired.[76] It reinforces the "prevalence paradox" of abortion: although it is very common, abortion is deeply stigmatized and thus hidden from public view.[77]

Ignorance about clandestine abortion is actively achieved through political choices. Ignorance is not a "simple omission or gap"; instead it can be "actively engineered as part of a deliberate plan."[78] Throughout this book, I show that states choose not to know about the extent of self-managed abortion with pills and choose not to act on that basis. Furthermore, it is often the case that different parts of the state differ in their approach to knowledge or ignorance about abortion. Elected representatives, health agencies, customs agencies, pharmaceutical regulators, police, prosecutors, doctors, and midwives might all take slightly different approaches to the level of knowledge they wish to acquire on clandestine abortion. As a result, they might find themselves with different levels of responsibility for acting on the issue of clandestine abortion if and when it is revealed.

Self-managed abortion can take on the status of a "public secret," meaning something that is "generally known, but cannot be spoken."[79] The public secret can become a powerful social force that implicates the community in forbidden knowledge and forces that community into a performance of not-knowing. By extension, revealing public secrets is transgressive. This observation resonates with the earlier discussion of social decriminalization. Revealing the prevalence of self-managed abortion is a transgressive act that activists do because they believe that forcing public recognition will change attitudes. This has generally been the case in the countries I discuss later in the book: public revelations about clandestine abortion, especially its criminalization, have often moved public attitudes toward greater acceptance of abortion. In some cases, they have also pushed political elites toward greater acceptance of abortion as a fact of daily life, as well as something that the state cannot effectively prohibit. However, this is by no means an automatic consequence of MA activism or public revelations about the scale of self-managed abortion. In some political contexts, even where public attitudes have become more accepting, the political and law enforcement responses are crackdown and criminalization.

It is difficult—but not impossible—for motivated law enforcement to criminalize self-managed abortion, and this book contains several accounts of investigations and prosecutions of people for supplying or using abortion pills. There are certain jurisdictions that actively attempt to criminalize abortion pill users, although even when they do, these cases tend to involve authorities going after individual pill users and their supporters, not well-organized activist groups who supply pills. Across the countries discussed in this book, prosecutions of abortion pill users remain rare. This is true even where states have managed to obstruct the movement of abortion pills into the country (see chaps. 6 and 7). Nonetheless, criminalization of pill users—and activists—occurs in small numbers (see chaps. 3, 5, and 8), and there are worrying signs that we could see more law enforcement crackdowns on self-managed abortion and MA activism in the future.

RESEARCH METHODS AND ETHICS

The practice of self-managed abortion is usually secretive as people who end their own pregnancies face social stigma and are sometimes criminalized for doing so. Likewise, the activists who help them get pills are usually breaking at least a few laws in the process, although whether they risk investigation and prosecution depends on the political context in which they live. Some activists revel in acts of public disobedience against the laws that they believe are unjust. Others prefer more secrecy, anonymity, and protection for their work. These different approaches come into conflict and sometimes cause serious disagreements. Online pill vendors also tend to prefer secrecy, although for different reasons. There is a lucrative market for abortion pills, but this market can only be supplied by vendors who know how to remain anonymous, how to locate their businesses in the right jurisdictions, and how to avoid detection of their products.

Conducting research on this topic with traditional social science methods is very difficult. Anti-abortion stigma is fierce, and enforcement of criminal laws against abortion pill users and activists is highly unpredictable. In researching this book, I have had to make some creative choices about where to look for relevant data, what to include or exclude, and how to protect informants. I have also had to make choices as a scholar-activist working in an abortion support organization. This book makes no pretense of neutrality on the issue of abortion, and it does not strive to present "both sides" of the issue by giving equal space to anti-abortion voices. This choice is the product of feminist political commitments but also academic judgments about the weight of evidence. Abortion is a social good, without which women and pregnant people cannot stand as equals in society. Political commitments aside, abortion is a fact of life that even its most committed opponents cannot eliminate, despite decades of trying.

This book is primarily drawn from eighty interviews conducted between 2017 and 2021 with activists, abortion providers, campaigners, lawyers, politicians, pill suppliers, and others in the medication abortion and abortion rights movements. A full list of interviews is provided in the appendix, along with more information on how interviews were carried out and anonymized. All interviews were conducted with informed consent by participants and approval from my university's ethics committee.[80] All interview participants are anonymous, except where they asked to be named. The book also draws on legislative transcripts, court documents, media coverage, social media discussions, and publicly available web material such as online pharmacy webpages and internet forums on using MA. In several chapters, I provide detailed analysis of illicit abortion pill vendors: GetAbortionPillsNow.com in chapter 1 and Organic Lifestyle Guru in chapter 3. These are pseudonyms. Where quoting from information that is publicly posted online by people who have used abortion pills, I have lightly edited the text so that it is not searchable.[81]

Writing this book involved a set of ethical choices. The book imagines a future in which abortion is safer, widely available, and not controlled by anti-abortion authorities. The ethical dilemmas arose when I confronted the reality of where we are right now: many of the activists interviewed in this book are currently engaged in work that is illegal. Writing a full account of their work could expose them to the risk of prosecution and imprisonment. At a minimum, it could expose their networks to law enforcement or anti-abortion groups that wish to disrupt the movement of abortion pills. For this reason, the information in this book about abortion pill networks and routes is purposely limited. Where I trace the specific logistical pathways through which pills move across borders, I provide detailed information only if it has already been made public in court documents or media accounts.

While many groups in this book remain anonymous, I do name several activist organizations that are central to the global flows of medication abortion. These groups are public about their work. Their names appear in nearly every chapter, so I briefly introduce them here. Women on Waves (launched in 1999) is a Dutch organization founded by Dr. Rebecca Gomperts. It came to global fame through its sporadic campaigns with a mobile abortion clinic onboard a ship that provides medication abortions in international waters. Women on Waves also uses technologies like drones and robots to move medication abortion pills across borders in protest actions, primarily to attract media attention; it does not regularly move pills with these technologies. Women on Web (launched in 2006) is the sister organization of Women on Waves, also founded by Gomperts. Based in Canada, it runs a global online service that sends medication abortion pills from India to people who cannot access abortions where they live. It provides medical consultation before and email support during the self-managed abortion. Aid Access (launched in 2018) runs a service identical to Women on Web but only serves people in the United States. Women Help Women (launched in 2014) is also a Netherlands-based global service providing digital consultations and sending medication abortion pills to abortion seekers. Women Help Women was formed when the majority of the Women on Waves/Web staff quit, over disagreements with Gomperts, and formed a new organization.[82] Women on Web and Women Help Women operate in similar ways, even using some of the same suppliers for medication abortion products, but the two groups have significant strategic differences.[83]

THE STRUCTURE OF THE BOOK

Abortion Pills Go Global examines Ireland, Northern Ireland, Poland, and the United States to answer questions about how abortion pills transform abortion access patterns and politics; it also uses data from India to answer questions about how abortion pills circulate around the globe. The decision to focus on these countries requires some explanation since there are many countries with restrictive abortion laws where people resort to self-managed abortion. First, they are united by the presence of a few sophisticated abortion pill activist networks that share strategies and comprise many of the same people. Second, the restrictive laws and uneven geography of abortion access in all four places has resulted in growing reliance on abortion pill products obtained online. Unlike many countries in Latin America, Africa, and Asia, misoprostol is hard to obtain in pharmacies in these countries, so transnational activist networks liaise between abortion seekers and suppliers that ship the pills from abroad.

Third, self-managed abortion and associated activism in these countries are under-researched. This is partly because Ireland, Northern Ireland, Poland, and the United States tend to be studied through the lens of domestic and international abortion travel. They either border countries with legal abortion or belong to larger territorial entities that have a patchwork of abortion laws, creating extensive abortion travel pathways. Abortion pill activism has been most extensively researched in Latin America because it is the cradle of clandestine self-managed abortion with misoprostol.[84] And fourth, the four countries in this study have seen major changes in their abortion laws since 2018: Ireland and Northern Ireland have recently liberalized their abortion laws, while the United States and Poland have made them more restrictive. A comparison of these countries—and their sharply diverging approaches to abortion—allows us to examine the prospects of and limitations on abortion pill activism.

The arguments introduced above appear throughout the book, but the chapters are organized geographically. We start, in chapter 1, in India. This chapter follows medication abortion pills from their production in the Indian pharmaceutical industry, from which most of the abortion pills discussed in the remainder of the book originate. From India, the book follows abortion pills as they move into countries with restrictive abortion laws: first to the United States, then to Poland, Ireland, and Northern Ireland.

In the United States, where abortion was constitutionally protected from 1973 to 2022, abortion rights are being rapidly rolled back. Medication abortion has been legally available in American abortion clinics since 2000, but the *Dobbs* decision of 2022 will make self-managed abortion outside of a clinic a main abortion method for Americans in the years to come. Chapter 2 addresses MA's official life in abortion law and medicine in the United States, illustrating the strategies that abortion advocates and opponents have used to expand and limit the availability of MA. Chapter 3 turns to MA's unofficial life outside of the medical system, before and after the *Dobbs* decision. It shows that numerous barriers to legal, affordable, local abortion have pushed US abortion seekers online, where there are two main methods for obtaining clandestine abortion: activist groups and online pill vendors. The chapter addresses the impacts of abortion criminalization and the prospect of further criminalization in the future in a rapidly changing legal landscape.

Chapters 4 and 5 turn to Poland. Like the United States, Poland has instituted more restrictive abortion laws in recent years, though it already had a near-total ban. Chapter 4 situates abortion pills in the context of the transformation of Poland's abortion laws since the 1990s from a system of legal abortion to a highly restrictive abortion ban, although abortion remained widely available in the underground. Poland's abortion geography has been reorganized again by MA. Chapter 5 maps the pathways through which people obtain MA, highlighting the ambiguous criminal status of self-managed abortion and the escalating legal threats activists face.

Chapters 6, 7, and 8 turn to the island of Ireland and explore the abortion geography of the Republic of Ireland and Northern Ireland. Chapter 6 illustrates how abortion pills helped catalyze the movement to repeal the 8th amendment in the Republic of Ireland because they offered safe abortion at home and reduced the number of people who traveled abroad to obtain an abortion. Chapter 7 examines the role of abortion pills in the 2018 abortion referendum in Ireland. It shows that abortion pills were central to changing the political consensus among Irish politicians, who came to endorse reform based on their understanding of how easily available and widely used abortion pills were despite Ireland's constitutional ban. Because the abortion pill networks on the island are closely linked in their operations and strategies, chapter 8 looks north to Northern Ireland. Activists working together across Northern Ireland and Ireland set up an underground distribution system, taking advantage of the soft border between the two territories and their separate customs agencies that took different approaches to the importing of abortion pills. This chapter follows abortion pills through Northern Irish politics, concentrating on state efforts to criminalize abortion pill users and activist strategies to achieve reform.

The final chapter returns the focus to the United States and discusses the possibilities and the limitations of medication abortion after *Dobbs*. In the short term, self-managed abortion with pills outside of formal medical settings will be a lifeline for Americans, as it is elsewhere. In the long term, medication abortion activism developed in clandestine contexts should inform the design and delivery of legal abortion services. Self-managed abortion practices, and the activist networks that facilitate them, show us the possibility of a future in which abortion is demedicalized, destigmatized, and decriminalized.

———————

People who self-manage illegal abortions engage in individual acts of resistance to anti-abortion laws. Thousands of people self-managing abortions, with the assistance of transnational activist networks, constitute a form of organized disobedience and defiance of unjust laws. Their actions have political power. This book asks what form that political power takes, how it is channeled by medication abortion activists, whether and how it translates into progressive reforms, and how countries with restrictive laws respond to it.

CHAPTER 1

How Indian Abortion Pills Travel the Globe

It's black market. Any pharmacy selling the abortion pill over the counter is doing it at the risk of their business, but they're doing it because there's definitely money to be made.

— Indian activist

Indian medication abortion travels the globe because it is cheap, plentiful, and easy to transport. To understand how this came to be, I trace MA from the point of manufacture to the point of use. I start with the pills rather than the story of a particular woman seeking an abortion in order to think differently about abortion, by setting aside the familiar image of the abortion clinic and considering instead the handful of tablets that arrive in the mail. Who makes them? Where do they come from? How do they travel? MA treads the fine line between what is informal, illicit, and illegal because of complex regulations on medicines. Legally produced in one place, good-quality generic abortion pills can nonetheless become tagged as fake drugs when they cross a border. Feminist activists supply generic Indian MA to abortion seekers, but so do many online pharmacies that recognize the enormous global demand for abortion pills.

Plenty of countries manufacture medication abortion. But I focus here on MA made in India because these are the products that abortion seekers discussed in later chapters most often obtain on the internet. The Indian online abortion pill vendors discussed here fit neatly into the existing academic literature on unregulated online pharmacies: they offer legally made but illicitly supplied medications without prescription to consumers across the world. However, I am reluctant to follow the scholars who call these pharmacies "rogue" vendors of "fake meds."[1] This implies an element of criminality and carries a misplaced sense of moral judgment. The online market in abortion pills is not reducible to heroic activists or criminal fraudsters. Online vendors sell pills at hundreds of times their wholesale price, but they still sell them for hundreds of dollars less than private clinics charge. Public conversations on illicit abortion pills can stoke anxiety about "risky" drugs bought online, but states that ban abortion put residents at far greater health risk than do online vendors of generic medication abortion.

As abortion pills move from producer to consumer, they travel through regulatory gray areas, navigating legal loopholes between countries, sometimes disguised as other products. Economic geography work on the "illicit" helps explain how different labels are attached to goods as they move across political and regulatory boundaries. "Illicit" is often used as a synonym for "illegal," but there is an important distinction: political and legal processes designate something as illegal, whereas social norms and attitudes determine what is illicit. Not everything illegal is subjected to social stigma or moral judgment. Meanwhile, not everything legal is socially acceptable. Something can be illegal and socially acceptable (marijuana use, for instance). Something can also be legal but socially unacceptable (tax avoidance, for instance). These categories can easily be scrambled as attitudes or laws change. Medication abortion activists' strategy of social decriminalization reflects this system, trying to change the social status of abortion from illicit to licit, even while it remains illegal.

Products acquire these different labels—legal, illegal, licit, illicit—at different times and in different places. Illicitness is not an intrinsic property but "a transient quality" that is linked to goods as they circulate.[2] At every step of a product's commodity chain— with suppliers of materials, producers of components, manufacturers of finished goods, distribution agents, transportation agents, retailers, and consumers—there is the possibility that these categories will intersect in different ways. Placing abortion pills within this framework is the most productive way to understand their status as they cross borders, because in each country where they land, abortion pills recombine these categories. In one country, they may be legal and socially accepted, while just over the border they might be illegal but socially accepted and widely used. The gaps that open up between legal status, political status, and social status present opportunities for change.

Medication abortion is transformative because it makes abortion mobile in new ways. This chapter begins to develop that argument by exploring the tangible, material qualities of medication abortion that make it cheap and easy to move. I start with the recent history of the drug, situating MA in the Indian pharmaceutical industry to understand how it came to be manufactured so widely there and how its production is organized today. Abortion pills move through the same transnational commerce pipelines that allow customers to get many products from across the world quickly and easily, but how? I follow its movements inside India and abroad and conclude with the distribution channels for MA, examining both the feminist activist networks and the online pharmacies that ship pills worldwide.

THE "UNPREGNANCY" PILL

Medication abortion is a combination of misoprostol and mifepristone. Although misoprostol was developed earlier, for a nonabortion purpose, mifepristone was deliberately designed to terminate a pregnancy. Mifepristone was developed in 1980 by a team of French scientists working for the pharmaceutical company Roussel Uclaf (so their creation was dubbed RU-486). Mifepristone is a progesterone antagonist; it blocks the hormone progesterone from acting on the uterus. In pregnancy, progesterone plays a variety of essential functions: it changes the lining of the uterus, helps the embryo implant, reduces the maternal immune system to prevent rejection of the embryo, and reduces uterine contractions that would expel the embryo. A progesterone antagonist prevents all these functions and makes the uterus unable to sustain the pregnancy.[3]

After a drug is developed, it enters clinical trials. If the trials find that it is safe and effective, national regulatory agencies can approve it and pharmaceutical companies can bring it to market. For a patented drug, only the pharmaceutical company that owns the rights can market it; once a drug's patent expires, other companies can manufacture and market it. Medications become available country by country when regulators approve them, patent holders license them, approved manufacturers produce them, and pharmaceutical companies market them. This creates a complex picture that varies between countries and even between states in federal systems. Existing national and subnational medicine regulations do not map neatly onto the transnational flow of pharmaceutical products that shape the way medicines move from producer to consumer. Every regulatory boundary creates opportunities for informal and illicit practices to circumvent it. Mifepristone's long journey from development to clinical use illustrates this dynamic.

After it underwent clinical trials, mifepristone was approved in France in 1988. However, it was quickly withdrawn by Roussel Uclaf in response to threats of boycott from anti-abortion groups in France and the United States. Under pressure from the French government, the company brought the drug back to market and eventually transferred all patent rights to single-product companies to market the drug.[4] While larger pharmaceutical companies could be pressured by threats of boycott against all their products if they continued to produce abortion pills, single-product companies are immune from such campaigns.

The makers of mifepristone anticipated a backlash to their abortion-inducing drug and tried to counteract it in the way they portrayed it. In his memoir, Étienne-Émile Baulieu, the scientist credited with developing mifepristone, tried to "diffuse the strength of the word abortion" by emphasizing mifepristone's effect in the very earliest stage of pregnancy. He advocated for mifepristone to be marketed as an "unpregnancy pill" or a "contragestive," to evoke its similarity to a contraceptive (if a contra-ceptive prevents conception, a contra-gestive prevents gestation).[5] Nonetheless, mifepristone met with opposition from anti-abortion groups. Their public messaging argued that abortion with pills was even worse than surgical abortion because it made pregnancy termination on a large scale too easy. Anti-abortion activists warned that medication abortion meant "chemical warfare."[6] Mifepristone generated an international controversy that entangled governments, pharmaceutical companies, international organizations, and civil society groups. Nonetheless, it was licensed across much of Europe during the 1990s, and by the mid-2000s, it accounted for the majority of abortions in some European countries.[7] Other countries where abortion was already legal but contested delayed its approval for decades (for instance, it was not licensed in Australia until 2012 or in Canada until 2015).[8]

ABORTION PILLS IN INDIA

Bypassing the corporate intellectual property battles ongoing in Europe and the United States, pharmaceutical researchers in Asia synthesized their own versions of mifepristone. Before mifepristone even came to clinical trials in France in 1983, Chinese pharmaceutical companies reverse-engineered the drug and began to produce their own version. China licensed its own mifepristone drug in 1988 based on this copy. Something similar happened in India.

In 1992, scientists at the Indian Institute of Chemical Technology in Hyderabad announced that they had "successfully developed a production process" for mifepristone.[9] Like the Chinese version of mifepristone, Indian mifepristone was a reverse-engineered copy of the Roussel Uclaf drug. Since 1970, Indian law had allowed patents on the method used to manufacture a drug but not the drug molecule itself; in other words, Indian companies could reverse-engineer an alternative manufacturing process and produce legal generic versions of patented pharmaceuticals sold by European and American manufacturers.[10] India allowed so-called process patents on drug manufacturing methods until 2005, when it came into compliance with international intellectual property treaties by ending process patents and permitting patents on finished drug molecules.

Between 1970 and 2005, India established a leading role in the production of low-cost generic medicines for export. During this time, its domestic industry was structured around the goal of reverse-engineering patented drugs and producing them at scale.[11] Domestic firms of all sizes—from the giants Cipla, Ranbaxy, Lupin, and Sun Pharma to smaller firms—relied on national research laboratories to identify new methods for manufacturing patented drugs. Once an alternative production process for a drug was developed, it could be patented by an Indian firm.[12] To name a well-known example, the Indian manufacturer Cipla came to global fame when it reverse-engineered the early antiretroviral known as AZT for the treatment and prevention of HIV. Cipla sold it at a fraction of the price charged for the branded version sold by the American company Burroughs-Wellcome.[13] Mifepristone is a lesser-known drug with a similar history. In fact, the Hyderabad research laboratory where AZT was reverse-engineered was the same that reverse-engineered mifepristone in 1992.[14]

Although Indian chemists reverse-engineered the process to manufacture mifepristone, the drug did not become available domestically for another ten years, when it was licensed in 2002. The following year, the Indian government modified the country's abortion law to allow providers of surgical abortion to prescribe medication abortion up to seven weeks of gestation (now extended to nine weeks). At that point, five companies in India were marketing mifepristone products.[15] This has since risen dramatically: in 2020, researchers from the International Planned Parenthood Federation identified at least twenty-seven brands of mifepristone produced in India alone, although this figure is almost certainly an underestimate.[16] Many of the MA products made in India are manufactured as combination packs—widely known as "combi-packs"—containing one 200 mg pill of mifepristone and four 200 mcg pills of misoprostol. This fixed dose of five pills is the quantity required for a first-trimester abortion, so these medications are packaged together in a single-use unit. Combi-packs with this fixed dose of mifepristone and misoprostol are manufactured and sold around the world, not just on the Indian market. Indian combi-pack products are marketed under a range of colorful names: "Unwanted" (Mankind Pharma); "Pregnot" (Lupin Ltd.); "Pregout" (Akums Drugs and Pharmaceuticals); "KillPreg" (PCI Pharma), and "Undo" (FDC Ltd.). The average pharmacy retail price for a combi-pack is ₹350 to ₹380 ($4.40–$4.75).[17] The combi-pack with a fixed dose of mifepristone and miso-prostol is the pharmaceutical product that I discuss throughout this book.

Abortion has been legal in India since 1971, but its federal system means that the availability of abortion varies significantly based on local regulations, authorities, and norms.[18] India's abortion law is "doctor-centric" in that it maintains criminal laws for abortions and does not establish a right to abortion but instead specifies the circumstances in which doctors can perform abortions without committing a crime.[19] MA accounts for 81 percent of abortions in India, and almost 75 percent of abortions take place with MA outside of a medical facility.[20] Medication abortion is available only with a doctor's prescription. However, in practice, MA can be purchased without prescription in some pharmacies and small shops.

The informal availability of MA in India is driven by a few factors. First, regulations on abortion providers raise the cost of abortion inside health clinics, creating a demand for over-the-counter abortion medications. Second, medication abortion is less widely available than surgical abortion in some healthcare facilities, despite a widespread preference for nonsurgical methods. Third, regulations of pharmacists are often weakly enforced, so there are many pharmacists who take a liberal view of the prescription requirement for MA in their facilities.[21] Fourth, there is wide geographic variation in how and where MA is sold because of different interpretations of regulations, confusion about the legal status of MA, and retailers' fear of falling afoul of drug inspections.[22] The nonprescription availability of this prescription-only drug, combined with the wide range of medication abortion products, creates a vast gray market for abortion pills in India and its neighbors. In Nepal and Bangladesh, an estimated 10 to 25 percent of MA drugs on the market are unregistered and smuggled across the border from India.[23]

Indian abortion politics look very different from those in the other countries studied in this book. Attitudes to abortion in India are shaped by competing norms: the celebration of fertility and the pressure to bear children combined with moral conservatism about sex (especially premarital sex) sharply constrain who is expected to bear children, when, and how many. Long-standing ideas about "overpopulation" and fertility control shape policy frameworks that encourage family planning and normalize abortion for married couples who already have children.[24] Indeed, Indian feminists have demonstrated that coercive population policies have been used there for decades and continue today, encouraged by international family planning organizations.[25] Dramatic inequalities along the lines of class and caste in healthcare shape the way that Indian people can access sexual and reproductive health: even abortions in government hospitals or MA bought over the counter can be unaffordable for the poorest.[26]

Anti-abortion stigma is pervasive in India and makes it difficult for people to find the abortion and contraception services that they need, but this is also compounded by a lack of information among abortion seekers and (in some cases) informal abortion providers.[27] India's legal context for abortion is markedly different from that in the United States, the Republic of Ireland, Northern Ireland, or Poland, and as a result, abortion activism in India takes a different shape. Abortion support activists in India engage in the work of providing practical, nonjudgmental information about how to obtain abortions that are legally protected but seem unavailable to the average abortion seeker. An activist in the south of India explains her work like this:

> I don't have a list of pharmacies that sell pills. In fact, even if I did have a list of pharmacies that sell pills, I wouldn't ever share it. What makes it easy for me is that I will be able to convince somebody: I have the resources—given that it is not illegal in this country—to help you access a safe means of abortion, secretly, without anybody even knowing. That's what I'm promising. That nobody will ever know.[28]

Stigma, lack of information, and financial barriers are the obstacles that she encounters most often. Informal routes to abortion outside of medical settings are popular because they are faster, more private, and sometimes cheaper but not because of the prevailing legal framework. In fact, the same activist tries to dissuade service users from pursuing informal routes to obtain medication abortion.

I will take you to a doctor, and we will get this sorted. Or you can go to this doctor, at a private clinic, you can get this sorted. . . . Basically I have to convince them out of trying to go find the pill in the black market. And I also have to warn them that finding the pill in the black market might cost them twice as much as going to a doctor, getting a consultation, and being prescribed the abortion pills.[29]

Abortion pills are available across India from a variety of retailers that sell them—illegally—to people without prescriptions. A relatively liberal abortion law, however, exists in a country of profound inequalities in access to healthcare where it can be harder to get the prescription than the pills. This economic context, combined with anti-abortion stigma and highly stratified fertility politics, means that there is a large gray market for MA inside India that leaks abroad.

INDIA'S PHARMACEUTICAL LANDSCAPE

After coming into compliance with international patent treaties in 2005, India became "the world's key geographic site for production and export of global generics."[30] Indian firms were attractive as acquisitions or subcontractors for global multinationals that wanted to outsource production, specialize in generics, and expand into new markets. Today India is the third largest source of global pharmaceuticals by volume.[31] India's pharmaceutical industry with specialization in the production of low-cost generics has been important in campaigns for global access to medicines, lending it the reputation of "pharmacy to the world."[32]

India's large pharmaceutical manufacturing sector is made up of a few different types of firms. The top tier comprises large Indian multinationals that produce generic drugs, like Cipla or Sun Pharma, as well as foreign multinationals that have outsourced some manufacturing to India or purchased Indian companies as manufacturing bases. Export-oriented firms must meet particular national manufacturing standards, depending on the country to which they export. One indication of this changing pharmaceutical geography is the regulatory presence of the US Food and Drug Administration, which opened permanent offices in New Delhi and Mumbai to inspect the many Indian firms that export to the United States.[33] The middle tier comprises firms that produce for the domestic market but do not meet the criteria for export. The bottom tier comprises small firms with less quality control and no export capacity.[34]

In practice, these different tiers may coexist within the same firm. For instance, firms might have multiple plants with different levels of export approval, or a firm might subcontract to a lower-tier manufacturer to increase its supply of a certain product.[35] The industry is structured by thousands of firms and tens of thousands of manufacturing units, all of which work with distributors to move their products to retailers. To add to this complexity, each Indian state has its own medicines control agency and the levels of regulation vary among them.[36] Indian firms concentrate less on producing active ingredients than on formulating the medicines in their final stage, for example, by combining active ingredients and bulking agents into pills.[37] Across all tiers of the industry, most of the active pharmaceutical ingredients are imported from China. Products that are manufactured in India thus might undergo the final stages of formulation there, but their ingredients will likely have been produced elsewhere.

Abortion pills are manufactured by numerous firms across the spectrum of the Indian pharmaceutical industry. Large Indian multinationals like Sun Pharma, Zydus Cadila, Nicolas Piramal, and Cipla have their own brands, as do numerous smaller firms that produce only for the domestic market.[38] The large multinational firm Sun Pharma, headquartered in India, markets a combi-pack called Medabon that is licensed for use in the United Kingdom, Romania, Tunisia, and Ghana, among other countries. The medium-size enterprise Alliaance Biotech exports a combi-pack called Mifekit for sale in West Africa. The small manufacturer Jaksh Pharma sells a combi-pack called Clearfast-Kit in the Indian domestic market only. In theory, each of these products has a distinct regulatory geography. In practice, all three of these kits are available to buy online from third-party vendors that ship worldwide.

Dozens of MA products are legally made in India for domestic and foreign markets, but anti-abortion stigma still shrouds the issue. In the course of this research, I sought interviews with every Indian pharmaceutical company whose products I could find advertised on online pharmacy websites. In the few instances that pharmaceutical executives agreed to be interviewed, they were reluctant to discuss the abortion pill products they manufactured. Some denied making any abortion pill products, despite clear evidence that they do so.[39] Several manufacturers explained that they make pills for export only, so any responsibility for inappropriately sold pills lies with the distributor and importer abroad.[40] In one interesting instance, a pharmaceutical manufacturer wrongly asserted that abortion was illegal in India, so his company could not make MA. After my research assistant persisted, indicating that he already knew about the legal status of abortion in India, the manufacturer loosened up and admitted that his company currently produced abortion pills but only for export.[41] Manufacturers' reluctance to discuss these medicines—licensed generics, legally produced in a country where abortion is legal—demonstrates the way that anti-abortion sentiment can blur boundaries between what is legal, illegal, licit, and illicit. Legally made products can appear socially illicit if they are stigmatized and surrounded by secrecy.

The public conversation about Indian pharmaceuticals in North America and Europe has often been dominated by suspicions about fake and counterfeit drugs. When I explain the different tiers of the pharmaceutical industry that make MA and the informal routes that MA takes, I do not mean to suggest that these products are of low quality or adulterated. In fact, the best available evidence suggests that Indian MA sold online is good-quality generic medicine. Only one study has attempted to understand the authenticity and quality of combi-packs sold online: in 2018, Chloe Murtagh and colleagues published the results of a "mystery shopper" study of online medication abortion products.[42] They chemically analyzed twenty abortion pill packs purchased from online pharmacy sites like AbortionPillRX.co and MTPkit24.com. All the products they received came from Indian manufacturers, and none were licensed for export to the United States (where the researchers received the packages). For a combi-pack that would have retailed in India for $5 to $10, the researchers paid between $150 and $350. When they tested the chemical components, Murtagh et al. found that all the mifepristone products contained the correct ingredients in adequate concentrations. They found that the misoprostol products also contained the correct ingredients, but some were degraded and contained less active ingredient than what was stated on the label.[43] If these products have a reputation for being fake drugs, that tells us something interesting about the categories that are used to label medicines as they move across borders rather than their chemical composition.

THE GLOBAL GEOGRAPHY OF MEDICINES

As goods cross borders, there are many different points where they can fall afoul of local regulations and become illicit. Legally produced but illicitly supplied medicine is a growing market. In fact, it is possible to move illicit pharmaceutical products across borders without committing a crime. When a buyer and a seller are located in different countries, they can circumvent certain national regulatory systems for medicines. A nonabortion example is Kamagra, a generic version of Viagra, which is no longer under patent. Kamagra is not licensed in the United Kingdom, but it is not a controlled drug prohibited by the nation's Misuse of Drugs Act. For this reason, someone in the United Kingdom could order Kamagra online from a pharmaceutical distributor in India without breaking UK laws, and the distributor could sell this product to a UK customer without breaking Indian laws. Selling prescription-only medicine without a prescription is a crime if the buyer and the seller are in the same country. But prescription-only medicines can be supplied from abroad without any criminal offense being committed.[44]

I emphasize the links between legally produced and illicitly supplied medications to show how abortion pills fit into broader conversations about economic globalization. The conventional analysis of illicit economies sees illicitness as a property of certain goods (e.g., counterfeit luxury fashion goods) or certain groups of people (e.g., organized criminal networks). This blinds us to the way that licit and illicit economies are intertwined. Scholars use terms like "deviant globalization" or "counter-geography of globalization" to evoke this relationship: informal or illicit economies use the infrastructure and regulatory structures of the formal economy, but they do so in a way that exploits gaps and differences in regulations across local, national, and regional boundaries.[45] Medications that are legally produced but illegally supplied illustrate this conceptual argument about globalization. Transnational flows of abortion pills via the internet, seemingly untethered to national regulations, are actually shaped by the physical infrastructures and national laws in the countries through which they move.

Goods like these can only move across borders with speed, ease, and anonymity because they are part of a larger system of borderless transnational commerce. The features of this system appear abstract, but they are the material vectors of economic globalization. Supply chain pipelines for goods move across national borders, creating new jurisdictions outside of state control.[46] Special economic zones facilitate these transnational pipelines, sitting within state territory but operating under a distinct set of laws and regulations. They attract business and investment by offering a less restrictive tax, labor rights, health, and safety environment than the state where they are located. Free ports and free trade zones allow commodities to transit with few restrictions and plenty of opportunities to disguise their origins.[47] The enormous quantity of cargo moving around the globe means that most of it is not physically inspected by regulatory authorities. Instead, when cargo crosses borders, regulators must trust that the description of the cargo is accurate.[48] Together, the infrastructure for cross-border commerce and the technologies to move goods quickly have transformed global production. This system is notable not just for its speed, but for its volume, which can overwhelm the institutions set up to monitor it.

HOW DO ABORTION PILLS MOVE?

Broadly speaking, there are two pathways for illicit abortion pills to move from Indian producers to consumers abroad. The first pathway is through transnational feminist networks that place individual or bulk orders for their service users. This method is often clandestine but relatively formalized, and the feminist networks inform their clients that they are obtaining "safe but illegal" medication. Here I illustrate the feminist networks' methods through the example of Women on Web (WoW) because that organization has been deliberately public about its process for obtaining pills.[49] The second pathway, discussed in the next section, is online pharmacies, a large and ever-changing group of vendors that sell prescription-only products directly to consumers. This method is also clandestine, but it is highly informal, and these vendors often misrepresent their services, their location, the status of their products, or the brands they supply.

Since 2006, WoW has supplied abortion pills to people through the postal system. When an abortion seeker contacts WoW, the help desk's shift doctor provides an online consultation. Next, the doctor writes a prescription and sends it to NN Agencies, a pharmaceutical distributor located in Nagpur, Maharashtra state, India. For individual orders, NN Agencies fills the prescription by sending a single combi-pack kit to the address provided by WoW. Often this is the home address of the recipient, but it might also be a holding address like a post office where the pills can be collected later. The drugs commissioner and customs offices in Mumbai clear pill shipments before they are dispatched.[50] WoW's service users often receive parcel tracking information so that they can follow the medications as they cross borders. For bulk orders, NN Agencies uses a similar process: when a purchase order comes in for a bulk shipment of combi-packs, the distributor applies for a no objection certificate from export offices in Mumbai or Delhi and then sends the shipments abroad. Mifepristone and misoprostol are not controlled substances in India, and there is no law prohibiting their export.[51]

When particular brands of abortion pills are publicly associated with feminist pill networks or when law enforcement agencies attempt to intercept shipments of pills, the pharmaceutical firms that market these brands come under scrutiny. In one such instance, a particular brand of MA and the pharmaceutical firm marketing it were named in court filings and contacted by a national drug regulatory agency. I interviewed the president of this firm shortly afterward. Although he expressed his support for the work of feminist pill networks "in principle," his response to the regulatory agency emphasized the many links in the chain between his firm and the person self-managing an abortion with his product.

> We let them know that we can't control it—the products that are being imported are [our products]. But we can't control who buys those products in India and puts them in a bag and ships them across the ocean. . . . We support the principles of what [the feminist networks] are doing, but we're not selling to [them]. We're selling to a distributor in India or to a pharmacy in India, and someone's walking in off the street and buying those products off the shelf in India and then doing what [the feminist networks] are doing. . . . They're going to commercial distributors, in India for the most part, and they're buying it. They know—because it's from [our company], because they know [us]—that it's good quality and the price is usually a very good price point. So it isn't that we're selling to them—they're doing that on their own.[52]

Feminist networks like Women on Web and Women Help Women use this regulatory ambiguity to supply pills to users across the world. Law enforcement agencies have occasionally succeeded in their efforts to stop the flow of abortion pills, but they are generally only able to stop pills when they intercept them at the customs border. American, Irish, or Polish authorities lack jurisdiction over Indian pharmaceutical manufacturers and the companies that market these products. Furthermore, the products that enter illicit abortion pill markets (online or offline) are the same as those that constitute the legitimate supply of abortion pill products. When supplied by a vendor that is not licensed or when not prescribed by a doctor, the combi-pack kit that the consumer buys might be understood by regulatory authorities as illicit or fraudulent. But it might be the very same brand that is licensed for sale in a different country and dispensed in healthcare facilities there.

ONLINE PILL VENDORS

An internet search for abortion pills returns dozens of sites built to sell one product: AbortionKits.com, AbortionPillRX.com, AbortionPills247.com, BestAbortionPill.com, BuyMifeprex.com, MifegestKit.com, MTPkit.com, RU486pills.com, and SafeAbortionRX.com, to name just a few. Sites like these sell abortion combi-packs made by middle-tier Indian manufacturers. How do these products move from the pharmaceutical manufacturers that are licensed to make them to online vendors that sell them abroad via unregulated channels?

Indian pharmaceuticals move from manufacturer to end user through a series of intermediaries. These drug distributors are the "invisible linchpin" connecting consumers and their medicines.[53] Manufacturers send their products to distributors in each state where the product will be sold. Distributors sell the products to stockists or wholesalers, which then sell the products to retail pharmacists. Retail pharmacists dispense the products to patients, either over the counter (if no prescription is required) or with a prescription. Scholarship on the pharmaceutical distribution system in India emphasizes its complex and leaky nature: as medicines move along the pipeline, crossing geographic and regulatory borders, they can be diverted and enter an illicit system of supply.[54] Dispensed medicines, unconsumed doses, and prescriptions might be traded or sold on.[55]

Suppliers and buyers of abortion pills engage in all sorts of illicit practices because, although abortion is legal in India and MA is cheap and mass produced, it can be difficult to obtain MA in the formal medical system. As a result, abortion pills are widely sold in informal ways, and stories about illicit abortion pill sales regularly make national headlines. In summer 2021, two states saw complaints, investigations, and arrests for the illegal sale of abortion pills. The first incident, in Maharashtra, concerned the sale of abortion pills without prescription through online platforms; the second incident, in Gujarat, concerned the falsification of purchase orders and the stockpiling of abortion pills by distributors. Neither raid was definitively linked to the abortion pill websites I discuss in this chapter. Nonetheless, the raids, their coverage, and the pill networks they exposed provide useful information about the routes that Indian abortion products take when they are diverted from the legitimate supply chain and sold by illicit vendors.

In Maharashtra, raids were triggered by sting operations conducted by pharmacists' associations. Powerful professional associations of pharmacists and druggists operate in India at the federal and state levels, mediating between pharmaceutical firms, government agencies, and retailers. Indian pharmacists had recently gone on strike to protest the rise in illicit online pharmacies and their impact on brick-and-mortar pharmacy businesses.[56] Pharmacists argued that online drug sellers operated with impunity and that the drug control agencies failed to enforce the laws.

As part of this wider campaign, pharmacists' associations ordered abortion pills from online platforms and then went public with the products they obtained. Giving false names, pharmacists from the Pune Chemists' Association obtained abortion combi-pack kits from Amazon, including A-Kare (marketed by DKT International) and Unwanted Kit (marketed by Mankind Pharma). Pharmacists sent the kits, with a complaint letter, to the state drug control agency and spoke to the press about how easily they had obtained the medications through the post without prescriptions.[57] A law enforcement official from the Maharashtra drug control agency who was involved in the raids explained that 50 to 60 percent of cases against illicit abortion pill vendors begin with complaints by pharmacists' associations. Law enforcement agents try to identify other "mediator agencies" that are engaged in this illicit trade by monitoring their advertisements in newspapers, on TV, and in other media. Frequently they find vendors selling abortion pills alongside products like Viagra, sleeping pills, and codeine syrup.[58]

This kind of media spectacle—and the public anxiety about illicit medicines that it generates—is not limited to abortion pills. Scandals about so-called fake drugs are regularly covered in the Indian press because of widespread public anxiety over the possible contamination of the drug supply with falsified and counterfeit products.[59] Drugs can acquire the label of fake or falsified products not because of problems in manufacturing but because of irregularities in packaging, distribution, regulatory authority, and mobility. Depending on its geography and the logistics of its journey, the same medicine "can be legal or illegal, cheap or expensive, considered efficient or dangerous," and so forth.[60] For this reason, scholars of pharmaceuticals challenge us to consider the way that the perceived quality or value of a drug is produced by what is outside the drug rather than what is inside it.[61]

We see this process at work in the responses to the Pune Chemists' Association complaint. As a Maharashtra drug inspector explained, medication abortion is not itself illegal. It is not a banned substance. When it is sold without prescription, he explained, it becomes illegal.[62] The Pune chemists obtained branded generics through Amazon, but there was nothing to indicate contamination or adulteration of these products. Nonetheless, the illicit abortion pill sales were covered in the press as acts of criminality that posed risks to public health. News reporting of the incident emphasized the danger of medical complications from abortion.[63] It is not illegal to obtain medication abortion with a prescription, so some of the anxiety reflected in this press coverage can be interpreted through what Julia Hornberger calls the "performative" world of drug security: this entails the public-facing pronouncements and activities where boundaries between "real" and "fake" drugs are produced and reinforced.[64] It also reflects the ambiguous status of abortion in India: abortion is legal but stigmatized because of its association with sex-selective abortion, skewed sex ratios, and the growing power of Hindu nationalist discourses on population and ethnicity.[65] Legal but often perceived and experienced as illicit, abortion is still a fraught subject in India.

The Gujarat incident sheds light on the way that abortion pills are diverted from the formal pharmaceutical supply chain into informal markets. In summer 2021, the Gujarat drug control agency raided four locations and seized 24,000 abortion combi-packs that were being sold online without prescription. Agency officers arrested several owners of a pharmaceutical distribution business that stored the products and the man responsible for selling them online. As the "kingpin" in the scheme, the agency named an employee of DKT India, part of DKT International, a nonprofit that is among the world's largest private providers of family planning products. Officials reported that the DKT India employee had pressured a pharmacist to write fake prescriptions for abortion pills and then sold those pills online.[66] Police charged one person in the scheme with selling 800 combi-packs through an online platform.[67] Gujarat officials identified a few brands in their raids, including A-Kare, marketed by DKT India, the employer of the man at the center of the diversion operation. A-Kare is one of the brands that WoW uses most often. The product took on a somewhat iconic status in Ireland when a member of Parliament brought a package of A-Kare into the debating chamber and campaigners for abortion reform posed outside the legislature with oversized A-Kare pill boxes (see chap. 7). Such a connection vividly illustrates the ambiguity of India's illicit abortion pill economy, where abortion pill supplies are diverted from the formal supply chain of branded and unbranded generics, into informal networks that sell them and ship them abroad.

GETABORTIONPILLSNOW.COM

The last piece of the distribution puzzle is the online pharmacies that sell abortion pill products directly to the consumer—without prescription and at a significant markup over retail price. Rablon Healthcare, an Indian company registered at an address in Mumbai, provides an instructive example here. In 2019, the US Food and Drug Administration (FDA) issued Rablon a warning letter, demanding that Rablon "immediately cease offering violative drugs for sale to U.S. consumers."[68] In its letter, the FDA accused Rablon of "offering 'Abortion Pill Pack' without requiring a prescription," in violation of US law. However, because the FDA lacked jurisdiction over the company, it could only "request" that the company cease its prohibited activities. The FDA identified eighty-seven Web domains that Rablon used to sell generic pharmaceuticals, including dozens of domains with names like Abortion-Online.com, FastAbortion.com, NoPregnancy.net, and AbortionKit.net. Most of these domains were taken down after the 2019 letter, but as of 2022, some of them still advertise prescription drugs, including abortion pills.[69]

Here I provide an analysis of twenty-nine online abortion pill websites, including those named in the FDA's letter to Rablon, Murtagh et al.'s 2018 mystery shopper analysis, websites used by activists I have interviewed, and websites that sold single pill packets to individual buyers I have interviewed.[70] Many of these sites represent themselves as located in Europe or North America, but they are likely based in India, or at least closely connected to India, because all of them share at least one of the following characteristics: they list an Indian phone number as their primary contact; they are listed as part of a company registered in India; they exclusively advertise Indian abortion pill products; they are part of a network of pharmacy domains in which some of them are registered at Indian addresses; or buyers of pills from these sites told me that their pills were shipped from India, based on their parcels' tracking information.

I collected the text and images from the pages of each site (About Us, How to Order, Shipping, Prescription Policy, etc.) and information about the abortion pill products they sold. Whenever these sites provided contact information, I attempted to contact them by email or by phone. Despite dozens of emails and calls over two years, I was only able to interview two people affiliated with these sites. My interview requests generally elicited skeptical responses. In one case, an abortion pill vendor assumed my request for an interview for this study was either a cover or a lie. The vendor responded, "How many kits do you want? Cut the crap and come to the point. We have FedEx, DHL, USPS delivery around the world." In the interviews with illicit vendors that I did obtain, the respondents were often cagey and misleading, sometimes giving me information that I knew to be false. This is understandable, because people running illicit pharmacy sites plainly have reasons to distrust strangers who ask questions about their business.

The online pharmacies that sell abortion pills are typical of what the criminologists Alexandra Hall and Georgios Antonopoulos call "rogue pharmacies": they are knowingly involved in the online sale of medications outside of law and regulation. Rogue pharmacies sell prescription-only medication without prescription or after asking customers to "virtually discuss" their health needs (in practice, this amounts to a prescription waiver). They typically own dozens of domains, all of which route to a few payment gateways. They use a few domain registrars that are known to ignore law enforcement requests. They often misrepresent their locations based on the customer group being targeted. For instance, a pharmacy targeting American clientele might pose as a Canadian business to capitalize on the association of Canada with low-cost pharmaceuticals. The products offered by the online pharmacies also vary depending on their customer base. Where healthcare is privatized, customers are likely to seek out prescription-only drugs that are expensive in their domestic healthcare system. Where healthcare is public and prescription-only drugs are cheap in the formal system, customers are more likely to seek out so-called lifestyle drugs, for example, anabolic steroids.[71]

My analysis of twenty-nine websites showed remarkable consistency across them. Rather than quantify their most common features, here I discuss one of the sites that is representative of the entire sample. I pseudonymously call it GetAbortionPillsNow.com. This site is part of a network of at least ten abortion pill domains, all of which are run by the same company. Other domains in the network advertise generic erectile dysfunction medications, generic chemotherapy medications, and generic psychiatric medications, with separate domains designed to sell each product to a different group of consumers. These sites regularly appear and disappear, reemerging under new URLs. Many of them appear to be run by a single entity with dozens of different domains.[72] This is common in illicit online pharmacy operations for any type of medical product: a single vendor might run hundreds of domains leading to the same payment portal.[73] GetAbortionPillsNow.com has numerous features that typify illicit online pharmacies in general: it displays dozens of customer testimonials, all written in ungrammatical English; it offers discounts for bulk orders; it displays an obviously phony address for the business; it requires no prescription; it promises anonymity and discreet packaging for the buyer; and it relies on payment intermediaries like PayPal and Bitcoin.[74]

GetAbortionPillsNow.com only sells abortion pill combi-packs made by Indian manufacturers. It advertises products like the Mifegest combi-pack made by the large multinational Zydus Cadila and the Mifepro mifepristone product made by HLL Lifecare.[75] The site elides the difference between the mifepristone product Mifepro (only licensed in India) and the US FDA-approved Mifeprex. Customers who are not wise to the dozens of mifepristone brands and their different approval statuses among countries might assume that Mifegest, Mifeprex, and Mifepro are the same product. Their confusion would be understandable: mifepristone is marketed in different countries as Mifeprex, Mifegyne, Mefaprix, Mifegest, Mifabort, and Mifeprin, among many other similar names.[76] GetAbortionPillsNow.com encourages this confusion by repeatedly touting its products as FDA approved. Visual cues, like American flags, stock images of doctors in white coats, and quality seals stamped "FDA approved" lend credibility to the site. Customers might also be persuaded of the authenticity of sites like this because they often contain pages stating their commitment to the right to abortion and they post blog entries deploring the lack of safe abortion around the world. I conducted an interview with the person who operates a network of similar sites, in which he reported that 95 percent of his customers live in the United States. As of 2020, before the *Dobbs* decision, he estimated two hundred to three hundred monthly customers in the United States for each website in the network.

Depending on the product, customers on GetAbortionPillsNow.com can choose from a variety of shipping routes. They cost between $65 and $110, but the cheapest option takes up to twenty-five days, compared to seven days for the most expensive option. For someone who urgently needs these pills to end a pregnancy, waiting three weeks or more is a risk. For the higher price of $110, customers are promised express delivery "from our USA warehouse." This "USA warehouse" is in fact a network of people who are recruited from among customers already on the site. GetAbortionPillsNow.com gives discounts to customers who order in bulk—known as "affiliates." When the site needs to fulfill an order with express shipping, it finds an affiliate who can dispatch the order from the supply they already hold in the United States through domestic mail. To ease their transportation process, these online vendors do not mark their products as pharmaceuticals when they are shipped, as other research has shown. Some vendors include small items like phone charging cables or necklaces in the packages to disguise their contents. Some ship pill packs that have been slightly damaged, with a pin prick in each sealed chamber of the blister pack, to make the medication harder to identify by postal workers or postal scanning equipment.[77]

The site I call GetAbortionPillsNow.com is only one vendor. Dozens of similar sites exist to serve the global market for self-managed abortion. As mentioned above, they disappear and reappear regularly as they seek to avoid scrutiny by law enforcement authorities. They operate in a gray area, selling legitimately produced medicines but in ways that are not compliant with regulations in their country of production and/or their country of consumption. Online vendors of abortion pills are ambiguous figures: they engage in deception and profiteering in some cases, but they nonetheless supply essential medicines to people with no other source for them. The products sold by these sites are easier to get in some markets than others because of differences in the way law enforcement authorities treat imported pharmaceutical products and the extent to which the sites market themselves to some countries more than others.

———————

When a package of abortion pills appears at the door, shipped from abroad, direct to the abortion seeker, it seems miraculous. The pills seem to have flowed easily across borders, part of pipelines of all sorts of goods that travel seamlessly from the site of their production to the site of their consumption. This is an illusion: like so many things that seem to move through a borderless, frictionless space of transnational commerce, abortion pills are produced in particular political and economic landscapes. They are materially shaped by the context of their production, as well as by the methods through which they are distributed. As the previous discussion of medication abortion—branded, generic, legally made, and illicitly sold—shows, a technology is never just a singular object with uniform features and a universal effect. Against the illusion that these pills freely flow across borders, transforming abortion access wherever they go, I will look closely at where they touch down. Each country, with its own social, cultural, political, and geographic context, interprets abortion pills and experiences their effect in a different way. Having traced abortion pills from the site of their production, across domestic and digital borders, I now follow them to destination countries to examine their impact. In the next chapter, on the United States, I show that abortion pills lived a double life long before *Dobbs*.

CHAPTER 2

Abortion Pills in US Clinics and Laws

We were so excited about this technology. My god! Abortion could be as easy as taking a pill? Think of what this would do for access for women, for empowerment!

— American activist

Abortion was established as a constitutional right in the United States in the 1973 *Roe v. Wade* decision. The 2022 ruling in *Dobbs v. Jackson Women's Health Organization* overturned *Roe* and removed constitutional protections for abortion. This decision accelerated changes that have been under way for years. States that have moved to ban abortion after *Roe* are those that had already made abortion as difficult to access as possible while *Roe* was in place. Without a constitutional right to abortion, some states will ban all abortions, including medication abortions. They will also attempt to institute laws that prevent people from obtaining medication abortion through the mail from another state; in some cases, they will try to pass laws banning people from traveling out of state to obtain abortion. The end of Roe has not ended abortion in the United States, but it has exacerbated the unevenness of abortion provision that already exists across states.

Anti-abortion laws in America have been enacted at a dizzying rate. They call to mind Gayle Rubin's comment about the "endless variety and monotonous similarity" of sexist oppression around the world.[1] Abortion restrictions in the United States exhibit endless variety, complexity, and creativity, with new innovations appearing all the time. Even so, they are monotonously similar in their relentless pursuit of reproductive control. Accounting for each type of restriction across all states is a mammoth task, which I do not attempt here; instead I concentrate on medication abortion and track its integration into (and obstruction) in US abortion practice. Advocates of medication abortion have seen it as an important tool to overcome the geographic obstacles that characterize US abortion provision. By contrast, opponents have folded medication abortion into their existing strategies for blocking abortions, taking steps to tether it to existing clinic spaces while working to eliminate as many clinics as possible.

This chapter deals with the official life of medication abortion in US law and abortion clinics. After MA was approved in 2000, it became available in many states, although it was subject to regulations imposed by federal and state governments. When people could not obtain MA through clinics, they developed alternative, unofficial routes for self-managed abortion, which are the subject of chapter 3. Here I look at how medication abortion was integrated into US abortion law and systems for clinical provision. Pro- and anti-abortion forces both employ geographic strategies in efforts to expand and contract the reach of medication abortion. I illustrate their competing strategies with a few detailed examples: first, through laws designed to anchor MA inside abortion clinics and ban the use of digital technologies to prescribe it; second, in my home state of Ohio, where medication abortion was slowly integrated into abortion practice despite years of legal challenges; and third, through online telemedicine abortion providers in abortion-friendly states. Online providers increasingly make use of border zones to extend access because state laws on abortion still strictly limit where medication abortion can be dispensed.

ROE AND THE ABORTION LAW LANDSCAPE

Roe v. Wade formed the basis for US abortion laws at the state and federal levels for nearly fifty years. In *Roe*, the Supreme Court struck down a Texas abortion ban and ruled that states could not outlaw abortion before fetal viability. The decision reasoned that the abortion right originated in the constitutional right to privacy because the abortion decision is a private medical choice and thus there are limits on what the state could do to restrict it. For a feminist analysis, this is an important caveat. The abortion right, as *Roe* established, protected the abortion decision as long as it was made in the context of the "private, confidential doctor-patient relationship." It did not establish a right to access this kind of medical care or a right to make an abortion decision outside of the medical system.[2]

From 1973 on, courts consistently ruled that abortion was a private right, so if someone needed financial support to exercise that right, the government had no obligation to provide it. Courts upheld laws that blocked public health-care programs from paying for abortion; while they acknowledged this was a barrier to abortion access, they ruled that it was not an unconstitutional barrier.[3] By upholding these kinds of restrictions, the courts have made clear that *Roe* offered only a negative right—limiting how states could criminalize and obstruct abortion—and did not entail a positive right to access abortion or other reproductive health services.[4] Legislation and litigation on abortion after 1973 whittled *Roe* down to "a bare negative contract right to buy a particular medical service" and meant, in practice, that abortion would only be available to those who could afford it.[5] Nonetheless, *Roe* meant that no state could ban abortion outright.

In *Planned Parenthood v. Casey* (1992), the Supreme Court did away with the viability line, instead allowing states to implement obstacles to abortion from the very start of pregnancy. The Court held that abortion restrictions were unconstitutional only when they posed an "undue burden" to access. *Casey*, and later judgments that reaffirmed it, showed anti-abortion activists that they could chip away at the right to abortion by introducing incremental restrictions that did not ban abortion but eliminated access in practice and the courts would uphold such restrictions. This strategy is known as anti-abortion incrementalism.[6] Many of the cases that followed *Casey* introduced restrictions in support of what the legal scholar Reva Siegel calls the "woman-protective anti-abortion argument," which purports to protect women's physical and mental health by limiting access to abortion.[7] The move to opposing abortion on women's health grounds has been part of a long-term shift in the anti-abortion movement, which sought to change the public's perception that it was violent and extremist by moving from moral or religious arguments to health and safety arguments.[8]

In *Casey*, the Supreme Court ruled that states could not impose an "undue burden" on the right to abortion, but lower courts disagreed on precisely what this meant, so Americans found themselves subject to "zip code jurisprudence" and wide variation in abortion laws across states.[9] Numerous state and local restrictions—and restrictions on federal funding for abortion—meant that abortion access was highly stratified by class, race, location, and other factors. These disparities have led US Reproductive Justice scholars to warn that the fixation on constitutional law had become a "dangerous preoccupation" in the fight for reproductive freedom because of the gulf between constitutional principles and the lived experience of people who cannot access abortion.[10]

They argued, in essence, that even while *Roe* and *Casey* stood for a constitutional abortion right, in practice, this right could not be exercised by many Americans.[11]

Nonetheless, *Roe v. Wade* and *Planned Parenthood v. Casey* stood as precedents until 2022, when they were both overturned in *Dobbs v. Jackson Women's Health Organization*. The majority opinion in *Dobbs* called *Roe* "egregiously wrong" from the start, finding neither a right to abortion in the Constitution nor a record of permitting abortion in US "history and tradition."[12] Without *Roe*'s constitutional protection for abortion, the question reverts to the states. States can ban abortion altogether, without exceptions, if they wish, or they can choose to expand abortion rights and accommodate abortion travelers from other states. Women, Justice Samuel Alito's majority opinion consoles, "are not without electoral or political power," so if they want abortions, they can lobby for state and federal laws to permit them.[13] With that, what was a constitutional right became a political preference that women may pursue with whatever political power they retain, in a country where they are no longer equal citizens.

By removing the constitutional right to abortion, *Dobbs* instantly changed the legal landscape. Within hours of the decision, some states began to enforce "trigger," or preemptive, abortion bans, set to come into force as soon as *Roe* was no longer law; several other states committed to passing abortion bans in the near future. Rather than try to predict what will happen to abortion laws in the coming years, I examine what impact medication abortion has had on abortion in the United States from 2000 to 2022. After *Dobbs*, the distinction between medication abortion in formal healthcare settings and clandestine or informal settings has blurred. The portability of MA and the flexible digital infrastructure that has been established to distribute it will challenge state efforts to ban abortion. Well before the *Dobbs* decision, MA in the United States has straddled the boundaries between formal/legal/clinical and informal/nonclinical/clandestine.

TRANSFORMING THE SPACES OF ABORTION CARE

Legal abortion in the United States was already established when mifepristone was developed in the 1980s. At the outset, mifepristone was mainly a regulatory matter for the FDA, which decides which drugs can be sold. Mifepristone was not approved for use in the United States until 2000, twenty years after it was first formulated and twelve years after it had become available in France.[14] The introduction of medication abortion—also known in the United States as RU486—generated questions about how this technology would change the practice of abortion, its accessibility, and its social meaning.

US advocates and opponents of abortion recognized the transformative potential of medication abortion when it first became available in Europe. Both sides saw that MA would change the spaces of abortion, its providers, and the nature of public debates about it, and they either supported or opposed the medication on these grounds. The most significant site of contention was the clinic. Supporters of abortion welcomed the potential for MA to introduce abortion into pharmacies, family medicine practices, sexual health clinics, and beyond. Removing abortion from standalone abortion clinic spaces was a major goal as they were the targets of violent confrontations and attacks by anti-abortion groups during the 1980s and 1990s.[15] Anti-abortion violence at clinics meant there was a basic safety rationale for moving provision out of clinics, but activists also saw a social rationale: making abortion available in a general practitioner's office or gynecology department at a hospital would help destigmatize it. It would reclassify abortion as a regular part of healthcare. Finally, decentering the clinic and multiplying the spaces where abortion could be accessed would expand the range of nonphysician providers and increase the number of abortion providers overall.[16]

Regulations on the spaces where abortion takes place also help determine the providers who are permitted to prescribe and dispense it. In the 1980s, when RU486 entered public debate, most US abortion restrictions regulated the conduct of physicians and, by extension, the spaces where physicians provided abortion. Medication abortion obtained through a nonphysician provider or used at home would undermine these restrictions, so anti-abortion groups strategized to concentrate MA inside clinical spaces. This spatial strategy was confirmed after a 1997 Supreme Court ruling on who could provide abortions, which national anti-abortion lobbying groups recognized as a "guarantee that states could channel abortions out of the home and into medical facilities."[17] Channeling abortion into standalone clinics made it easier to regulate providers, easier to target abortion clinics by protesters, and easier to restrict clinic operations through a variety of legal and extralegal measures, like those that increase clinic operating costs.[18] The anti-abortion incrementalist legislative strategy is fundamentally geographic: targeted regulations of abortion providers deliberately impose so many restrictions on abortion clinics that they force clinic closures, reducing abortion's availability and expanding the areas without a single provider.[19]

As early trials on MA showed that it changed the way abortion was experienced, making it more analogous to a menstrual period or a miscarriage than surgery,[20] abortion supporters sought to reframe the public conversation. MA was used in the early stages of pregnancy and therefore presented a contrast with the "very icon" of the anti-abortion movement, the late-term fetus. Anti-abortion groups also modified their messaging to oppose MA. Although they used familiar arguments about the purported physical and mental health risks of abortion that were leveled against any abortion method, they also developed arguments specific to medication abortion. Anti-abortion groups labeled MA a "death pill" and "human pesticide."[21] They argued that it was even worse than surgical abortion because it made abortion more convenient. They called it "guilt-free, responsibility-free, carefree living—better killing through chemistry."[22] If technologies come to be understood through narratives about the people who use them, this message makes it clear how MA and its users were portrayed by the anti-abortion movement: as a dangerously easy to use drug that would allow careless women to have abortions more often and with less suffering. By and large, anti-abortion narratives about MA folded the new method into existing arguments about the social harms of abortion in general, building on the incrementalist "woman-protective anti-abortion argument" that worked to chip away at abortion rights in the name of protecting women.[23]

BUYING, MAKING, AND TESTING MIFEPRISTONE

Mifepristone's pharmaceutical geography posed problems for US advocates who wanted to see it integrated into clinical practice. The FDA requires US clinical trials before approving a drug, and it refused to accept the available French clinical trial data on mifepristone. US MA advocates attempted to initiate clinical trials, but they were delayed by the French manufacturer, which in 1989 pulled the drug from US trials under pressure from anti-abortion groups. Further clinical trials were effectively halted when the Republican presidential administration issued an import ban on mifepristone the same year.[24] With the European manufacturer unwilling to participate in US clinical trials and US authorities empowered to seize all shipments of mifepristone, activists sought to obtain, test, and study the medications themselves.

Advocates of MA pursued a strategy of scientific knowledge production. They did so because the FDA required US clinical trial data but also because US abortion jurisprudence was increasingly based on competing narratives about the science of abortion.[25] The issue of abortion in the United States typifies both the "scientization of politics," in which science is used as a resource to promote consensus, and the "politicization of science," in which different groups bolster their arguments by providing competing scientific experts.[26] These are linked, of course: bringing in technical experts to settle political questions can mean that each group presents its own experts, and public trust in the value of such expertise is eroded. Contesting scientific evidence about the safety of abortion became even more effective for anti-abortion groups after 2007, when the Supreme Court upheld a ban on one particular abortion method. The Court ruled that the science of abortion safety was uncertain, so states' abortion restrictions that promised to protect women's health were constitutionally protected, whether or not there was evidence to support their health claims.[27]

MA advocates sought to use science to settle the matter of mifepristone's safety and acceptability to patients and thereby persuade the FDA to approve the drug, but they also recognized the extent to which scientific research on abortion was polarized and constrained by corporate interests. One strategy was to publicly violate the ban on private individuals importing mifepristone, in order to test the law enforcement response and galvanize public support for MA approval. In 1992, activists found an American woman, Leona Benten, pregnant and seeking an abortion, who was willing to fly to England to obtain MA from an unnamed doctor. Benten had notified US Customs in advance of her return, and Customs seized her abortion pills when she reentered the United States. Her lawyers challenged the mifepristone import ban, and a district court judge sided with Benten.[28] The US Supreme Court overturned the lower court and refused her request to return the pills, but in the meantime the case garnered national media attention and mobilized support for making MA available.[29] Public support notwithstanding, the obstacles to integrating MA into practice were regulatory and political: the FDA, political authorities, and pharmaceutical companies saw much to lose and less to gain by championing a medication that would antagonize the anti-abortion movement.

On the testing front, US groups like the Abortion Rights Movement tried to develop and synthesize their own mifepristone, based on the Chinese copy of the French original, in an "underground lab" in Upstate New York. They also obtained donated pills for use in US clinical trials from sources abroad, including the United Kingdom and China, but supply problems delayed clinical trials in the 1990s. Relationships with Chinese manufacturers became important for American supplies of the drug, as no US manufacturer could be found.[30] Larger trials of mifepristone started after the US government's import ban was removed and the French pharmaceutical company that held the patent was persuaded to transfer it to the Population Council, which, along with private foundations, funded the clinical trials beginning in 1994.[31]

Pro-choice feminists were themselves polarized over MA technology and the wisdom of seeking fast-track approval of the drug. Feminist groups of the abortion rights establishment pursued patent rights so that clinical trials could begin, partnering with the Population Council to this end.[32] By contrast, some feminist health and racial justice activists expressed concern that accelerated efforts to approve MA could lead to unintended health harms. They feared it could become a coercive tool of fertility control in marginalized communities that faced pressures not to give birth and parent.[33] This dispute about medication abortion is representative of the larger fault line between the reproductive rights and justice movements; broadly, reproductive rights groups have prioritized the right to abortion, while reproductive justice groups have fought to position coercive fertility control and sterilization abuse alongside abortion in a broader spectrum of reproductive activities.[34]

Based on the clinical trial data from the partnership between the Population Council and private foundations, a new drug permit was sought in 1996 and finally granted by the FDA in 2000. After tentative approval was granted, no company was willing to bring the drug to market, so a single-product company called Danco was established. Danco operated with an unusual level of secrecy because of threats of anti-abortion violence: it was registered in the Cayman Islands, its investors remained anonymous, its employees worked from an unlisted office in New York with an unlisted phone number, and it contracted with a manufacturer in Shanghai.[35] Mifepristone was its only product. When news of the Chinese mifepristone supplier broke, anti-abortion groups called it an "outrage" that put patients at risk "because China is a major source of impure drugs" that cannot be closely regulated by the FDA.[36] No US manufacturer agreed to supply the drug, ironically, because of the threats of those same anti-abortion groups.

FDA approval came after fifteen years of sustained debate about mifepristone.[37] When it approved mifepristone, the FDA imposed an unusual set of extra restrictions on it. It required providers to stock the mifepristone that they supplied, barring pharmacies from carrying it. It also required abortion providers and patients to sign long agreements certifying the provider's medical qualifications and the patient's knowledge of fourteen points about the drug protocol. The restrictions placed on mifepristone resemble those placed on controlled substances like narcotics, not essential medications of comparable safety to mifepristone.[38] The restrictions imposed on mifepristone made its integration into regular abortion practice and broader medical practice more difficult. General practitioners who wanted to provide abortions, for example, would have to acquire a certification and arrange a relationship with a surgical abortion provider in order to do so. They would also have to personally order the drug from the manufacturer and stock it in their offices. Surgical abortion providers already possessed the necessary qualifications to dispense the drug, but many were dissuaded by the cumbersome regulations on ordering, stocking, and dispensing the medication inside their clinics.[39]

LEGAL LIMITS ON MEDICATION ABORTION

It would be difficult to "find another drug that had undergone as long, sustained, and partisan a barrage" as mifepristone.[40] The restrictions on MA imposed by the FDA, as well as state-level restrictions on its use, meant the medicine was slowly integrated into abortion practice over time. In the first year it was available (2001), medication abortion accounted for 6 percent of all abortions. By 2014, it accounted for 31 percent, and by 2020, it accounted for a majority—53 percent—of all abortions carried out in the United States.[41] However, as with abortion access more broadly, medication abortion has been taken up unevenly across the country because it is encumbered by a wide range of restrictions. Laws that lower the gestational age for legal abortion do not always have an impact on its use since the FDA approved it only for abortion in the first trimester, but some general abortion restrictions, like mandatory waiting periods or multiple clinic visits, pose obstacles to both surgical and medication abortion. Medication abortion has also been the target of specific restrictions to constrain it spatially.

Even before mifepristone's FDA approval, federal legislators sponsored dozens of bills, amendments, public hearings, and petitions on mifepristone, most of which were aimed at preventing and/or suspending the drug's approval; none were successful, and the terms of mifepristone's approval were expanded over time. When they could not pass anything at the federal level, legislators moved to introduce mifepristone restrictions at the state level. Without federal laws setting national standards for abortion, the laws that matter most for whether or not people can access abortion have been those passed by state legislatures. Ohio was the first to pass its own mifepristone restriction in 2004, followed by Oklahoma in 2010. The midterm elections of 2010 ushered in the "Tea Party Wave," which gave Republicans power in statehouses across the country and bolstered the anti-abortion legislative agenda.[42] State lawmakers broke records in 2011 by passing the largest number of abortion restrictions ever in a single year, not to be exceeded until the 2021 session.[43] Restricting MA was a major goal: between 2011 and 2017, twenty-eight states passed laws designed to limit MA specifically.[44]

Restrictions on medication abortion at the state level generally fall into three categories: mifepristone protocols that regulate dosage and clinic visits; physical proximity requirements that regulate the physician-patient interaction; and telemedicine bans that prohibit MA from being prescribed by phone, video, or online consultation. These restrictions embody the anti-abortion strategies outlined earlier: on their face, they use woman-protective reasoning and tropes of scientific uncertainty to argue that medication abortion is untested and dangerous to abortion seekers but preferred by profiteering abortion providers. A 2012 report by the anti-abortion group Americans United for Life (AUL) offers an example (here, like many anti-abortion groups, they refer to medication abortion as "chemical" abortion): "The chemical abortion revolution has meant more than changing definitions. In the name of 'access' (which not so coincidentally translates into profits for abortion providers and drug companies), the chemical abortion revolutionists are bypassing, and outright attacking, important health and safety laws and regulations for RU-486."[45]

Rhetorically, MA restrictions are framed as protecting women. Practically, MA restrictions pursue the goal of channeling all medication abortion into brick-and-mortar abortion clinics and anchoring them to supervision by physician abortion providers. In the pre-*Dobbs* era, when they could impose restrictions but could not ban abortion outright, anti-abortion incrementalists used piecemeal restrictions to erode *Roe* without directly challenging it.[46] As part of a broader incrementalist anti-abortion strategy, concentrating medication abortion in abortion clinics accomplished a few goals. First, it maintained the importance of clinic spaces as sites where the anti-abortion movement can concentrate protests and intimidation. Second, it furthered the strategy of imposing numerous incremental restrictions on abortion clinics that can effectively prevent them from offering legal services. To this end, anti-abortion incrementalists worked to tether MA to abortion clinic spaces while pursuing measures that eliminate abortion clinics one by one.

MIFEPRISTONE PROTOCOL LAWS

Early state efforts to reduce the use of MA used mifepristone protocols to limit how the medicine was prescribed or dispensed. They did this by preventing abortion providers from prescribing MA off-label. Prescribing off-label means prescribing an FDA-approved medication in a dose or for a purpose that is not explicitly detailed in the FDA's approval documents. When it approves a drug, the FDA specifies the dosing regimen used in the clinical trials the agency used to make its approval decision, but this does not require providers to adhere to this regimen. Off-label prescribing is common and is not unique to abortion medication: an estimated 21 percent of prescriptions are off-label.[47] In fact, misoprostol is always used off-label when it is prescribed with mifepristone for a medication abortion because misoprostol is FDA approved only for gastric uses.

Prohibiting providers from off-label prescribing was especially problematic for medication abortion: the FDA's approved dosing regime was already outdated by the time approval was granted in 2000 as it did so with clinical trial data from the mid-1990s. This clinical trial data did not reflect best practice among abortion providers at the time. Mifepristone protocols that required providers to adhere to the FDA's 2000 approval documents—and outlawed the newer prescribing practices—reduced the window when MA could be used (from nine weeks to seven weeks), required more in-person clinic visits, and raised the dosage of mifepristone.[48] In effect, they raised the financial cost of MA by increasing the dosages, compounded the logistical burdens of MA by increasing clinic visits, and decreased the number of people who would be eligible to use MA by limiting its use to very early pregnancy. Mifepristone protocol laws became largely obsolete in 2016, when the FDA updated its approval label for mifepristone to reflect many of the changes in the newer evidence-based dosing regimen. By this point, however, they had already been superseded by more popular restrictions on where doctors could prescribe MA.

PHYSICAL PRESENCE REQUIREMENTS

A second group of mifepristone restrictions took up a different strategy to anchor medication abortion in brick-and-mortar clinics. These laws mandated that the abortion provider be in the same room as the patient when prescribing and dispensing the medication. Physical presence requirements emerged in response to telemedicine abortion systems that some clinics began to adopt from 2011 on. Many states have laws that specify that only physicians may prescribe mifepristone, so telemedicine abortion was developed to multiply the clinics that could offer abortion, allowing one physician to remotely prescribe for patients in other locations.[49] Early forms of telemedicine abortion used partial telemedicine. The patient would visit a nearby healthcare facility (which did not provide abortion) for preliminary tests. At this local facility, they would speak with an abortion provider in a different part of the state by phone or video. The abortion provider would remotely prescribe MA, to be dispensed at the patient's local facility. The patient would take the mifepristone, sometimes while still on the video call with the abortion provider, and keep the misoprostol for use at home later. Telemedicine was first introduced into abortion provision in the United States around 2008, by Planned Parenthood of the Heartland (Iowa),[50] but it came to the attention of the national anti-abortion movement after it was "exposed" by the anti-abortion group Operation Rescue in 2010.[51]

Laws with physical presence requirements effectively prohibit telemedicine abortion, although they do not always explicitly name telemedicine. Instead they use language about the physical proximity between doctor and patient to ban remote prescribing, illustrated in the four excerpts presented in table 1.

These laws closely resemble each other because many of them are adapted from the AUL model bill on medication abortion. AUL, a powerful anti-abortion group with federal and state chapters, focuses on drafting model legislation opposing abortion, assisted dying, and embryonic stem cell research. AUL's model legislation is highly influential in anti-abortion policy in part because it reduces the amount of work that each state needs to do to introduce a new policy. Legislators who want to introduce anti-abortion legislation frequently turn to the "ready-to-go, easily adaptable" model bills offered by groups like AUL.[52] In its annual compendium of model legislation, AUL has produced model bills designed to prohibit "the use of teleconferencing systems to dispense abortion-inducing drugs without a physician's examination (i.e., 'telemed abortions')" since at least

TABLE I   STATE LAWS WITH PHYSICAL PRESENCE REQUIREMENT FOR
MEDICATION ABORTION

North Dakota Century Code §14-02.1-03.5 (Added 2011)	North Dakota mandated that the "abortion-inducing drug or chemical . . . must be administered by or in the same room and *in the physical presence* of the physician who prescribed, dispensed, or otherwise provided the drug or chemical to the patient."
South Dakota Codified Laws §34-23A-56 (Added in 2011)	South Dakota prohibited any "surgical or medical abortion . . . except by a licensed physician and only after the physician *physically and personally meets* with the pregnant mother, consults with her, and performs an assessment of her medical and personal circumstances."
Wisconsin Statutes and Annotations §253.105 (Added in 2011)	Wisconsin prohibited "a person from giving a woman an abortion-inducing drug unless the physician who provided the drug for the woman *performs a physical exam* on the woman and *is physically present in the room* when the drug is given to the woman."
Missouri Revised Statutes §188.021 (Added in 2013)	Missouri required that "the initial dose of the drug or chemical shall be administered *in the same room* and *in the physical presence* of the physician who prescribed, dispensed, or otherwise provided the drug or chemical to the patient."

SOURCE: Compiled by the author from state bills and laws.
NOTE: Emphasis added.

2010.[53] AUL's own publications announce that laws like North Dakota's, excerpted in table 1, are "substantially based" on their model law that uses a physical presence requirement to ban "webcam abortions."[54]

Physical presence laws are also part of the state-level legislative pushback against newer telemedicine services that send pills through the mail. The partial telemedicine model of visiting a local facility for a video conference with a doctor and dispensing the medication in person became outdated as technology developed and research showed the safety of "no touch" protocols without any abortion clinic or healthcare facility visits. This change was accelerated by the COVID-19 pandemic, when even a single in-person visit to a doctor's office posed a public health risk. In response, abortion providers with brick-and-mortar clinics began to introduce no-touch abortion services in which a remote consultation with a doctor takes place by phone or email and medication arrives a few days later by mail. Other online-only services launched with no brick-and-mortar facilities.[55]

Anti-abortion legislatures responded by expanding physical presence requirements to prohibit all forms of remote prescribing and dispensing. For example, in 2021, Texas added new restrictions to its telemedicine abortion ban. Previously, the law required that the physician must "examine the pregnant woman in person" before providing any "abortion-inducing drug." In 2021, it added a new restriction: "A manufacturer, supplier, physician, or any other person may not provide to a patient any abortion-inducing drug by courier, delivery, or mail service."[56] The Texas abortion law already mandated in-person counseling and a twenty-four-hour waiting period between counseling and the abortion, necessitating at least two trips to the facility.[57] As of April 2022, shortly before the *Dobbs* decision, twenty-one states had physical presence requirements for medication abortion.[58] Many of these have since been superseded by post-*Dobbs* abortion bans.

TELEMEDICINE ABORTION BANS

While physical presence requirements effectively ban telemedicine abortion without naming it, outright telemedicine bans are also a common form of MA restriction. From 2011 on, anti-abortion groups began to mobilize against telemedicine abortion and states began to pass explicit telemedicine abortion bans. Telemedical technologies for remote consultations, prescriptions, and even surgeries are widely used across many different fields of medicine to improve access to healthcare in rural areas.[59] Telemedicine abortion bans, however, demonstrate the familiar fact of American "abortion exceptionalism" whereby abortion is singled out for unique restrictions that are not imposed on medical treatments of equivalent safety.[60]

States ban telemedicine abortion in two ways: by explicitly prohibiting telemedical prescribing in laws that regulate other aspects of abortion practice or by specifically outlawing abortion in laws regulating the practice of telemedicine. For example, Indiana's Senate Bill (SB) 371 (2013) included a physical presence requirement alongside a direct telemedicine prohibition: "A physician shall examine a pregnant woman in person before prescribing or dispensing an abortion inducing drug. As used in this subdivision, 'in person' does not include the use of telehealth or telemedicine services."[61] By contrast, Idaho's Telehealth Access Act (HB 189, 2015) on telemedicine services contains the following exception in its regulations on prescribing: "No drug may be prescribed through telehealth services for the purpose of causing an abortion." Idaho's law opens by celebrating the power of telemedicine services to "address an unmet need for health care by persons who have limited access to such care due to provider shortages or geographic barriers."[62] These are precisely the kinds of barriers faced by people trying to access abortion in the United States. Nonetheless, Idaho's law explicitly prohibits telemedicine abortion.[63] Both Indiana and Idaho implemented near-total abortion bans after the *Dobbs* decision came down.

MEDICATION ABORTION IN OHIO

In practice, the laws described above overlap and work together to constrain medication abortion. Ohio's regulation of MA illustrates this dynamic. An important swing state in presidential elections, Ohio has long been seen as a political bellwether at the national level, but it has been governed by Republicans for several decades. On abortion, Ohio encapsulates broader trends in abortion-restrictive states across the country.[64] Ohio has imposed many anti-abortion restrictions, including in-person state-directed "counseling" (using an anti-abortion script), a twenty-four-hour waiting period, parental consent for minors, a mandatory ultrasound scan, a mandatory test for fetal heartbeat, a twenty-week gestational limit except in cases of threat to life, blocks on insurance coverage for abortion, and several targeted regulations on abortion providers and facilities.[65] On top of these, Ohio enacted a series of medication abortion restrictions from 2004 on. These laws—in force during the period when *Roe v. Wade* was still the law of the land—did not ban MA outright. Instead, they tethered it to clinical space in order to stymie the creation of alternative models for abortion provision that could rearrange its geography and expand access. They mandated more in-person visits, prohibited remote prescribing, and fixed the spatial boundaries of the physician-patient relationship.

Ohio was one of the first states that "effectively banned" medication abortion through the mifepristone protocol described above. Ohio's mifepristone protocol law required doctors to use the outdated dosing regimen, reducing the number of weeks into pregnancy when MA could be used, prohibiting telemedicine by mandating extra clinic visits, and increasing the price of an abortion by mandating higher doses of medicine.[66] This law was challenged in the courts from 2004 until 2016, when the FDA updated its mifepristone rules. The FDA's update effectively made the Ohio law moot, because Ohio's law relied on the FDA's 2000 approval documentation and criminalized doctors who deviated from it. After this change, medication abortion as a share of abortion began to rise quickly: from 6 percent of all abortions in Ohio in 2015, MA accounted for 48 percent of abortions by 2020 (fig. 1).[67]

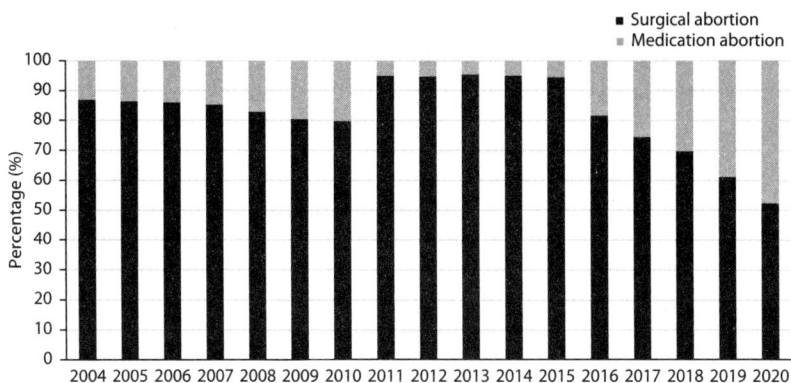

FIGURE 1. Method of abortions in Ohio, 2004–2020. Source: Data compiled by the author from Ohio Department of Health reports.

When the FDA updates made their mifepristone protocol obsolete, Ohio legislators moved to introduce new restrictions in order to reimpose limitations on medication abortion and telemedicine that could not be undermined by the FDA. SB 260 adopted a physical presence requirement, mandating that the physician be "physically present at the location where the initial dose of the drug or regimen of drugs is consumed at the time the initial dose is consumed." The bill's sponsor, Republican Steve Huffman, explained that his bill would prohibit physicians from providing abortion through "webcam exam, audio, or any other telecommunication platform." The bill also imposed felony criminal charges for medical providers who provided medication abortion through telemedicine. SB 260 was signed into law but enjoined by the courts, so in early 2022, Senator Huffman introduced a new bill to require an in-person physical examination by a doctor for medication abortion.[68]

The Dobbs decision, however, allowed anti-abortion legislators to go much further: in 2022, legislators outlawed abortion after fetal cardiac activity. In practice, this law amounts to a six-week abortion ban.[69] Ohio's law requires two sonograms, twenty-four hours apart, to detect fetal cardiac activity, plus mandatory counseling to discourage the abortion. It permits medication abortion to be provided using the FDA protocol, up to a point: while the FDA authorizes medication abortion up to 70 days (10 weeks) into pregnancy, in Ohio this medication will only be available to people 35 to 42 days (5 to 6 weeks) into pregnancy depending on their sonogram. As of early 2023, the six-week abortion ban was blocked while a legal challenge proceeded. Ohio's

SB 260 is also blocked in the courts, but if allowed to go into effect, it would ban all telemedicine abortion in the state, even for abortions before 5 to 6 weeks.[70] Ohio has not (yet) passed a total ban and still permits abortion, including medication abortion. Nonetheless, anti-abortion forces in the state are pursuing a familiar set of medication abortion restrictions that aim to prevent any expansion in abortion that telemedicine services would enable.

ABORTION IN THE BORDER ZONE

Under *Roe's* and *Casey's* constitutional protections, states were prohibited from banning pre-viability abortion inside their territories. This meant that even the most abortion-restrictive states had at least one operational abortion clinic (in 2021, there were six states with only one clinic).[71] In large states, obtaining an abortion at this lone clinic could still require numerous journeys of hundreds of miles.[72] People might choose to travel out of state if a neighboring state's laws made it easier to get an abortion. Much of this activity has been concentrated in border zones where neighboring states have drastically different abortion laws. For example, the greater St. Louis area encompasses Missouri and Illinois. Even before Missouri instituted its post-*Dobbs* trigger ban, thousands of Missouri residents bypassed the St. Louis Planned Parenthood clinic and crossed the river to obtain abortions in Illinois. While Missouri mandated a 72-hour waiting period, anti-abortion counseling, a pelvic exam at each visit, and parental consent for minors, Illinois had no such requirements.[73] In 2020, while abortion remained legal in Missouri, only 167 Missourians obtained abortions in their own state, while 9,800 traveled to Illinois or Kansas for an abortion.[74] Given how widely used this abortion-travel workaround became, it is no surprise that Missouri legislators have been at the forefront of attempts to criminalize abortion travel to other states (see chap. 3).

After the *Dobbs* decision, some states began to ban abortion altogether. As a consequence, there are enormous geographic areas without legal abortion. There are also a few important border zones where states with abortion bans meet states with relatively liberal abortion laws, including laws protecting telemedicine abortion. In these border zones, activists and providers see opportunities to transform the geography of medication abortion in the United States.

Since the federal government relaxed some of its medication abortion regulations during the COVID-19 pandemic, a growing number of no-touch full telemedicine services operate in abortion-friendly states. They offer remote consultations with doctors and dispense medication through the mail without any requirement for in-person visits. However, these digital health services are still physically tethered to particular state territories with laws that permit telemedicine abortion.[75] For all the technological potential of digital abortion services, abortion seekers from out of state are required to physically travel into a state where telemedicine abortion is legal before they can have a consultation with a no-touch telemedicine service. A telemedicine abortion provider licensed in New Mexico, for example, may not be able to treat a resident of Texas unless they are physically present in New Mexico.[76] This means that abortion travel has taken new spatial forms. The Texan may not be able to order pills from their home, but rather than drive to a New Mexico clinic for an in-person consultation, they can now drive just across the state border in order to be physically present in New Mexico while they conduct the online consultation call with a New Mexico–licensed doctor.

Telemedicine abortion providers in the United States face legal risk if they treat people in states with restrictive abortion laws, so they take steps to limit their services geographically. Telemedicine services use software to detect the caller's location and confirm that they are in a state where abortion is legal.[77] A caller whose location shows they are in Texas, for example, might be asked to call back from New Mexico. They must return to that same state to collect medications, although they need not reside there. Early evidence suggests that MA activists in the United States are already engaging in the kind of cross-border work that characterized the Republic of Ireland and Northern Ireland and continues to flourish in Poland. In the United States, people use post office boxes in border towns to collect pills or mail-forwarding services to ship their pills via abortion-friendly states. They use telemedicine abortion services that do not monitor the caller's location, or they use abortion activist services that provide information about how to give an alternative address. The legal risks of providing information about abortion are serious—but uncertain—so medication abortion activists set out procedures for moving pills between states in a detached, third-person tone: "Rosa lives in Texas where the law makes it hard to find pills by mail. Here is how she used a telemedicine service in another state and a mail forwarding service to get pills mailed to her home."[78] The site details Rosa's options in a descriptive—never directive—manner.

Some telemedicine abortion providers are developing mobile clinics that will offer services over the border of abortion-hostile states, like the Texas–New Mexico or Illinois-Missouri borders.[79] In the United States, mobile clinics have so far been a tactic of the anti-abortion movement, whose "crisis" pregnancy vans skirt state regulations as they move between different jurisdictions.[80] Mobile clinics for medication abortion in border zones raise the possibility of new geographies of access and new services that can respond more quickly to legal change. They also, however, raise questions about how anti-abortion legislation might constrain abortion travel to other states.[81] Ultimately, mobile clinics in border zones do not address the fundamental geographic problem of abortion travel: it requires time, money, support, and mobility, among other things. Traveling just across the border for a telemedical consultation and then again to collect medication might reduce an abortion journey by a few hundred miles, but it may do very little to mitigate the "tyranny of distance" in the abortion journey.[82]

Every advance in medication abortion and telemedicine technology has been met with a raft of restrictions that reduce the possibilities for medication abortion to expand access and to address socioeconomic and geographic inequalities. The "dire and ecstatic" predictions about mifepristone in the 1990s have not become reality. Although medication abortion made up the majority of abortions in the United States by 2021, changing people's abortion experiences and restructuring the landscape of abortion care, it has not radically transformed clinical abortion care to the extent that was hoped.[83] Medication abortion access is growing in states with few abortion restrictions overall, as no-touch services expand. States that target surgical abortion for restrictions do the same with medication abortion, so people in abortion-restrictive states generally cannot access medication abortion more easily than they can access surgical abortion (at least through legal channels).[84] The same goes for abortion bans after *Dobbs*: abortion bans do not differentiate between methods, so they ban doctors in a state from providing both surgical and medication abortion.

Laws to limit abortion, or to ban it outright, operate on the assumption that increasing the cost of abortion, reducing the number of clinics that provide it, or imposing other barriers will eliminate abortion. This assumption is wrong. Self-managed abortion existed when abortion was legal in all fifty states but hard to access in many of them. It will continue to grow in importance for US abortion seekers who live in hostile legal climates. After 2022, when many states have banned abortion, state authorities' efforts to limit surgical abortion are likely to be more successful than their efforts to limit medication abortion. Small, cheap, easy to move, and supported by digital information and networks, medication abortion travels in ways that surgical abortion cannot.

CHAPTER 3

How to Self-Manage an Abortion in America

They've been closing down clinics, but how do you close down everybody who's got access to a mailbox and the internet?

— American activist

Self-managed abortion is transforming access in places where abortion is banned by law. In the United States, it might be tempting to think of self-managed abortion as something that took place before *Roe v. Wade* made abortion a constitutional right in 1973 and will return after the ruling was overturned in *Dobbs* in 2022. But this is not true. The promise of *Roe* has been illusory for many, and self-managed abortion has been widely practiced despite the constitutional protection of legal abortion. The unevenness of abortion access, even when abortion was a constitutionally guaranteed right, meant that medication abortion lived a double life. Officially, it was available in every state through abortion clinics, though it was restricted by many barriers. Nonetheless, major obstacles to accessing abortion in clinical settings meant that the uptake of medication abortion was much slower in the United States than in other countries. Obstacles to obtaining MA in clinics also pushed Americans to obtain MA through illicit means. Unofficially, it was available through clandestine networks of activists and online pharmacies.

As I write shortly after the *Dobbs* decision, the US abortion law landscape is chaotic and rapidly changing. Anti-abortion states are passing draconian restrictions to limit their residents' access to abortion in or out of these states, pro-abortion states are passing laws to protect providers and abortion travelers, the federal government is acting in a limited capacity to protect some abortions, and lawyers are engaged in heated debate about whether any of these efforts will stand up in court. I offer no predictions. Instead this chapter deals with the unofficial life of medication abortion in the United States: outside of formal healthcare spaces, online, and/or through activist networks. The practical difficulties of obtaining in-clinic abortions had already resulted in widespread use of pills to self-manage abortion before *Dobbs*. The structure of clandestine abortion in the United States up to this point can help us understand what might follow *Dobbs*, when self-managed abortion becomes the default option for many more people. Reliance on self-managed abortion will grow, and activist infrastructures for supporting self-managed abortion will expand, but these will not need to materialize as a response to the fall of *Roe*. They already exist.

Accounting for secretive self-managed abortion practices takes some creativity. I illustrate its past in the feminist DIY reproductive health movement and its present in the case of a pseudonymous abortion pill seller who operated in the United States during the late 2010s. Offering a wide-ranging exploration of self-managed abortion practices in the country today, where the legal climate is increasingly hostile, I address two further practical questions: How do the medications move into the United States? And how often are pill users criminalized for self-managing abortion? The chapter shows, in short, that self-managed abortion is already in widespread use and is set to expand in the coming years.

SELF-MANAGED ABORTION BEFORE *ROE*

Self-managed abortion is not a new phenomenon. When abortion was criminalized across the United States—from the mid-nineteenth to the mid-twentieth century—illegal abortions were widespread. The "back alley butcher" remains a "vibrant cultural icon" and a widely used justification for retaining legal abortion, but this image is not representative of abortion in that earlier period.[1] In fact, illegal abortion before *Roe* was obtained, for the most part, through a "white coat underground" (to borrow the Polish term) of doctors, nurses, and midwives who offered illegal abortions in private practice for a fee.[2] Self-managed abortion methods were also used, but in the era before abortion with pills, self-managed abortion was a far more dangerous proposition: women douched with toxic substances, ingested abortifacients, or used sharp instruments.[3] Self-managed abortion accounted for a minority of illegal abortions in the years before *Roe* but a majority of the injuries and deaths from illegal abortion.[4] The so-called back alley butcher came to stand in for all illegal abortion in public discourse, but it was actually dangerous attempts to self-induce abortion that caused the most injury and death, not procedures done by clandestine abortion providers.[5] As an illegal abortion from a qualified provider was expensive, the ability to obtain a safer abortion varied by class and race: women who were white, wealthy, and urban were more likely to obtain a physician-provided abortion; nonwhite women and low-income women were more likely to resort to self-induced abortion.[6] Legal abortion was also easier for the wealthy to access because people who could pay privately for medical care were more likely to find a doctor who would certify that they met the medical or psychiatric indications for a "therapeutic" (i.e., medically necessary) abortion.[7]

In addition to illegal physician-provided abortions, groups of women in the self-help reproductive health movement offered abortion services. They were part of a feminist movement that set out to challenge the production of knowledge and provision of services about sex, reproduction, and women's health. They wanted individuals—not the "state, experts, or market forces"—to hold power over their own reproductive health.[8] Groups like the Abortion Counselling Service of Women's Liberation, better known as the Jane Collective (1969–73); the Society for Humane Abortion (1962–79); and California Women's Health Centers (1970s) provided services that included illegal abortions without physician involvement and/or outside of medical settings. These groups were limited geographically, providing abortions in Chicago and California only, and should not be understood as representative of the whole country. However, these feminist groups were significant because they challenged the medico-legal paradigm of abortion: they showed that illegal abortion could be safely provided by laypeople.[9] The Jane Collective started as a referral service that gave information only, but its members soon learned that abortion could be safely provided by a trained nonphysician. By the time Jane's services closed, three-quarters of the collective had learned medical skills for performing abortions, of which they did three thousand per year.[10] Similar networks arose in Italy and France to offer referrals to reliable doctors who would provide clandestine surgical abortions, but as the groups expanded they also learned to perform abortion themselves.[11]

These groups, and the facilities they ran, assembled a "mobile set of practices" that could be moved, altered, and spread to other groups of women. This included instructions on how to build the Del-Em Menstrual Extraction device, a homemade manual vacuum aspiration technology.[12] It worked like this: a small tube inserted in the uterus was connected to a syringe that acted as a pump, so that by pumping the syringe, a vacuum suctioned all the contents of the uterus into a small jar. Using the homemade vacuum aspirator, the activists would undertake a process called "menstrual extraction" through which "all of the menstrual fluid incident to a normal monthly 'period' may be removed."[13] The device could be assembled from everyday supplies bought from grocery, hardware, and pet stores. Activists saw productive ambiguity in the blurry line between menstrual period, very early miscarriage, and induced abortion. If the earliest sign of pregnancy was a missed period, they reasoned, bringing on a period by manual intervention could ensure that no pregnancy existed without having to test for it first. The movement for menstrual extraction developed what Michelle Murphy calls "protocol" feminism: it sought to develop protocols (information, instructions, experiences) that could move across national and transnational boundaries and be reassembled in different places, according to their political contexts.[14]

The feminist self-help movement saw medical institutions and practitioners as systems of patriarchal control that subordinated women, but it did not see all things medical and technological as tools of patriarchy; these tools, practices, and technologies could be taken up by women, who would determine their use on their own bodies.[15] The movement's ethos was, in short, "Why ask permission for something you can do yourself?"[16] For a short time, they effectively built a "rival set of institutions" to meet some people's need for abortion by means that were safer and cheaper than available alternatives. At a time of growing mobilization for abortion reform, self-help activism in the women's health movement illustrated that the criminal laws against abortion were unenforceable.[17]

Feminist groups providing illegal abortion services in the years before *Roe* engaged in a variety of tactics, all of which are visible today in self-managed abortion groups around the world. They shared information about abortion providers in foreign countries; they developed rating and review systems to refer people to the best providers and help them avoid providers with bad reputations; they negotiated with abortion providers to lower prices for their service users; they raised funds to cover abortion costs for low-income people; they provided logistical, emotional, and financial support through lay volunteers; and they provided information on how to safely self-manage an abortion.

After the 1973 ruling in *Roe v. Wade*, some of the feminist movement providers attempted to establish legal abortion services with a feminist self-help ethos that preserved the movement's belief in demedicalized and egalitarian methods of practice. Two obstacles stymied this goal: first, extensive bureaucratic regulation of abortion providers made it impossible to operate along feminist principles;[18] and second, the growing militance of the anti-abortion movement meant that abortion providers worked under the constant threat of violence, so clinic life became oriented around concerns about security and preserving basic operations. These pressures meant the end of the "era of radical experimentation" in clinical medicine spaces for reproductive and sexual health.[19] This is not to suggest that the feminist self-help movement ended after abortion legalization or that abortion providers are not committed feminists. Rather, it is important to note that later groups operating according to self-help principles to facilitate clandestine self-managed abortion are not the same people working as medical professionals and staffing abortion clinics. The differences and disagreements between these groups would emerge again over the question of self-managed abortion with mifepristone and misoprostol.[20]

COUNTING SELF-MANAGED ABORTIONS

One question emerges across every country studied in this book: How can we count clandestine self-managed abortions? The nature of clandestine abortion (sometimes illegal, often secret, almost always stigmatized) means it is a shadowy and amorphous subject for study. People who successfully self-manage an abortion without accompaniment or medical intervention will usually be invisible to researchers because they will not come to the attention of doctors, police, or government statisticians.[21] Pathways for accessing self-managed abortion are diverse and enroll a wide variety of feminist networks, friends, family, health workers, websites, pharmacists, and other informal providers.[22] In this and later chapters, I show how it is possible to roughly estimate the demand for self-managed abortion using a few different measures: how many pill requests the feminist pill networks receive, whether there is a notable decrease over time in people presenting at abortion clinics domestically or internationally, and the number of abortions obtained before a restrictive abortion law came into force, compared to officially recorded abortions obtained after it. Uncovering these data is rarely straightforward.

Pathways for self-managed abortion in the United States are diverse: Americans report that they self-manage abortion with pills ordered from online pharmacies, with misoprostol bought in Mexico, and with abortifacients they source locally.[23] For this reason, most studies that have attempted to estimate the prevalence of self-managed abortion in this country have done so by asking people directly about their knowledge and experience of self-managed abortion. Estimates vary but show growing knowledge and experience of the topic: while a 2017 study estimated 1.4 percent of US women had attempted to self-induce an abortion, a 2020 study of women in Texas found that 13 percent had sought or attempted to self-manage an abortion and 30 percent had prior knowledge of self-managed abortion.[24] A 2022 study found that 28 percent of people who sought in-clinic abortion care had tried self-managed abortion first, the majority of whom had first tried dangerous and ineffective methods, including herbal abortifacients, large doses of contraceptive pills, and self-harm.[25] As pharmaceutical products and information about self-managed abortion circulate online, measuring online searches for terms like "DIY abortion" also shows the scale of abortion demand and its geography.[26] Studies of online data show that people in states hostile to abortion are much more likely to carry out internet searches for self-induced abortion than are people in states where abortion is more easily accessible and that search rates for self-induced abortion increase during years when more abortion restrictions are passed.[27]

There is another way to gauge the prevalence of self-managed abortion on a larger scale: between 2011 and 2017, the number of abortions recorded in the United States fell by 19 percent.[28] This dramatic decline might be caused by wider access to contraception, uptake of more effective contraceptive methods, or more state-level abortion restrictions. It might also be caused by people looking outside of the medical system and thus procuring abortions that do not show up in official data.[29] Considering how effective abortion pills are and their growing availability in the United States, it is possible that the number of people who successfully self-manage an abortion outside of a clinic may "vastly outnumber" those who later seek medical care and thus show up in studies of failed self-managed abortion.[30] Existing methods for estimating the prevalence of self-managed abortion may underestimate it because improved access to safe medicines and high-quality information makes it less likely that people will require follow-up care that would bring them into contact with medical institutions.[31] This difficulty will be exacerbated as more states ban abortion. Studies estimate that states with post-Dobbs bans will see their abortion rates drop by 32.8 percent, but this only accounts for the decline in abortions reported by medical facilities.[32] That figure is easy to measure, but the corresponding rise in self-managed abortions, or births after not obtaining a wanted abortion, will be nearly impossible to know.[33]

Available data indicate the growing prevalence of self-managed abortion in the United States, but they present a familiar dilemma. Safe self-managed abortion that occurs without the knowledge of law enforcement, and without the need for follow-up medical care, will remain officially invisible. At an interpersonal level, this can perpetuate the stigma and silence that surrounds abortion.[34] At a policy level, this can mask the extent of noncompliance with restrictive abortion laws and can lend false credibility to anti-abortion policy makers who claim to have eliminated abortion by passing bans.[35]

BUYING AND SELLING ABORTION PILLS ONLINE

Americans take numerous routes to self-managed abortion. One route is to buy abortion pills online from online pharmacies and other small-scale vendors. To illustrate this phenomenon, I delve into detail about one such vendor who came to public attention when she was prosecuted for selling abortion pills. To protect the anonymity of the people who bought pills from her, some of whom I discuss below, I refer to the vendor and her blog by a pseudonym, Organic Lifestyle Guru (OLG). This blog, business, and court case present a fascinating window into self-managed abortion in the United States. OLG was the personal blog of an American woman who wrote about topics such as homeopathic remedies, wellness, sexuality, and parenting. In the early 2010s, she published a post explaining how she had self-managed an abortion with medications she bought online, in which she discussed the advantages of self-managed versus in-clinic abortion. Her post began to attract attention from commenters, who wrote to ask how to get abortion pills for themselves. The OLG blog came to function as an informal web forum where people gathered to share information about where to buy pills, which sites to avoid, how to obtain genuine pills, and how to self-manage an abortion, among other things. In 2016, OLG herself opened an online shop where, for the next three years, she sold abortion pills for less than half the price that most online pharmacies charged. OLG was later raided by law enforcement authorities, indicted, and pleaded guilty to one count of conspiracy to defraud by selling misbranded drugs from India. She was sentenced to probation, a fine, and forfeiture of tens of thousands of dollars she earned selling abortion pills.

Organic Lifestyle Guru imported abortion pills in bulk from a few online pharmacies located in India, received the packages at her home, and then shipped individual MA doses across the United States through domestic mail. At the peak of demand, she was filling orders for three thousand to four thousand customers each year.[36] OLG obtained her products from the online pharmacies discussed in chapter 1. The online pharmacies advertised Mifeprex, the FDA-approved mifepristone product, but when the pills showed up at her home, they were products from various Indian manufacturers: Misoprost (mifepristone) manufactured by Cipla and Mifegest (a combi-pack with mifepristone and misoprostol) manufactured by Zydus Cadila, among others.[37] OLG bought in bulk from the same sites that her customers could buy from as individuals, but she negotiated lower rates with the vendors when she started purchasing in larger quantities. OLG was selling each combi-pack for $70 to $80 plus domestic shipping charges, while the sites she bought from would sell the same product for $200 to $300 plus international shipping. Once her online store was established, she became a preferred vendor for abortion seekers and even advocacy groups that helped people find reputable pill suppliers.[38] OLG was not the only one to run this kind of business, but she was the first to be caught and prosecuted.[39]

Commenters on her blog included people who bought pills from the Indian pharmacies that OLG recommended and who bought directly from OLG herself. I collected and analyzed the 827 comments that were posted between 2012 and 2020 below the original blog post about how to self-manage abortion. I also conducted interviews with two people who publicly posted on the blog about their search for abortion pills. People who gathered in the comments section developed a repertoire over time: commenters would initially post about their unplanned pregnancy, asking for advice on where to get pills; they would often follow up with comments about where and how they purchased pills, returning to post updates on their anxious wait for the pills to be shipped or to clear customs; and finally, many of them posted long narratives about their experience using the pills, offering advice and support for others about to go through the same thing. Some commenters tried to find instructions for using MA in medical journals: when they hit journal paywalls, they extracted the available information from article abstracts and shared it with others in the forum. Because of the social stigma and legal risk of self-managing an abortion with medications bought online, there were few other places where women could gather to share advice on how to do this or discuss their personal experiences.

Commenters provided numerous reasons for seeking out MA online. The most frequently cited reason was cost. Although they knew of clinics where abortion was legally provided, they could not afford them. Prices varied. At the low end, one commenter reported that she found a "reliable" clinic that would charge her $375, a price she still could not afford without applying for help from a local abortion fund. At the high end, another explained that none of her nearby clinics offered medication abortion, so she would have to pay $1,200 for a surgical abortion. The average price for a medication abortion quoted by commenters who had contacted their local clinics was $626.

The second most frequently cited reason for seeking out MA online was the distance between home and clinic. Commenters were distraught about the hundreds of miles they would need to travel to the nearest clinic, sometimes more than once and sometimes with their children in tow. Distance was compounded by the need to make numerous trips to accommodate a mandatory waiting period. Others spoke about negative experiences they had at abortion clinics in the past, mainly involving feeling judged by clinic staff and harassed by protesters outside. Two commenters explained:

> At five weeks along, I would have thought going to the clinic would be more afford- able for me. Instead, I got a quote for $730! And only upfront, no payment plans available. It also meant several trips to the clinic with someone accompanying me. As you can guess, I don't want anyone else to be involved in this. All these differ- ent things made it basically impossible for me and this was just to get the pills! I was totally shocked. I felt trapped, like I had no options.

> A few years ago, I had an abortion with pills at a local clinic. The thing I remem- ber very clearly from that time is the pro-life people standing across the street yelling at the women going into the clinic and videotaping us. I was a strong person—I still am—but that really shook me![40]

The numerous obstacles to abortion led commenters on OLG to search for advice about where and how to buy abortion pills from online vendors. For many commenters on OLG, abortion pills represented a last resort after other methods had failed. Commenters reported trying other methods, unsuccess- fully, before finding OLG's blog or webstore: they used herbal abortifacients that they learned about online, for example, ginger and dandelion teas, Vita- min C and parsley, cinnamon, neem, cotton root bark, blue cohosh, black cohosh, pennyroyal, and tansy. These were all well-known "emmenagogues" in nineteenth-century America that were widely used to "restore" the men- strual flow before the medicalization and criminalization of abortion but had fallen out of use for the most part in the twentieth century.[41] Other OLG commenters reported driving to Mexico to buy misoprostol in pharmacies just over the US-Mexico border. When they could not get to Mexican pharmacies for misoprostol, they asked elderly grandparents to call up nearby pharmacies to see if they could obtain misoprostol without a prescription. This is a tactic also used in Latin America, where it is easier to buy misoprostol over the counter if you read as male or postmenopausal.[42] Some commenters on OLG reported that they had tried to purchase veterinary-grade misoprostol from veterinary supply stores: misoprostol is used in dogs, cats, and horses for the same reasons it is used in humans (to treat ulcers and end pregnancies). Although far from mainstream, the practice of converting veterinary misoprostol into a format that can be distributed to human abortion seekers is an ongoing project among some activist groups.[43]

After OLG's webstore was shut down by federal authorities, her blog remained up. Commenters continued to post there with messages of desperation and confusion. In the absence of OLG's shop, scammers appeared in the comments of the blog with offers of pills. One woman, who I will call Tracy, had an experience that illustrates the practical obstacles of self-managing an abortion online. Tracy was a mother of two young children living in a southeastern state where abortion was available but expensive. The price of an abortion, plus the idea of protesters "yelling at you when you're walking inside," scared Tracy and gave her extra motivation to find abortion pills online.[44] After "a lot of digging," she found a website on which activists listed reputable abortion pill vendors. OLG's website was highly ranked, so she bought pills from the OLG online shop, and they were shipped from within the United States in a small envelope stuffed with bubble wrap, a necklace, and then two blister packs containing the mifepristone and misoprostol discreetly tucked in extra layers of packaging material.

A few years later, Tracy needed an abortion again and returned to OLG's site only to find that the online store had closed. She posted in the comments to ask for help to obtain medication abortion, and another commenter offered to sell her pills. It turned out to be a scam: the commenter took the money and never sent the medication. Tracy found the fake vendor's information online but was too afraid to contact them. As she explained, "I figured I was doing something illegal anyways, and I didn't need to dig myself any deeper." After losing money to the scam, Tracy obtained an abortion in a clinic in her home state, for which she paid $800. OLG's online store was a relatively small-scale operation, and the community of commenters that emerged on the site represents just a few hundred people among the many hundreds of thousands who seek out an abortion in the United States each year.[45] Ultimately, in the United States, as in other countries where self-managed abortion is a lifeline, there can be no single, straightforward explanation for how to securely get abortion pills into the hands of people who need them: much depends on their local geography, the political context in which they live, their social networks, their socioeconomic status, their race or nationality, and their access to technology, among other factors.

The reasons for seeking medication abortion, barriers to in-clinic abortion, and routes to obtaining self-managed abortion that OLG commenters discussed are consistent with a growing body of public health research on self-managed abortion in the United States. Studies of Aid Access (Women on Web's US service) show that the main reasons that Americans turn to abortion pills online are the high cost of in-clinic abortions, state-level restrictions that create barriers to access, the need for secrecy because of an unsupportive partner or family, the distance to the nearest abortion clinic, and the preference for a self-managed abortion at home. Financial factors are the most important in shaping the decision, and the comparatively low cost of MA online motivates people to seek out care from online providers, whether feminist networks like Aid Access or foreign pharmacies selling direct to the consumer.[46] Financial hardship not only shapes how people seek out abortion, but also why they seek it: a 2015 study found that 40 percent of women seeking abortion in the United States were motivated to end their pregnancies because they could not afford to raise a child.[47]

ABORTION PILL ACTIVISM OUTSIDE THE LAW

After medication abortion was approved in the United States, extensive regulation prevented it from achieving the kind of transformation of abortion that activists had hoped for in the 1980s and 1990s. Meanwhile, US activists watched as other countries used mifepristone and misoprostol to expand the geography of safe abortion. One activist reported to me:

> We started noticing everywhere we went—the last three countries were Ethiopia, Ghana, and Nigeria—you could go to pharmacies in these places, like the highlands of Ethiopia, and you could get mifepristone and misoprostol, or "the abortion kit" as they called it. . . . So we would see that you could get this abortion kit in

Ethiopia and we'd come back and there would be news about Texas—"We just lost more access to services in another state." We just got frustrated![48]

Reproductive health professionals and campaigners worked to expand the use of medication abortion, drawing on expertise from previous campaigns on hormonal contraceptives and emergency contraception.[49] At the same time, US abortion advocates saw the expansion of feminist MA services like Women on Web and Women Help Women abroad and began working to introduce that model in the United States. Coalition building for such an effort was difficult, however, because any entities involved in providing legal abortions in the United States or any entities connected to organizations that received funding from the US government risked legal action or loss of funding if they were associated with illegal abortion.[50] Information about how to safely use mifepristone and misoprostol was plentiful, but information about precisely how to obtain it in this country was not. Collecting and publicizing information on reliable online pharmacies and pill vendors was a significant step in this process undertaken by organizations like Plan C. However, questions about the legality of sharing information on self-managed abortion delayed activist efforts and fractured the coalition of organizations. The threat posed by the well-funded and highly litigious US anti-abortion movement, and its allies in positions of authority, meant that many in the pro-choice movement instead wanted to focus on preserving the services that already existed.[51]

Activists who had hoped medication abortion would transform the US abortion landscape were demoralized by clinic closures and restrictions on medication abortion. Reflecting on its approval and integration into clinical practice, they saw the limitations of working within hostile anti-abortion structures. MA had the potential to radically transform access, but activists felt that "we lost that battle by medicalizing and regulating it so badly that the empowering aspects, the ease of the technology, they got completely destroyed."[52] Twenty years after medication abortion was approved by the FDA, the pace of adoption had been slow and limited by the regulations that anchored it inside a diminishing number of abortion clinics (e.g., physical presence requirements, discussed in chap. 2). For some activists, the time for compliance had come to an end, and they decided that facilitating widespread illicit use of medication abortion was the only way to achieve change. An activist who had been involved in decades of public policy campaigning work explained this change:

There's absolute outrage! Our strategy is: let's build that outrage, let's take advantage of that outrage. Let's spread the knowledge, and people are going to take it into their own hands. There's going to be so much happening in the public that there is strength in those numbers. There's protection in those numbers, and that will eventually push the regulatory situation. Maybe not to full over-the-counter access but to something that's a lot more convenient and accessible.[53]

Small-scale vendors like OLG sold abortion pills, as did various online pharmacies, but no formalized system for telemedicine-supported self-managed abortion existed in the United States until 2018, when Aid Access launched. Aid Access was founded by Rebecca Gomperts, of Women on Web and Women on Waves. Aid Access extended the WoW service model to the United States but it did so as a separate legal entity that would not jeopardize its sister organizations if it were to be shut down by US authorities.[54] Up to that time, Women on Web, Women Help Women, and Safe2Choose had not provided medication abortion in the United States for fear of legal reprisals from the well-funded and highly motivated anti-abortion movement; Women on Web had, and still maintains, a stated position of not supplying abortion pills in countries with legal abortion.[55] Nonetheless, Gomperts and staff launched the separate US service in 2018, and it received 57,000 requests in its first two years of operation.

Aid Access introduced a two-track model of provision for self-managed abortion in the United States. For abortion seekers in states with liberal abortion laws, Aid Access works with US doctors who operate no-touch telemedicine abortion services and can ship the medicines from within the country. For abortion seekers in states that are hostile to abortion, Aid Access uses doctors located abroad, in countries where the doctors doing remote prescribing are legally protected. To supply MA in abortion-hostile states, Aid Access liaises with the same Indian pharmaceutical distributor that ships medications abroad for WoW (including the Republic of Ireland, Northern Ireland, and Poland). Aid Access's precise practices became public knowledge in 2019, when the FDA issued a letter ordering the organization to stop its operations in the United States; Aid Access refused to stop and filed a suit on behalf of Gomperts and her patients against government officials.[56] FDA attention to Aid Access and the FDA's demand that it cease its operations have coincided with some periods of interruption of the service when packages are seized. Nonetheless, logistical difficulties and legal uncertainties mean the US government has not been able to stop Aid Access from delivering pills.[57] Before the *Dobbs* decision, Aid Access received around 82 MA requests from the United States every day. Two months after the decision was announced, this figure had risen to around 213 MA requests every day. Requests for MA increased most dramatically in states that immediately banned abortion after *Dobbs*.[58] Aid Access is able to move pills into the United States, in apparent violation of federal regulations on mifepristone and misoprostol, because of the position of medication abortion within the wider economic geography of US pharmaceuticals.

IMPORTING MEDICATION ABORTION

Aid Access and Organic Lifestyle Guru's methods for providing illicit medication abortion inside the United States illustrate one of this book's key arguments: abortion pills move like other prescription pharmaceuticals, from the same manufacturers, distributors, and infrastructures. They are therefore difficult to stop for states whose publics are used to obtaining medicines through the mail. The no-touch telemedicine services also use the US postal system to ship medications to their clients, but these services are different from those like Aid Access. Telemedicine abortion services in the United States—like Abortion on Demand, Hey Jane, or Just the Pill—operate only in states where medication abortion is legal and only ship pills inside those states. Unlike Aid Access, they do not ship pills into states where abortion is banned, where medication abortion is severely restricted, or where telemedicine is banned. People living in those states have another source for medication abortion through the postal service in Aid Access, but it occupies a legal gray area. The medicines it supplies are essentially the illicit equivalents of medicines that people obtain through legal telemedical services in other states. In this regard, illicit MA is much like the prescription medications that many Americans order from abroad through the postal system.

American healthcare is notoriously expensive: the same high prices that deter people from obtaining in-clinic abortions push many Americans to seek out other medications and treatments online. As a matter of law, it is illegal for Americans to import prescription medications from outside the United States, regardless of whether the medication is approved by the FDA. When Americans do import medications, and these products are identified by customs, the FDA has discretion over whether to seize them.[59] There are certain circumstances under which prescription medications can be imported, known as the "personal-use exemption," but this exemption is at the discretion of FDA agents and is not codified in law. The personal-use exemption allows residents to import a small quantity of medication for personal use (not for resale) when the treatment was started abroad and the FDA agrees that the products "do not represent a significant health risk."[60] The personal-use exemption for medicines was introduced in 1989 at the behest of HIV/AIDS treatment activists and buyer's clubs who wanted treatments that were not yet approved by the FDA.[61] Although people do import prescription drugs for treatments that are not available in the United States, evidence suggests that most people who import their prescriptions from abroad do so because of price. Foreign versions of FDA-approved medicines are usually cheaper than the brands marketed in the United States.[62]

As a matter of practice, prescription drugs are widely imported and prohibitions on the import of such drugs for personal use are rarely enforced. This is partly a result of the particularities of the US healthcare system: 62 percent of US adults take prescription drugs, yet 29 percent of adults report that they have skipped doses or stopped filling their prescriptions due to costs.[63] Many Americans depend on cheaper prescription drugs purchased abroad, evidenced by the expanding federal agency and state programs being set up to facilitate the import of drugs from Canada. In a 2016 poll, 8 percent of Americans reported purchasing drugs from Canada or Mexico, in violation of the law.[64] Nonetheless, the FDA rarely stops people entering the United States with personal prescription drugs bought abroad, and it seizes only a small fraction of drugs purchased from online pharmacies. Stringent enforcement of the legal prohibition on importing prescription drugs would likely prompt a backlash among consumers as many Americans rely on cheaper foreign versions of FDA-approved medicines.

Regardless of its legal position on illicit medications entering the country, the FDA practically lacks the enforcement capacity to stop them. International mail moves through nine service centers in the United States, with the New York facility processing 60 percent of international packages.[65] At the entry point for international mail, US Customs and Border Patrol processes goods and designates items that require further inspection by the FDA (for noncontrolled substances such as wrongfully imported or counterfeit medicines) and the Drug Enforcement Administration (for controlled substances such as narcotics).[66] As e-commerce grows, packages make up a larger share of international mail, at almost half of all items in 2016.[67] In 2017, when 275 million packages came into the country through the US Postal Service, the FDA had only twenty-two import investigators responsible for covering its nine international mail facilities.[68] Even as the use of the US Postal Service to import fentanyl, fentanyl analogues, and novel psychoactive substances to the United States has generated alarm in recent years among regulators and legislators, regulatory agencies are "already overwhelmed by the number of incoming packages."[69] The FDA estimates that it can inspect less than 0.18 percent of the packages assumed to contain drugs that pass through international mail facilities.[70]

When law enforcement agencies want to intercept abortion pill packages, they often have limited success, as actions against Aid Access and Organic Lifestyle Guru show. Pharmaceutical distributors like the Indian companies that distribute abortion pills via feminist networks operate within the legal framework of India, not the country to which they export. US agencies do not have jurisdiction over manufacturers and distributors of medication abroad, but they can restrict the flow of abortion pills into the United States to a certain degree.[71] Customs agents can intercept incoming packages at the border (when they can identify them), and the FDA can target internet service providers that host such sites or the US-based platforms that earn advertising revenue from them with requests to cease their operations, as with the Rablon network of online pharmacy sites that the FDA unsuccessfully tried to close. As a consequence, the criminalization of people who self-manage abortion is much less likely to happen when they are ordering the medications and much more likely to happen after they have used them.

THE CRIMINALIZATION OF SELF-MANAGED ABORTION

Abortion restrictions have historically worked by regulating doctors and the practice of medicine. When the abortion seeker is also the abortion provider, it raises questions about if, when, and how the criminalization of abortion might change. To what extent do states have the capacity, and the willingness, to enforce restrictive abortion laws by criminalizing individual abortion pill users? The answer to this question varies by country context: differences in history, political culture, institutional structure, and public attitudes all shape the state's position on criminalization of abortion. The United States has seen a growing movement to pass laws that treat fetuses as people in need of protection from the women and pregnant people who carry them.[72] The issue of abortion criminalization is closely linked to the creation and enforcement of these laws, because fetal rights measures have been used to prosecute people for illegal abortions. The two topics should also be examined together because the patterns of pregnancy criminalization to date indicate what we might expect to see if abortion criminalization post-*Dobbs* were to escalate.

Criminalization of abortion and conduct during pregnancy has the greatest impact on communities that are overpoliced. In this regard, pregnancy and abortion reflect broader trends in criminalization, where minority groups are disproportionately penalized for activities that are evenly distributed across racial groups (e.g., drug use).[73] The criminalization of abortion sits inside the existing architecture of the US criminal legal system. As a result, surveillance, prosecution, and incarceration of pregnant people for crimes related to pregnancy and abortion fall disproportionately on poor women of color. This is worth emphasizing because public conversations about abortion restrictions tend to obscure their uneven impact. New anti-abortion measures are frequently met with talk about a "war on women" or the claim that "we are living in the *Handmaid's Tale*," in reference to Margaret Atwood's famous reproductive dystopian novel.[74] These responses evoke, as Sophie Lewis has observed, the old feminist illusion that women are "united without regard to class, race, or colonialism ... [against] evil religious fundamentalists with guns."[75] Abortion criminalization, as it is lived in the United States, vividly illustrates the problems with such a narrative because it demonstrates the stratified impact of abortion restrictions.

Few abortion pill packages are actually intercepted in transit. The criminalization of self-managed abortion generally takes place after the abortion (or attempted abortion) when the person presents for medical care or when fetal remains are discovered. As a result, people are more likely to be criminally investigated and prosecuted if they are poor: they face steep financial barriers to in-clinic abortion, they may delay their abortion because they cannot afford care, and they may be participants in public programs that subject them to more government observation. This interplay of "regulation, discrimination, and exposure" means abortion criminalization disproportionately falls on already disadvantaged groups.[76]

In practice, criminalization of self-managed abortion is more likely to affect people later in pregnancy who could not obtain abortion pills before the twelve-week mark, when services like Aid Access stop providing them. A lawyer who advocates for the decriminalization of self-managed abortion explains it in frank terms. Campaigning against the criminalization of self-managed abortion can be difficult because the people being prosecuted have generally attempted to self-manage abortions in their second trimester.

> It's not a nice white college girl who got her pills directly from Rebecca Gomperts. That's just not who is being criminalized. It's people who are living in poverty, it took them four months to get the pills, and they don't know what to do with the fetal remains. That's something that's important to keep in mind in the policy work.[77]

Methods for criminalizing self-managed abortion, miscarriage, and behavior during pregnancy exhibit what the legal scholar Michele Goodwin calls "troubling legal innovation."[78] Legal techniques to criminalize self-managed abortion are varied and, as with all things about abortion in the United States, heavily dependent on the state and local context in which a person lives. A few states have laws that explicitly criminalize self-induced abortion (many of them archaic laws reminiscent of the 1861 Offences Against the Person Act discussed in later chapters on the Republic of Ireland and Northern Ireland). Without laws that explicitly ban self-managed abortion, anti-abortion prosecutors make use of roughly forty types of laws that can be used against people who self-manage abortion and those who help them.[79] This legal tool kit includes laws against homicide, feticide, assault with a weapon, abuse of a corpse, concealing a birth, unlawful practice of medicine, and unlawful practice of pharmacy.[80]

Because data on criminalization of self-managed abortion are scarce, data on criminalization of pregnant women who miscarried or were perceived as risking harm to fertilized eggs, embryos, or fetuses provide a useful indication of trends.[81] Among the four hundred criminal cases brought against pregnant women between 1973 and 2005, studies show stark racial and geographic trends. The majority of criminal cases against pregnant women originated in southern states, with cases concentrated in just a few states, a few counties within those states, and a few hospitals within those counties. South Carolina accounted for 22 percent of all recorded cases, of which one-third were initiated by a single South Carolina hospital. In Florida, 42 percent of cases originated in just two hospitals. Not only were criminal cases geographically concentrated, but they disproportionately targeted Black women. In Florida, where 15 percent of the population is Black, 75 percent of criminal cases against pregnant women were brought against Black women. In South Carolina, where 30 percent of the population is Black, 74 percent of cases were brought against Black women.[82] For many, it was interaction with healthcare professionals that resulted in their criminalization. Where researchers could identify how cases became known to law enforcement, 40 percent of arrests resulted from disclosures made by hospitals, healthcare, or drug treatment programs.[83] Private hospitals are less likely to perform drug tests on mothers or newborns that would lead to arrests, so criminalization is more common at hospitals whose patient populations use public healthcare. As a result, Black women, who are more likely to use these services, are disproportionately criminalized.[84]

The "dramatic pattern of selective law enforcement" against self-managed abortion is a hyperlocal issue. A state's laws, its political climate, its local medical culture, and its prosecutors' attitudes to abortion all profoundly shape if, when, and how investigations will be undertaken and prosecutions will be brought.[85] Prosecutors motivated to bring charges can often find a legal pretext to do so; where they concentrate efforts to criminalize pregnancy and self-managed abortion is shaped by the fundamental inequalities that already shape American life (class, race, geography). State-level abortion bans in the wake of the *Dobbs* decision will widen inequalities in abortion access. They will also expand the spaces where self-managed abortion with pills is the only option, regardless of the uncertain legal risks that it carries.

When asking who is most likely to be criminalized for self-managed abortion, data on pregnancy criminalization indicate that long-standing trends will persist, disproportionately targeting the poorest groups in society. In states that ban abortion entirely, we can expect to see the escalation of surveillance of people seeking post-miscarriage care and the criminalization of miscarriage because it can be difficult to discern whether someone had an induced or spontaneous miscarriage.[86] When asking how people will be criminalized for abortions obtained in another state, answers are more speculative. This is because anti-abortion legislators are devising novel ways to criminalize abortion. It is unclear whether these laws will stand up in court, whether authorities will choose to prosecute people under them, and whether prosecutions will be possible practically. Nonetheless, in the context of so much uncertainty in the United States, we must seriously consider how abortion criminalization might proceed after *Dobbs*.

The most restrictive anti-abortion states—which have already instituted abortion bans within their territories—are now looking for ways to prevent their residents from obtaining abortions elsewhere. The criminalization of cross-border abortion travel is the subject of debate today: lawyers disagree about whether states can prosecute a resident who travels to a different state and engages in conduct that is a crime in their home state. As anti-abortion states try to pass laws that would make it a crime to have an abortion elsewhere, pro-abortion states are working to pass shield laws that would protect their doctors and clinics from criminal and civil suits. Anti-abortion states that want to prosecute for abortions obtained elsewhere will find it difficult to prove that they have jurisdiction, showing exactly where the "crime" took place and providing sufficient proof of any crime having been committed. These are the same problems that have made it impossible (so far) for federal and state governments to stop Aid Access from prescribing to Americans and delivering MA from abroad.[87]

For novel technologies like no-touch medication abortion via telemedicine, novel laws are being devised to criminalize them. A 2021 Missouri bill (introduced but stalled in committee) gives an indication of the strategies that lawmakers might use to exert extraterritorial control over citizens who obtain abortions elsewhere. Missouri's SB 603 attempts to expand the reach of the state's abortion laws by applying them to a much wider range of people and places. Who is subject to Missouri's abortion laws, according to this bill? Anyone with "a substantial connection" to Missouri; anyone who works there; anyone who resides there, including "an unborn child who is a resident"; anyone who would otherwise give birth in Missouri if they could not obtain an abortion; anyone who conceived their pregnancy in Missouri or "may have" conceived in Missouri by having sex there around the time they got pregnant; and anyone who sought prenatal care in Missouri. SB 603 proposes that Missouri's abortion laws should apply to all these people, even when they are seeking an abortion outside of the state.

SB 603 also seeks to apply Missouri abortion laws to MA, even when prescribed and dispensed in another state. It suggests that an abortion in which pre- or post-abortion counseling, payment for the abortion, or "advertising or solicitation" takes place in Missouri would be subject to Missouri laws, likely including remote counseling delivered via phone or email, digital payment for abortion services, or information about abortion travel accessed within the state. Nor can a Missourian travel out of state to take the mifepristone but bring the misoprostol home for later use: If the first medication is administered outside the state but the second dose is "administered or expected to be administered . . . within the state," that abortion would also be subject to Missouri law and therefore become illegal.[88]

Missouri legislators are also following in the footsteps of the Texas "Heartbeat Act" (SB 8) to develop an alternative legal strategy for burdening abortion providers and abortion seekers. This Texas law, effective as of September 2021, introduced the theory that abortion laws could be delegated to private individuals for enforcement, meaning state agents like police and prosecutors are not responsible for investigating and prosecuting individuals who violate the law. Instead, private citizens are expected to enforce the law by bringing civil suits for money damages. Laws of this type create financial deterrents, because abortion providers—even those providing legal abortions—could be bankrupted if they have to repeatedly face down lawsuits.[89] In Missouri, this strategy has been adopted in proposed bills that allow private parties to sue out-of-state doctors who perform abortions on Missouri residents (or anyone else who "aids and abets" the abortion).[90] Missouri House Bill (HB) 1987 proposes a civil liability mechanism for self-managed abortion: it allows private parties to file for damages against anyone who attempts to self-manage an abortion, anyone who "knowingly aids or abets" another person to do so, and anyone who provides an "instrument, device, medicine, drug, or any other means or substance" for self-managed abortion. This includes using "speech or writing" to "influence another person to undergo a self-induced abortion," a measure that presumably aims to ensnare medication abortion activists who provide online information about how to obtain pills for a self-managed abortion in every US state.[91]

The Missouri bills above have not, at the time of writing, become law. However, they represent a significant and expanding strategy that anti-abortion legislators are deploying around the country.[92] Missouri had a trigger law in place to ban abortion as soon as *Roe v. Wade* was overturned, so its attorney general signed an order to enact this abortion ban minutes after the decision in *Dobbs* was announced. Even before *Dobbs*, abortions in Missouri were almost totally unavailable and most Missouri abortion seekers obtained abortions out of state. In the eyes of anti-abortion forces in Missouri, its own abortion ban is incomplete without measures to criminalize abortion travel out of state and criminalize anyone who assists with self-managed abortion for Missourians.

The criminalization of self-managed abortion in the United States is likely to escalate in the context of post-*Dobbs* abortion bans. The available evidence suggests, however, that law enforcement efforts to prevent self-managed abortion with pills are largely futile. Medication abortion moves in ways that make it difficult to detect and intercept. The transnational pipelines that move goods from one country to another have reduced the significance of physical borders and contributed to the mobility of pills. It is easier than ever to buy medication abortion online, whether from online pharmacies or telemedicine abortion providers based outside of the United States. As in other countries, MA activists in the United States are piecing together pathways for expanding the practical accessibility of this medication, at different scales. Sometimes this means referring individuals for consultation with a foreign doctor who can write a prescription and liaise with an Indian distributor to ship a single combi-pack of MA. In other cases, it means purchasing MA in jurisdictions where it is legal (in the United States or abroad) and physically moving it across the border into abortion-hostile places. The systems for facilitating self-managed abortion with pills, outside of the law, had been well established in the United States before 2022 because of the numerous intersecting obstacles that abortion seekers faced in the era of *Roe*'s protections. They have also been established in other countries with restrictive abortion laws, where activist networks operate clandestine but highly organized systems to facilitate self-managed abortion. We can anticipate the future of clandestine abortion in the United States by looking abroad—first to Poland.

CHAPTER 4

The Geography of Clandestine Abortion in Poland

The abortion underground is part of a national hypocrisy. It's fine as long as we don't talk about it!

— Polish activist

In 1964, the "Poland Affair" sparked a scandal in Sweden. Sweden's prosecutor general announced his intention to prosecute Swedish women who had traveled to Poland for abortions. Poland allowed abortion on request, whereas Sweden allowed abortion only in cases of medical necessity when certified by a doctor. The prosecutor's threat caused a national uproar and a groundswell of support for abortion reform in Sweden, eventually contributing to legal change in 1974.[1] Today it is Poles who travel to Sweden when they need abortions. Poland's abortion geography has undergone such a dramatic transformation over the past fifty years that it has become a state from which abortion seekers flee.

Unlike most abortion-restrictive states, Poland had legal abortion for several decades before it adopted a highly restrictive abortion law. This is an unusual trajectory: most countries move from more to less restrictive abortion laws over time. Yet while its legal status has changed in Poland, abortion has remained available through a shifting set of underground institutions. Poland has seen major shifts in the geography of abortion: legal to illegal, hospital to private clinic to private home, home to abroad to home again, surgical abortion provided by doctors in the underground to self-managed abortion with pills supported by activists.

This chapter explores the political and legal context for abortion in Poland; the next chapter delves into self-managed abortion there. Medication abortion has prompted a major reorganization of clandestine abortion in Poland, although the state has been unable and unwilling to eliminate clandestine abortion, preferring instead to ignore the extent of the demand for abortion. The issue of abortion has consistently stoked debates about the meaning of these political changes, so I start with the politics of Poland since the end of state socialism and the democratic transition. I then move to the contemporary political context, addressing questions about knowledge and ignorance of abortion, including the extent of clandestine abortion, state efforts to manage abortion data, and the growth of self-managed abortion with pills.

ABORTION DURING AND AFTER SOCIALISM

From shortly after World War II until 1989, Poland was a satellite state of the Soviet Union governed by a centralized Communist authority. Abortion was legal in Poland from 1956 until the early 1990s, during the years of state socialist rule. Poland's abortion law was shaped by this wider political context; when the USSR implemented abortion liberalization in 1955, it triggered similar reforms across the bloc. From 1956, Poland made abortion available on the grounds of "difficult living conditions," and from 1959, it permitted abortion on request.[2]

Permissive abortion laws in the Soviet Union and its satellite states were part of a broader pro-natalist policy agenda to shape women's role in the family and economy. In the context of centralized economies where population and labor force were seen as synonymous, states actively cultivated control of population through control of fertility. Decrease in population could be managed by restricting abortion, just as rapidly growing population could be managed with more liberal abortion laws (or so states assumed). Soviet-aligned socialist states took an active role in providing services like maternity leave, maternity loans, child benefit payments, child care, and access to abortion. The state provided these services to free women for participation in employment outside the home. Accordingly, reproductive policies "fluctuated in response to labor force requirements and demographic trends."[3] Across the entire Soviet bloc, contraceptives were in short supply, so abortion was heavily relied on as the main method for controlling fertility.[4] Provision of reproductive and family benefits had another function: these services diminished women's dependence on a male breadwinner and increased their dependence on the state. This caveat is important because it situated liberal abortion laws in their political context. Abortion policy under state socialism was not premised on state commitment to the feminist principle of bodily autonomy but on a particular vision of the role of the state in women's family, economic, and reproductive lives. Under Polish state socialism, women came to be seen as a "special object of state policy" and therefore as allies of the socialist regime.[5] This is a perception that continues to shape ideas about women, feminism, and abortion in Poland today.

Abortion occupied an important place in the Polish political landscape during the tumultuous 1970s and 1980s, when the socialist regime faced opposition and escalated its use of authoritarian tactics to stay in power. The role of the Catholic Church in Polish politics also contributed to the importance of the abortion issue. During the most repressive years of state socialist rule, opposition groups sought protection from the Catholic Church, which took on a symbolic role as protector of the Polish people against the regime. It acquired political power as the de facto mediator between the regime and the Solidarity opposition movement.[6] As the church gained power during the 1980s, it took a hard line on issues related to sexuality and reproduction, opposing the more abortion-permissive policies of the state. This stance was also reinforced by Catholic healthcare professionals who were important leaders of the anti-Communist opposition and campaigned for abortion restrictions.[7] Faced with this pressure, the regime sought to appease the church and its power base by making concessions on abortion.[8]

The regime instituted incremental restrictions on abortion throughout the 1980s, including mandatory counseling before abortion and greater scope for doctors to refuse to provide services.[9] In 1990, government funding for abortion was removed, additional doctor approvals were required to certify a legal abortion, gestational age limits were reduced, and protection of conscientious objection was expanded. One year later, the National Assembly of Doctors introduced a code of ethics that prohibited all abortions except in cases of rape and threat to life. Entire hospitals began to declare themselves conscientious objectors to abortion. By 1991, the doctors' code of ethics made abortion practically unavailable in the public health system. As restrictions mounted in the late 1980s, Poland began to see the return of deaths from complications of self-induced abortions, after twenty years without a single such death.[10]

Poland's socialist regime collapsed, and a democratic transition followed in 1989–90, marked by a backlash against all things associated with state socialism. The Catholic Church emerged from the political transition with enormous public support and power over politicians, who courted its favor by pursuing church-approved policies like restrictions on abortion and contraception.[11] The new democratic government immediately introduced anti-abortion legislation when it took power in 1990 and eventually, in 1993, passed the Act on Family Planning, Human Embryo Protection, and Conditions for the Lawful Termination of Pregnancy. For the sake of brevity, I refer to it as the 1993 law. This law was widely interpreted as an effort to "repay" the Catholic Church for its support of the Solidarity movement against the former socialist regime, although it is also true that leading members of the new government were devoutly Catholic and anti-abortion.[12]

The resurgence of antifeminist conservatism in Poland at the time cannot be explained by the power of the Catholic Church alone. The moral climate of the postsocialist transition period must be understood as a legacy of what came before: the ideas, policies, and structures associated with the socialist state profoundly shaped the gender politics of postsocialism. A backlash against gender equality and reproductive freedoms swept across the region. Feminist scholars refer to this process as the "re-masculinization" or "re-traditionalization" of public discourse and gender roles in postsocialist states. It was a process that was not limited to Poland but took place across central and eastern Europe after state socialism.[13] The transition to democracy was marked by forceful efforts to reposition women in the private sphere of the home, eliminate them from public life, and jettison the social and family policies associated with the former regime.[14]

Reproductive politics played a key role in this re-masculinization process. The Polish government implemented a pro-natalist policy agenda with the aim of "returning" to a traditional ideal of Polish womanhood, in a broader context of economic transition from a command to a market economy and austerity policy. In practical terms, this meant the elimination of child care services, cuts to maternity and paternity leave, cuts to family benefits, removal of insurance coverage for contraceptives, and reduction of healthcare subsidies. Cuts in social services associated with the former regime changed the composition of the workforce and altered gender relations in homes and communities, pushing women out of work or into poorly paid precarious work.[15]

The abortion law that governs in Poland today is—for the most part—the same law that was passed shortly after the democratic transition. The 1993 law is known as the "abortion compromise" in political circles, because it restricts abortion without banning it entirely.[16] This law made termination of pregnancy illegal except in three circumstances: when the pregnancy presents

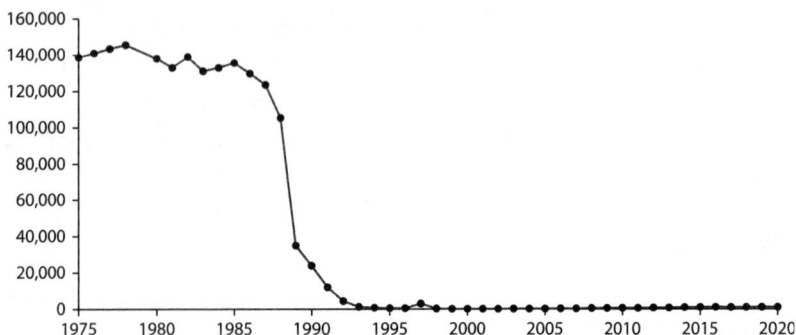

FIGURE 2. Abortions in Poland, as recorded in Polish government data, 1975–2020. Source: Data compiled by the author from UNFPA and Polish government reports. Note: This chart excludes 1997 because the law temporarily changed in 1996 to permit abortion on the ground of "hardship." This ground was quickly removed, and by 1998, the number of abortions had fallen back to 1996 levels. I exclude 1997 data to show the general trends without that distortion.

a threat to the life or health of the woman; when the pregnancy results from rape (provided this crime has been certified by the police and the abortion takes place before the twelfth week of gestation); and when there is a "severe and irreversible" fetal anomaly. However, abortion on the grounds of severe fetal anomaly was ruled unconstitutional by the Constitutional Tribunal in 2020. At present, abortion in Poland is legal only in cases of rape or threat to life and health.[17] The 1993 law makes performing or "assisting" an illegal abortion punishable with up to three years in prison, though it does not include criminal penalties for the person who obtained the abortion.[18] The law concretized numerous restrictions—legally imposed by the state on doctors and professionally imposed by doctors on their own practice—that had already steeply reduced the abortion rate since the mid-1980s. In 1992, one year before the new law was enacted, official records showed abortion numbers were only 3 percent of their 1982 levels (fig. 2).[19]

The 1993 law effectively criminalized 97 percent of abortions in Poland, because only 3 percent of the abortions carried out in the 1980s would have been permitted after its passage. Compared to the system that preceded it, the 1993 law marked a dramatic restriction in abortion access. It significantly changed the way that people accessed abortion, but it did not end the need for abortion or the system for providing it: instead it merely drove demand underground, generating complex clandestine abortion pathways through Poland and across its borders.

THE "WHITE COAT UNDERGROUND"

Restrictive abortion laws do not eliminate abortions. Some people still need abortions and other people still provide them, regardless of the legal risks they face. Poland's unusual abortion trajectory—from free and legal to almost totally prohibited—created a distinctive system for clandestine abortion after the highly restrictive 1993 law came into force. During the 1990s, clandestine abortions in underground clinics were mostly provided by trained gynecologists who had practiced abortion legally before the law changed.[20] This so-called white coat underground of working doctors providing illegal abortions was shaped by the social, economic, and professional context of postsocialist Poland.

Poland's law effectively banning abortion came into force during a time of shock therapy economic reforms, as the state moved from a socialist to a capitalist economy. It coincided with public spending cuts and restructuring of the Polish health system, when doctors saw cuts to their salaries; some sought to make up for lost wages by providing abortions after hours to fee-paying patients.[21] Doctors charged between 2,000 and 4,000 złoty ($450–$920) for an illegal abortion, equivalent to double or quadruple the average monthly wage at the time; as a result, those working in the white coat underground could draw many times their ordinary wage from providing illegal abortions.[22] Abortion providers offered their services in the white coat underground not only because it was lucrative but also because abortion became highly stigmatized within the medical profession. Being associated with abortion was a professional liability. For abortion providers and abortion seekers, clandestine abortion was often the easiest option.

Although the 1993 law dramatically changed the status of abortion in Poland, the practicalities of obtaining an abortion remained similar. When abortion was legal in Poland (1950s–1980s) some gynecology services were already privatized, so legal abortions were often carried out in private facilities for a fee rather than in public hospitals.[23] Outside of hospitals, abortion was obtained in clandestine settings and outpatient facilities. Such an abortion underground had existed before abortion legalization in the late 1950s and continued during the period when abortion was legally available.[24] Because it was fragmented across several different services with different reporting requirements and it was socially stigmatized, the rate of abortion was generally underreported (even when legal) before 1993.[25]

After the 1993 law banned the vast majority of abortions, illegal abortion was widespread. The infrastructure for abortion in private clinics was already well established, and doctors often had clinics attached to their homes where patients could be treated discreetly.[26] For many Poles, abortion services had a semiclandestine status even before they were criminalized because they were split between public and private, formal and informal. This generated confusion for some abortion seekers regarding whether abortion was indeed illegal or whether it was legally available in private clinics alone;[27] for others, it reinforced the tacit understanding that abortion would be available only to those with the money to pay for it. As in many abortion-restrictive countries, Polish women operated informal whisper networks to share information about which doctors would perform abortions or provide referrals.[28] Abortion in 1990s Poland was situated in a postsocialist health system where informal payments for treatment were "virtually mandatory" in order to access better and faster services.[29] In the case of abortion, informal payments to a private doctor could secure a referral or a termination, depending on the doctor. At the same time, professional medical bodies and prominent doctors were allied with powerful anti-abortion elites, so doctors who were known to have pro-choice views were professionally ostracized.[30]

The culture of anti-abortion stigma worked to "enforce and obscure" the commercialization of clandestine abortion, in the words of the anthropologist Agata Chełstowska.[31] The 1993 law imposed criminal penalties on the abortion provider if they could be caught "in the act" of providing an illegal abortion. Underground providers announced their services by posting euphemistic newspaper advertisements for "full spectrum" gynecologists who offered "all services" in "discreet" settings.[32] Posting such a newspaper advertisement was not enough evidence to prosecute a doctor for providing illegal abortions, so law enforcement relied on witnesses who would testify against the doctor: disgruntled partners or family members of the abortion seeker or the abortion seeker if she could be compelled to denounce the doctor.[33] Investigations and prosecutions of underground abortion providers were rare and usually resulted only in fines or suspended sentences.[34] The risk of criminalization did not deter doctors, for the most part, from providing this service. In the context of healthcare restructuring and wage cuts, the small risk of prosecution was outweighed for many doctors by the financial incentives.

The doctors who operated the white coat underground had trained before the 1993 law came into force, so, lacking knowledge of and equipment for more modern methods, they generally relied on older abortion methods. In both legal and illegal settings, doctors used dilation and sharp curettage (emptying the uterus by scraping it with a sharp implement) rather than vacuum aspiration (emptying the uterus with a suction device).[35] Dilation and curettage is considered an outdated method by the World Health Organization, which recommends vacuum aspiration instead because it carries fewer risks.[36] The use of outdated methods in Poland also helps explain the high cost of an illegal abortion: surgical abortion in an underground clinic required a gynecologist, an anesthetist, and a driver, among others.[37] Fewer doctors providing clandestine abortions also meant higher prices for illegal abortion in Poland compared to legal abortion abroad.

By the mid-1990s, at least twenty companies in Poland operated as abortion referral and travel agencies, facilitating more than sixteen thousand abortions abroad per year. The pathways for abortion travel abroad from Poland were shaped by the interplay of class and geography. Wealthier women who could afford more expensive services traveled to the Netherlands, Germany, Belgium, or Austria, where abortion services were considered higher quality; those who lived in the south or east of Poland and could not afford to travel west could go to Ukraine, Lithuania, Belarus, the Czech Republic, or Slovakia to obtain an abortion. Abortion travel services ranged from referral agencies that could connect abortion seekers with clinics abroad to full-service travel companies that arranged bus trips from Polish cities to clinics in bordering countries. These services dwindled after some abortion referral agencies were prosecuted and the people involved in running them jailed.[38] As organized travel services declined, abortion travel came to be oriented to private clinics in countries on Poland's western and southern border and to arrangements by individuals organizing abortions for themselves.

GENDER IDEOLOGY AND THE LAW AND JUSTICE PARTY

Since the end of state socialism and the transition to democracy, Polish political debates have evoked abortion as a yardstick to measure how far the country has transformed itself.[39] During the 1990s, debates on abortion regulation became venues for parties to set out opposing views of Polish identity after socialism: opponents of abortion argued that liberal abortion laws were anti-Polish, imposed by oppressive foreign communist rulers; advocates for abortion argued that anti-abortion restrictions were reminiscent of the repressive tactics of the old regime. Debates about reproduction have been, and remain, central to politics in central and eastern Europe because they are sites where "coded arguments" about state, society, morality, and political authority play out.[40]

The issue of abortion in Poland today has, however, been reframed as part of a larger culture war led by the Law and Justice party, the government, allies in various branches of the state, and civil society groups. The Law and Justice party—in Polish, Prawo i Sprawiedliwość, or PiS—is best characterized as a populist, nationalist, and right-wing party. It was founded by former members of the anti-Communist Solidarity movement as a law-and-order political party dedicated to expelling former Communists from Polish public life and politics.[41] PiS governed from 2005 to 2007 and came to power again in 2015 with strong support from the Catholic Church.[42]

PiS is staunchly against abortion, and its stance on the issue is part of a wider agenda to combat what it calls "gender ideology." This is a broad signifier: it includes specific things like feminism, abortion, sex education, and LGBTQ+ rights, but it also signifies a general dissatisfaction with the current socioeconomic order. Opponents of gender ideology present themselves as protectors of the family and children from cosmopolitan elites who wish to corrupt them.[43] Populist and nationalist parties across Europe mobilize their followers and draw support by opposing gender ideology, although PiS has been uniquely successful in Poland, where it has made this anti-gender campaign into state policy.[44] Opposition to gender ideology is context-specific, so Poland's anti-gender movement differs in important respects from similar movements in Italy or France, for example. In Poland, gender ideology is equated with Marxism (pulling Poland back into the Communist past), secularism (attacking the institution of the Polish Catholic Church), and the European Union (eroding Polish sovereignty through European integration).[45] PiS campaigns against gender ideology with the support of allied civil society groups like Ordo Iuris, which are especially influential on the issue of abortion. Ordo Iuris is an ultraconservative Catholic pressure group that functions as a legal think tank, intervening in litigation, issuing legal interpretations in support of PiS, and publicly campaigning against abortion, LGBTQ+ rights, and other issues they identify as "gender ideology originating in Marxism."[46]

PiS came to power in 2015, winning both the presidency and an absolute majority in parliament on a platform of nationalism, populism, and opposition to gender ideology.[47] After taking power, PiS went about implementing its anti-gender agenda through the following measures: changing emergency contraception to a prescription-only medication, so it became extremely difficult to access in a timely manner; introducing abstinence-only sex education and limiting access to sex education; reducing state funding for assisted reproductive technology; cutting government funding to women's rights organizations; and authorizing raids on charities that work on gender equality and domestic violence issues. PiS also tried to withdraw from an international treaty to prevent violence against women and proposed a law that would redefine domestic violence to exempt "first time" offenders.[48] Informally, PiS rule has had a chilling effect on reproductive healthcare, with growing numbers of doctors invoking conscientious objection to refuse prenatal testing or contraceptives services since 2015.[49]

PiS and its allies also took action to further restrict abortion in 2016 and 2018, triggering mass protests known as the Black Protests—the largest demonstrations since the Solidarity protests of the 1980s.[50] Many thousands of Poles mobilized in 2016 against a bill titled "Stop Abortion" that was being considered in Parliament. The bill was the product of a citizens' initiative led by Ordo Iuris. It proposed to define life as beginning at the moment of conception and to ban abortion altogether. It also proposed to criminalize the person who gets the abortion and anyone who helps. A coalition of pro-choice groups launched a civic initiative called "Save the Women" in response, proposing legal abortion on request up to twelve weeks, but this was immediately rejected by Parliament.[51] Mass mobilization against the 2016 "Stop Abortion" initiative led the PiS government to eventually reject the bill, but parts of it came back in later citizens' initiatives in 2018. That Polish feminists felt compelled to oppose a total abortion ban with a proposal for a twelve-week on-request period (and that the twelve-week proposal was still rejected outright in Parliament) speaks to the extremely anti-abortion political context. While some polling suggested that abortion attitudes in Poland were becoming more conservative at the time PiS returned to power, polling conducted after the Black Protests of 2016 and 2018 suggests that a majority support abortion on request up to twelve weeks into pregnancy.[52]

Civic initiative bills like "Stop Abortion" had reached Parliament in previous years, but they had never met with the support of the ruling party. The party in power in 2007–15 preferred to preserve the so-called abortion compromise of 1993 and did not support further restrictions. However, when PiS came to power in 2015, the political climate changed. By 2016, with the populist conservatives of PiS in power in the presidency and Parliament, proposals for a near-total abortion ban were met more favorably and rejected only after public protests.[53] Ultimately, by rejecting both the "Stop Abortion" and "Save the Women" bills and preserving the 1993 law, the government was able to position itself as embracing the old compromise. Anti-abortion groups took an incrementalist approach that one activist calls "the salami method": slicing thinly and attempting to pass the desired measures one small piece at a time.[54]

Anti-abortion measures like those in 2016 and 2018 are pieces of a larger agenda to curtail the reproductive rights that remain in Poland. While the Black Protest mobilizations against the "Stop Abortion" bill forced the government to vote down the proposals, opponents of abortion in the legislature retained measures that they could "pull out of the drawer" at any moment, as one former member of the Polish Parliament explains.[55] This is effectively what happened in 2020: members of Parliament from PiS and other right-wing parties appealed to the Constitutional Tribunal to strike down the part of the 1993 abortion law that allowed abortion in cases of severe fetal anomaly. Political machinations in 2015–17 had already packed the Constitutional Tribunal with PiS-appointed judges, who worked to facilitate its legislative agenda in the courts.[56] The Constitutional Tribunal ruled that abortion in the case of severe fetal anomaly was unconstitutional. Its decision provoked large street protests when it was announced in October 2020, although it did not officially come into force until January 2021.[57] Nonetheless, hospitals immediately began to conform to its restrictions by refusing to provide legal abortion care.[58] The Tribunal's ruling drastically reduced the availability of legal abortion because abortions granted on grounds of severe fetal anomaly accounted for the vast majority of legal abortions obtained in Poland—an average of 95 percent of those performed in hospitals every year between 2008 and 2020.[59] This discussion of official abortion data, however, is only a small piece of the true picture of abortion in Poland.

THE POLITICS OF POLISH ABORTION DATA

Silence and stigma are key to keeping abortion "illegal but accessible" in Poland today.[60] Officially, very few abortions take place in the country; unofficially, hundreds of thousands of Poles resort to clandestine abortion at home or travel abroad for an abortion. To illustrate Poland's abortion landscape today, and situate MA in this context, I now turn to the topic of how data on abortion—illegal, legal, and somewhere in between—are developed, framed, and managed. I show, drawing on the sociology literature on strategic ignorance, that official data intentionally underestimate the demand for abortion and the numbers of people who access abortion (whether clandestine inside Poland or abroad). Official ignorance is not just the absence of knowledge but instead can be "an actively engineered part of a deliberate plan."[61] Ignorance has strategic advantages because acquiring knowledge can have repercussions. If an institution can protest its ignorance, it is more difficult to hold it accountable for failing to take action on a problem.[62] On abortion, specifically, states deliberately choose to remain ignorant about the extent of noncompliance with their abortion laws as a way of mediating tensions in their policies.[63] Choosing not to acquire knowledge about clandestine abortion can relieve states of pressure to act against people who flout the abortion law or any obligation to reform the abortion law when it loses public legitimacy. In this way, institutions can divest themselves of responsibility for providing legal abortion by choosing to remain ignorant of the demand for it or the extent of requests denied.

Official government data on abortion in Poland offer one (partial) way to understand the impact of the 1993 abortion law. Hospitals are required to report their annual abortion numbers to the government, so the annual reports published by the Ministry of Health provide an official count of how many abortions take place in Polish hospitals. They paint a dire picture. At the lowest point, in 2001, only 123 legal abortions were carried out. In the twenty years since, the number has slowly risen, reaching a high of 1,076 in 2020. This rise has been driven by growing numbers of terminations granted on the grounds of severe fetal anomaly. By 2020, abortion on these grounds accounted for 97.8 percent of legal abortions in Poland.[64] Accordingly, after abortion for severe fetal anomaly was ruled unconstitutional in 2020, official abortion figures plummeted: the following year the Polish government announced that only 107 abortions had taken place.[65]

Clearly, these figures do not represent the true number of abortions in Poland or among Poles who seek abortion abroad. Given that figures in the 1970s and 1980s hovered around 140,000 (officially recorded) abortions, post-1993 data showing between one hundred and one thousand abortions per year are implausibly low for a population that hovers around 37 million (see fig. 2).[66] Demographers argue that this figure is also extremely low when compared to other countries in the region. Postsocialist countries in central and eastern Europe are the best comparators for Poland because they share important pieces of reproductive history: in postsocialist states where abortion was legal and freely available and where modern contraception was very difficult to access, abortion rates were high.[67] Many countries with this history continue to experience high abortion rates and low rates of contraceptive use. Indeed, Polish women use modern contraception at lower rates than do women in other European countries.[68] Nonetheless, neighboring countries report abortion rates anywhere from thirty-five times higher (Slovakia) to eighty-two times higher (Belarus) than Poland's official rate.[69]

Poland's 1993 abortion law criminalized roughly 97 percent of the abortions that had taken place in previous years. But there is evidence that the state undercounts even the extent of demand for abortions legally permitted under the 1993 law because authorities take steps to prevent abortion requests from appearing in official records. The production of ignorance on abortion takes place at different scales, implicating individual doctors as well as officials who collect and manage data. In her work on the sociology of ignorance, Linsey McGoey names this dynamic the interaction of "micro" and "macro" ignorance. For ignorance to become entrenched at the level of policy, it must be sustained on a daily and individual basis.[70] Individual acts of ignoring (micro ignorance) become cemented into ideological positions and policy frameworks that obscure the faulty assumptions on which they are based (macro ignorance).

Micro ignorance of abortion is a daily practice in Polish hospitals. Hospitals that are legally obliged to perform abortions under the 1993 law frequently report that they do not perform any abortions because no patients ask for them.[71] Hospitals minimize the number of abortions requested in their facilities using the following tactics: they issue verbal denials without written confirmation, they refuse to record abortion requests in official documentation, they mislead patients as to whether they qualify for a legal abortion, or they order additional tests in order to exceed the legal time limit for an abortion.[72] Beyond giving verbal refusal only, hospitals are known to refuse patients by giving inaccurate information about the legal grounds for their abortion, the availability of hospital personnel, or the availability of medical equipment for abortion.[73] With these tactics, hospitals can informally avoid performing any abortions without explicitly refusing and thus report that no requests have been made. Advocates for abortion seekers have developed strategies to combat official refusal to acknowledge abortion requests. They coach clients on how to make a formal abortion request at the hospital. For example:

She should bring a file with her, with the request for abortion. She should have two copies of each, one for the hospital and another as proof—with the signature and the stamp with the date—that it was filed, that she submitted the request for abortion. Once they have this document, that's proof she wanted an abortion. Because otherwise they lie! [They say,] "We don't have any such cases or any women asking us for abortion."[74]

Obstructive doctors and hospital staff refuse patients' requests for legal abortion in ways that circumvent the requirement to record their refusals in official statistics. Although this violates hospitals' legal obligations, pro-choice lawyers report that once refused by doctors, abortion seekers are often reluctant to pursue legal challenges against the institutions that refused them. The extent of anti-abortion stigma presents a high barrier: people obtain the abortion abroad and then "forget about it."[75] Many of these Poles, refused abortion at home, are referred through legal support and activist networks to hospitals abroad where they can obtain abortions covered by European health insurance.[76] Official reports of legal abortions in the hundreds do not reflect the need for abortion in Poland, but they instead reflect a system designed to deny abortion requests and push abortion seekers out of the formal medical system.

Deliberate decisions to ignore and obscure abortion requests may also explain why legal abortions recorded in the case of rape are vanishingly low: over the ten years between 2008 and 2018, there were only ten abortions granted for this reason. This is despite three to four thousand reported rapes— itself a notoriously underreported crime—filed with the police every year.[77] Ministry of Health officials have publicly claimed that Poland has such vanishingly low rates of abortion in cases of rape simply because people do not request an abortion in these circumstances.[78] Government data that show zero or few requests for such abortions reflect the faulty data compiled and reported by hospitals. Monitoring efforts by civil society groups illustrate a similar strategic ignorance, with high levels of nonresponse or claims that no abortion requests—for any reason—are received.[79]

These daily acts of micro ignorance on abortion demand accrete over time into policy or ideology in institutions that officially provide legal abortion. According to data compiled by nongovernmental organizations (NGOs) between 2013 and 2017, only two doctors out of three hundred Polish hospitals had formally declared themselves conscientious objectors to abortion.[80] Twenty-two hospitals reported they had not received—and therefore not refused any abortion requests. The extent of informal refusal is much greater: in practice, before the restrictions added in 2020, it was estimated that only 10 percent of hospitals in Poland performed abortions.[81] Minimizing the number of requested abortions is another way to suggest that Poland's abortion ban is obeyed and supported by the public. Efforts to distort the numbers of requested abortions, by refusing to collect and publish data, all serve the political fiction that Poland's abortion ban stops abortion. This is belied by the widespread use of medication abortion to self-manage in clandestine settings.

COUNTING CLANDESTINE ABORTIONS

Official data on abortion in Poland deliberately undercount the number of people who want, and get, abortions. But how many abortions really take place in Poland each year? And how can we count them? The Federation for Women and Family Planning (Federa), a prominent Polish reproductive rights NGO, has consistently estimated that Poles have between 80,000 and 200,000 "illegal" abortions each year. Federa arrives at this estimate based on demographic data, comparisons with countries with similar demographic structures, and historical data on pregnancy termination.[82] A United Nations report similarly estimates between 80,000 and 180,000 abortions per year.[83] Estimates of the number of Poles who seek abortion abroad each year ranges from 40,000 to 100,000.[84] Public polling also shows the prevalence of clandestine abortion: a 2013 poll found that at least one in four and nearly one in three Polish women had had an abortion in their lifetime.[85] Polling on this question is practically difficult, however, because the extent of anti-abortion stigma means people are reluctant to admit that they had an abortion—even anonymously.[86]

Medication abortion pills are, by all available evidence, the main way that clandestine abortion takes place in Poland. MA first came to widespread attention in Polish media in 2003 when Federa invited Women on Waves to sail its abortion ship to Poland. Three years after this ship campaign, in 2006, Women on Web began operating its pill service. In its first years, the group received the majority of its pill requests from people in Poland.[87] The same year that group launched its online pill service, the Polish activist Justyna Wydrzyńska established an online forum for discussing abortion, contraception, and sex education. At the same time, Poland's white coat underground had become a less appealing place for clandestine abortion, as fewer doctors offered abortions and prices rose. People began to seek out abortion abroad as information about foreign clinics became more available online and as they realized that legal abortion across the border was less expensive, and less risky, than clandestine surgical abortion at home.[88] Self-managed abortion at home with pills also became an attractive option for people who sought out alternatives to illegal surgical services.

The secretive nature of self-managed abortion makes it impossible to precisely track how demand for pills rose over time. Anecdotal reports, however, confirm a growing interest in pills in the years after Women on Web launched. An activist on the staff of a women's rights group in the early 2010s explains how she realized MA was becoming a preferred method:

> [My job] was to give information about what's legal and illegal. But I realized it was changing because more and more people started to ask me, "OK, is this organization good for pills? What's going to happen? What do they look like? When are they going to come? What's the risk? What will it look like? Can I go to work afterward?" . . . So I realized, at some point, that it was shifting.[89]

MA became more available to Poles as WoW established its services in the mid-2000s and public awareness about medication abortion grew. Poland's abortion geography shifted again as growing numbers sought MA or abortion abroad. Like the other countries discussed in this book, it is nearly impossible to accurately account for the number of people using abortion pills to self-manage abortion in Poland. This is because pills come in through different routes and different suppliers, as I illustrate later, some of which are feminist networks that publicize their data and some of which are secretive for-profit groups selling pills online. The feminist pill networks Women on Web and Women Help Women do not release annual data on the extent of pill requests from Poland.[90] However, Women on Web, which intermittently publishes its data for Poland, reports 200,000 visits to its website from Poland each year.[91] In the first six months of 2016, 1,220 Poles ordered pills from the site.[92] During a six-month period between 2020 and 2021, Women Help Women reported that it had supplied 10,000 people in Poland with pills.[93]

The Polish government is required to produce an annual public report about the implementation of the 1993 law, in which it publishes data on legal abortions only.[94] The Polish government does not collect information on what it calls "the extra-legal phenomenon" of clandestine abortion inside Poland, explaining in a 2019 monitoring report that "this phenomenon is difficult to study."[95] Nor does the government collect data on abortions that Poles obtain abroad.[96] When pressed by European Union officials, the Polish Ministry of Health offered an estimate of 10,000 clandestine abortions per year.[97] This acknowledgment of clandestine abortion by the state is partly the result of advocates' work publicizing it in the international media as acknowledging clandestine abortion runs counter to the interests of the state. Denial of the abortion underground—and underestimation of its scale—serves a political purpose, shoring up anti-abortion institutions that describe the law as a "very good compromise" that is effective at eliminating the need for most abortions.[98]

Anti-abortion groups offer very low estimates for illegal or clandestine abortions, but they do not deny their existence entirely. Anti-abortion groups like the Polish Association of Human Life Defenders estimate 7,000 to 14,000 per year, an estimate that they use to disavow the "myth of the abortion underground."[99] Opponents contest the scale of clandestine abortion in Poland, but they also refuse to concede that the existence of clandestine abortion should prompt policy reform. They draw parallels between illegal abortion and other forms of criminality that the state cannot tolerate, arguing that abortion, like the crime of theft, should not be legalized simply because it continues to occur when it is treated as a crime. Polish anti-abortion groups warn that "overstating" the extent of the demand for clandestine abortion is a familiar "tool in the political struggle."[100] As we will see in Ireland, Irish conservatives also branded medication abortion a red herring in debates about law reform in order to argue against liberalization.

While institutions take deliberate steps not to collect data on the extent of requests for abortion, clandestine abortion, or use of extraterritorial abortion services, Polish authorities have recently moved to collect additional forms of pregnancy data. In 2022, the Polish minister of health signed an order requiring doctors to register the pregnancies of all their patients on the national medical record database.[101] Self-managed abortion and spontaneous miscarriage are not crimes in Poland, but the introduction of a data collection system that might detect them with greater frequency and makes data about them available to more authorities will likely have harmful consequences and could escalate efforts to criminalize those who assist with abortion.

———

Clandestine abortion in Poland has taken many forms over the decades. When abortion was legal under state socialism, it was often quicker and easier to seek out a gynecologist in the private sector. These private providers were pushed underground through mounting restrictions in the 1980s. Once the political transition occurred, and abortion was severely restricted by the 1993 law, private abortion providers became a crucial resource for abortion seekers, who could obtain an illegal but generally safe surgical abortion if they could pay for it. Others could travel to countries just across the border or farther afield, depending on their situation and financial resources. The introduction of MA in Poland prompted another reorganization of the clandestine abortion pathways there. Pills changed some aspects of abortion in Poland, but the essential feature stayed the same: abortion in Poland remains heavily stigmatized and clandestine, yet widely available in practice.

Abortion pills have become more widely available and more important for clandestine abortion in the context of an emboldened anti-abortion movement in Polish politics. There is an important caveat to the claim that self-managed abortion is available, in practice, for many people in Poland. Even as MA becomes more widely available in clandestine settings and through activist networks, the practical lack of abortion services in Polish healthcare institutions is deadly. Three Polish women died in hospitals between 2020 and 2022 when they were denied life-saving abortions.[102] Their deaths demonstrate that self-managed abortion can only facilitate safe abortion for a portion of the people who require it, and it cannot eliminate the need for safe, legal, and local abortion services with medical support. Government officials denied that the deaths were caused by the abortion law, arguing instead that medical malpractice was the cause and that life-saving abortion remains available in Poland.[103] (Some of the doctors involved even faced charges of manslaughter by malpractice.) On the contrary, these deaths demonstrate that Poland's law is, in effect, a total ban on abortion. Nevertheless, as we have seen, this ban is circumvented and challenged every day through the activities of MA networks inside Poland and across its border.

CHAPTER 5

Abortion Pills in the Polish Abortion Underground

People can think we are crazy or whatever, but when the police actually come after us, people are gonna wake up! If that happens, it happens. We're not afraid of that.

— Polish activist

In April 2022, the activist Justyna Wydrzyńska went on trial in Warsaw. Wydrzyńska had been contacted online by a woman in an abusive relationship who was desperate to end her pregnancy but was prevented from having an abortion abroad by her husband. The woman turned to the internet. Wydrzyńska sent a package of her own abortion pills, but the woman's husband intercepted the pills and contacted the police, who then raided Wydrzyńska's home. After a year-long trial, she was convicted of breaking Poland's 1993 abortion law, which criminalizes anyone who "renders assistance to a pregnant woman in terminating her pregnancy in violation of the law."[1] Outside the courtroom, speaking the language of social decriminalization, Wydrzyńska framed her own prosecution as part of a larger social change:

> I don't regret what I did. I would love it if people could support each other, could share pills, could be with each other. I hope that this case will be a breakthrough and the fact that we share abortion pills will be a reflex of empathy and understanding for the needs of another human being.[2]

Wydrzyńska became the first activist in Europe to be prosecuted for facilitating an abortion with pills. The year before, Wydrzyńska's organization and its allies in Abortion Without Borders had helped 34,000 people from Poland obtain abortions. Around a thousand of these people traveled to clinics abroad, but the vast majority obtained pills inside Poland to self-manage their abortions with information from support groups.[3] Wydrzyńska's conviction signals increased efforts to criminalize abortion, but it also illustrates the broader contradiction of abortion access in Poland. An activist directly facilitating one abortion is a crime, but the same activist indirectly facilitating tens of thousands of abortions is not a crime. In fact, it is the basis for abortion access in Poland today.

For nearly thirty years, Poland's abortion ban has been evaded and defied. This defiance has taken different shapes over time: the Polish abortion underground now involves fewer doctors, fewer surgical abortions, more lay activists, and more self-managed abortions with pills. In Poland, abortion pill use has transformed the practical accessibility of self-managed abortion—making it cheaper, more widely available, and more protected legally—all while the political momentum moves in the opposite direction. A political context of extreme anti-abortion hostility exists alongside strategic ignorance over the extent of clandestine abortion and a legal context of decriminalized self-managed abortion.

This chapter discusses the pathways and sources through which people obtain and use pills in Poland, each of which offers a different level of support, reliability, and risk. Polish abortion activism works on the principle of enabling practical access now to achieve reform later, a strategy that is made possible by the ambiguous legal status of self-managed abortion. However, accessing pills is not easy or straightforward because the abortion ban, the high level of demand for abortion, and misinformation about abortion continue to create opportunities for profitable scams. I explore the legal status of self-managed abortion, and the extent of its criminalization, by tracing pills through three pathways: doctors, transnational activists, and online pill vendors.

THE LEGAL STATUS OF SELF-MANAGED ABORTION

Like all abortion bans, Poland's law causes harm to people who end their own pregnancies. Unlike many abortion bans, however, Poland's law does not criminalize the person who ends *their own* pregnancy. It criminalizes anyone who terminates someone else's pregnancy with the consent of the pregnant person (article 152), as well as anyone who causes someone else to have an abortion through the use of violence, threat, or deceit (article 153).[4] It requires all legal abortions to take place in public hospitals, with medical grounds certified by multiple doctors, and it prohibits abortions in private clinics. The law concentrates on limiting doctors' ability to provide abortion.[5] This model of criminalization reflects the system for abortion at the time: when abortion meant surgical abortion carried out by someone else, criminalizing anyone who provides an abortion would effectively criminalize all abortions. With the emergence of medication abortion, which allows the pregnant person to be their own abortion provider, the law's distinction between the pregnant person and the abortion provider is anachronistic.

Other legal provisions that facilitate self-managed abortion relate to the importation of medicines. A person can bring in medication from abroad—in person or via the internet—because it is not a crime to bring medications into Poland for personal use, even if these medications are not sold inside Poland.[6] Mifepristone is not registered for use in Poland, and misoprostol is sold in pharmacies for gastric uses, although it is only available with a prescription.[7] Buying these medications and supplying them for another person to use can be considered "assisting" with abortion, as the conviction of Justyna Wydrzyńska shows, but abortion seekers themselves can legally buy medication abortion pills abroad. Ultimately, it is not a crime for a person to end their own pregnancy with pills in Poland, provided they are fewer than twenty-two weeks into pregnancy.[8]

As self-managed abortion with pills becomes a greater share of clandestine abortions in Poland, this means that a growing number of abortions are not illegal, because they do not violate Poland's 1993 abortion law. Advocates of self-managed abortion use this to dispute the oft-repeated claim that 200,000 "illegal abortions" take place every year and, by extension, the claim that 97 percent of abortions that take place in Poland are illegal. Clandestine self-managed abortion falls between these categories because it is not a legal abortion provided in a hospital, nor is it a crime. According to a lawyer and activist, "What's illegal is a doctor or someone performing an abortion on someone. [Self-managed abortion with pills and abortion travel abroad] are not illegal. . . . They are, of course, in the shadow of the formal system, but they are not illegal."[9] This is not to say that abortion with pills is decriminalized in Poland. On the contrary, people who assist with abortion are at legal risk, including people who provide MA and facilitate abortion by paying for its related costs. People who order abortion pills for themselves are subjected to police harassment, even if they have committed no crime, because abortion seekers are often unaware of the precise legal status of the medicines they have obtained. Anti-abortion groups are actively working to devise legal theories that would extend the state's power to criminalize self-managed abortion. Although self-managing an abortion is not a crime for the person who uses pills to end their own pregnancy, to get to that point, at least one other person (in Poland or abroad) will be involved. There are a few different pathways that people use to obtain medication abortion inside Poland: elements of the white coat underground who moved into pill provision, the activist groups working in Poland and with allies across Europe to supply pills, and the online pill vendors who supply misoprostol for a price.

THE WHITE COAT PILL UNDERGROUND

The white coat underground for surgical abortion has diminished, as the doctors who comprised its workforce retired and stopped practicing in their private clinics. When abortion was all but prohibited, abortion care was removed from the medical curriculum, and Polish gynecologists no longer received training in it.[10] Abortion providers from the pre-1993 cohort aged out and retired without being replaced by a younger generation.[11] The decline can also be explained by cultural changes in the Polish medical profession. Surveys of Polish doctors show that the post-1993 generation holds more conservative anti-abortion views and tends to see clandestine abortion providers as profiteers rather than advocates for patients. Polish doctors report that they fear being professionally associated with abortion—even legal abortion. They fear being denied career opportunities, being ostracized by colleagues, or being exposed and denounced from the pulpit, as has happened to doctors who were publicly named as abortion providers.[12] The white coat underground for surgical abortion became less appealing to abortion seekers as well, because it relied on outdated abortion methods and charged high prices. However, the decline of the white coat underground providing surgical abortion for a fee has not meant the end of Polish doctors' involvement in underground abortion. Rather the way they are involved has changed.

Despite the conservatism that is widespread in the profession, doctors still have economic incentives to provide clandestine abortion services.[13] Agata Chełstowska calls this the process of "turning sin into gold": though stigmatized and criminalized, abortion in Poland is also thoroughly commercialized.[14] This intense stigma leaves abortion seekers vulnerable to authority figures who would exploit them. Abortion clinics on Poland's border in Slovakia and the Czech Republic increasingly target Polish patients with

Polish-language advertisements, websites, phone lines, and, occasionally, travel services that collect patients from Polish cities and take them directly to the clinic and back again. Nonetheless, abortion seekers without access to this information may still turn to their local doctors. Doctors can profit from anti-abortion stigma and misinformation by charging patients for "referrals" to foreign clinics, although these referrals amount to little more than publicly available contact information. A translator who previously assisted Polish women in an abortion clinic in Vienna provides one example of this trend. Her clinic was visited by Polish women who had been "referred" by a gynecologist in a border city in the south of Poland:

> He was giving women a piece of paper with our clinic's name and email address under the table. He charged 400 zł [$100] for that. And then we had two women from [that city] in a row. . . . I called him later, because I felt that his charging those women for nothing was completely unacceptable. He started shouting at me that I shouldn't call him because anyone could be listening to his phone.[15]

Abortion clinics outside of Poland typically do not require a referral from a patient's local doctor; at most, they require an ultrasound scan to date the pregnancy, but this can be obtained without disclosing the desire for an abortion.[16] Many abortion seekers do not know this, of course. They rely on knowledge shared within social networks or posted online, but, though information is plentiful, it is unreliable. People searching for Polish-language abortion resources online can easily find advertisements for all manner of "providers" because the newspaper advertisements of previous decades now exist in online classified ads. They use familiar euphemisms for abortion. Searches carried out in 2020 returned dozens of results advertising clandestine abortion in barely disguised terms (table 2).

To study these pill sources in more depth, I worked with a Polish-speaking researcher, Zosia, to contact the sellers who advertised online.[17] Zosia called the publicly advertised phone numbers for twenty pill vendors like those listed in table 2. During the calls, she posed as a woman living in Łódź who was six weeks' pregnant and trying to obtain pills. She asked the pill vendors the kinds of questions that any abortion seeker who found their numbers online would ask. She did not ask any of the vendors about their identity or precise location. One of these calls reached a man who identified himself as a practicing doctor working in central Poland. He told Zosia that she had to travel to his office to collect the pills:

TABLE 2   ADVERTISEMENTS FOR CLANDESTINE ABORTION SERVICES IN
POLAND, 2020

Northern Poland	"A–Z Gynecologist—Full range. Pharmacological recovery of menstrual cycle, ultrasound scan. Contact 24 hours."
Southern Poland	"Gynecologist, full range of services. Pharmacological recovery of menstrual cycle, ultrasound scan, free consultation, attractive prices."
Central Poland	"Full range of gynecologist services and procedures. Non-invasive recovery of menstrual cycle. Discrete recovery of menstrual cycle. Surgical procedures in professional setting with gynecologist and anesthesiologist care."
Southern Poland	"I care about women with unwanted pregnancies. I guarantee a safe and natural miscarriage. Call me. . . . There is also the option to perform the procedure in the clinic."
Western Poland	"Tablets helping to bring back menstrual cycle. 300zł ($70)"
No region indicated	"Painless pharmacological removal of unwanted pregnancy. Success rate: 98% until 10 weeks, 91% until 10–14 weeks. Full discretion is ensured."

SOURCE: Compiled by the author and a research assistant from Web material.

Do you want to come by train or car? We need to arrange it in advance, as I have my hospital practice and quite a lot of work in surgery. . . . I still need you to go to a gynecologist in Łódź to confirm the pregnancy and tell you exactly how many weeks you are. If they want to start a pregnancy card—usually they don't do it during the first visit, but they might—don't panic. When everything is over, I will tell you exactly what to say to them, so it looks like a natural miscarriage.

A pregnancy card is used by doctors to monitor visits, tests, and interventions during pregnancy. The doctor assumed she would be worried about this because it would create an official record of her pregnancy with her local doctor and thus raise eyebrows the next time she returned, no longer pregnant.[18] When Zosia asked the doctor about payment, he explained that he charged 1,500zł ($380)—cash only—for the abortion pills. But he explained that this high price was justified by the quality of the products:

You will find adverts out there for 300 to 400zł [$75–$100]. The internet is full of ridiculous advertisements from people who know nothing! You will see the "1+12" nonsense. I had patients who did that, and then the tablets were not genuine. I had to help them. I charge more, but I will be in contact with you throughout the whole time, and you can feel safe with me.

When the doctor mentioned the unreliable 1+12, he was referring to the kinds of online pill vendors that I address in detail later in the chapter. When he touted the quality of his products to Zosia, the doctor justified his higher price and reassured her about his motives: "I am not doing this for the money, believe me. I have enough work, but to be able to help long term I need to charge, as it costs me as well. And I have too much to lose here." Zosia ended the call by saying she would follow up with him, but she did not call again. The person who Zosia reached, if he was truly a doctor, was putting himself at some considerable risk by selling MA to people who contacted him by phone. The information gleaned from Zosia's conversation is consistent with information provided by interviewees and NGOs monitoring the abortion underground.[19] Some doctors continue to provide clandestine abortion by selling MA, though they rarely face law enforcement sanctions for doing so. Convictions of doctors for illegal abortion usually result in fines and/or temporary bans on practicing medicine and only occasionally result in suspended prison sentences.[20]

Fewer doctors provide clandestine surgical abortion than in previous years, but there are still significant economic incentives for those who want to sell abortion information and referrals. The experience of another Polish clinic worker in Vienna illustrates this system. The clinic worker regularly sees Polish patients come to the clinic after multiple unsuccessful attempts to use pills bought online. In one instance, the clinic worker was able to verify that faulty pills had been sold by a practicing gynecologist in Poland: the patient "paid for tablets twice, 1,200zł each time," but they did not cause an abortion. When the patient reported the pills had not worked, the gynecologist "told her that she just needed to buy another set!"[21] Patients like this woman who can pay for treatment in a private clinic in Vienna, where abortion costs at least €600, tend to be wealthier on average.[22] For others, buying multiple rounds of faulty pills at 1,200zł each will likely have exhausted their resources and left them without the funds to pursue an abortion abroad.

This illustration of the ways that some Polish doctors profit from turning "sin into gold" should not be interpreted as a blanket indictment of Polish doctors. There are, of course, profiteers and obstructors, but there are advocates and allies who engage in clandestine abortions driven by a conscientious commitment to reproductive freedom. They face significant risks. Surveys show widespread anti-abortion conservatism among the medical profession in Poland today. The doctors who speak publicly on abortion are mainly powerful anti-abortion conservatives whose views have a chilling effect on the attitudes and actions of the profession at large.[23] Their anti-abortion stance creates pressure on pro-choice doctors to keep silent; they are reluctant to get publicly involved in debates about abortion or to be identified by their colleagues as pro-abortion. Association with abortion can result in public denunciation, professional marginalization, and financial consequences for their practices.[24] On the whole, Polish doctors choose "political nonengagement" with abortion because they fear stigmatization more than they fear criminalization.[25]

The obstacles faced by pro-choice doctors are illustrated in the story of the activist group Lekarze Kobietom (Doctors for Women). This group formed in 2017 after the Polish legislature enacted a law banning the sale of emergency contraception over the counter and making it available with a doctor's prescription only. The waiting time for an appointment with a public gynecologist is eighteen days on average.[26] Emergency contraception is effective up to three days after unprotected sex, so in practice this change made emergency contraception unavailable for people who could not afford to pay privately for a speedy doctor's appointment. Lekarze Kobietom was founded by several doctors and medical students who were committed to keeping emergency contraception available in light of the new restrictions.

Initially, the group wanted to write prescriptions for emergency contraception themselves, but they were advised they could lose their licenses if those prescriptions were investigated. As a safer mode of working, they gathered information about primary care doctors around the country who were willing to prescribe contraception. This was challenging because of the number of doctors who declare themselves conscientious objectors and refuse to prescribe emergency contraception.[27] Fear about professional consequences, legal risk, workload, and conservatism in the medical system all constrained the doctors' activist work. A founding member of Lekarze Kobietom explained, in late 2019, that she had largely ceased her activism because of hostile conditions at the hospital where she was employed. Pressure from her superiors, who knew about her reproductive rights activism and discouraged her from continuing, combined with long shifts, unpaid overtime, and the prevailing political climate, took their toll. Feeling unable to continue her activist work and bullied at work by anti-abortion superiors, she considered emigrating. It is impossible, she explained, to be "both a doctor and an activist" in Poland.[28] Her account illustrates, in brief, why abortion pill activism in Poland tends to be concentrated in feminist networks, with professional medical supporters based in countries where their activities are not legally or professionally risky.

POLISH ABORTION PILL ACTIVISM

Abortion pill activists operate across Poland and beyond its borders in transnational networks that facilitate abortion for people who can use abortion pills at home and people who have to travel to other countries to access abortion (usually those who are later in pregnancy or have medical complications). As we will see, Polish abortion pill activism works in ways that are recognizable in other countries, including the Republic of Ireland and Northern Ireland, because pill networks in those countries involved some of the same actors, particularly the feminist networks that supply MA (Women on Web and Women Help Women). Below I discuss the networks that currently operate, based on interviews with abortion pill activists in Poland, Germany, the Netherlands, England, Austria, and the United States. Individuals and organizations are only named in association with information that they have already chosen to make public.

Polish abortion pill activists work in a uniquely restrictive context in which a legal loophole for self-managed abortion coexists with a hostile political climate where officials have shown willingness to investigate and criminalize activists, as well as others who support family and friends with abortions. Poland had legal abortion in the 1950s through 1980s, but the years since the democratic transition have been marked by relentless efforts to restrict abortion. This includes the so-called compromise of 1993 and the efforts since 2016 to go further and ban abortion altogether.[29] Perhaps unsurprisingly, Polish abortion activists are cynical about the possibility that their political institutions can be persuaded to make progressive changes in the short term. Echoing activists in other countries who advocate for social decriminalization as a driver of legal decriminalization, a Polish activist explains:

> Many people think that the law is more important than access, and law creates access, but in my opinion it's totally different. Access creates law. It should create law. . . . We have been lobbying to change the law for many years, and it's pointless. So we decided to work on different ground, to support people, to encourage them to tell their stories, to show what abortion looks like. I think that this is a chance to change the situation. And maybe someone will take advantage of our work and change the law someday, but we don't even have time to lobby.[30]

Working with the principle of access now and legal reform later, Polish abortion pill activists see their work as operating at the "edge of the law."[31] When a woman contacts Polish pro-choice activists on the phone or through social media, she goes through a sort of geographic and gestational triage. How far along is she? Where in Poland does she live? If she is more than around twelve weeks' pregnant, can she travel? If she is under twelve weeks, can she receive a package at her home? If she is over twelve weeks and cannot travel, can someone support her to self-manage the abortion at home? Can she afford to pay a €75 donation? On the basis of that assessment, those who are early enough in their pregnancy to use MA have two main ways to acquire it: shipped from abroad through the post or supplied by local activists who maintain pill stockpiles.

This system of abortion pill provision works through a complex constellation of activist groups who operate across the country and in varying degrees of secrecy. Some groups, like the Abortion Dream Team, speak publicly in the Polish and international press about their work, providing information about where to obtain abortion pills and how to self-manage abortion with pills.[32] In an effort to destigmatize abortion, they appeared on the cover of the women's magazine *Wysokie Obcasy* (High heels), published by the liberal daily *Gazeta Wyborcza*. The cover showed them smiling in front of a bright pink background wearing T-shirts that read, "Abortion is OK."[33] The activists who engage in this work of public provocation are taking calculated risks because, as evidenced by the prosecution of Abortion Dream Team member Justyna Wydrzyńska, they are the most likely to attract attention from police and prosecutors. The wider network of activists who are not publicly visible also take substantial legal risks by personally obtaining, storing, and distributing abortion pills where they are needed.

Public-facing groups like Abortion Dream Team provide information about how to safely obtain and use such medications. The legal basis for their activities is this: it is not a crime for people to obtain abortion medication for themselves, nor is it a crime to self-manage an abortion, so information-sharing activities are constitutionally protected under freedom of information. While activists like members of Abortion Dream Team argue that providing information on self-managed abortion is not illegal, anti-abortion groups advocate for an alternative interpretation that would make this a crime. Anti-abortion campaigners also advocate for the criminalization of web forums like Kobiety w Sieci (Women on the Net, not affiliated with the Dutch group Women on Web). They do so by submitting information to prosecutors, usually notices of "suspicion" that the web forum is committing a crime by helping a woman end a pregnancy with her consent in violation of article 152 of the penal code. The anti-abortion legal think tank Ordo Iuris and its allies also monitor the work of abortion pill activists and ask prosecutors to open investigations. They copy discussions from the Kobiety w Sieci forum and publicize them, posting screenshots of the site and accusing the forum's administrators of "encouraging" women to end their pregnancies.[34]

While it is not a crime to purchase MA online, it is not easy or straight-forward to get the medication inside Poland: there are a variety of obstructions that make this process challenging, stressful, and slow. There is enormous regional variation in the way that Polish customs treats MA. In some provinces, pills are routinely stopped; in others, they are routinely allowed to proceed to recipients. As particular regions or methods of shipping come under scrutiny and are more often intercepted, activists change their tactics and routes.[35] Customs and postal decisions are unpredictable and sometimes pose serious problems for the reliable shipment of pills. In 2017, for example, the Polish Postal Service announced that it had "lost" several hundred shipments of MA ordered from Asia. Because it did not register these packages as having entered the country, recipients could not request information on the whereabouts of the packages or challenge decisions regarding the shipment.[36] In other instances, there have been more direct forms of intervention by customs officials to obstruct the movement of MA through the post. In 2019, at least four people in northern Poland who ordered pills from a feminist network received their packages only to find that each of the blister packs had been opened and the pills crushed.[37] Online, activists and supporters engage in monitoring and mapping work to update pill users on where to direct their deliveries, based on which customs regions are least likely to interfere with pill shipments from pharmaceutical distributors abroad.

When abortion pill shipments from Women on Web or Women Help Women are delayed or detained, people can contest the decision on the basis of the legal status of imported pills for personal use and even employ a form letter drafted by an NGO to contact customs authorities.[38] Of course, intense anti-abortion stigma and fear of criminalization—by people who do not know that they are not committing a crime by ordering pills for themselves—present major disincentives to questioning customs decisions. Abortion seekers can try to order again, using a different route. If they have the money, they can travel abroad for abortion. Some abortion seekers are so fearful of delays in waiting for pills or the interception of pills ordered online that they choose to travel abroad for MA, where they must pay three or four times the online price to obtain the same abortion pills in a clinic.[39] Others who cannot afford to wait longer for pills and cannot afford to travel can pursue alternative pill sources through a domestic pill underground. (Most who travel abroad for abortion opt for surgical abortion because it is much faster.)

The most visible of the Polish abortion pill activists, who speak publicly and receive media coverage of their activities, are by no means the only people working in this area.[40] Many people can order pills online through the feminist pill providers Women on Web or Women Help Women, but people who are close to the end of the first trimester may not be able to wait for a package to arrive, especially if they face uncertain shipping delays. To meet their needs, a network of activists around Poland connects people who urgently need pills with people who hold emergency supplies of them. Such stockpiles are secretly held across the country, in small towns and big cities. Difficulties accessing emergency contraception quickly are also addressed through these groups, which often hold stocks of both MA and emergency contraception.[41]

Supplies of pills are replenished by a network of activists across Europe. In countries where packages of abortion pills are reliably delivered, activists order in bulk and then ship smaller parcels to countries where they are needed. Pill supplies inside Ireland and Poland were filled simultaneously, for instance, by an activist working in a country in western Europe where she could receive large pill shipments and then transfer the pills to discrete packaging, without pharmaceutical marking, for onward delivery.[42] Supplies can also be refreshed by Poles living abroad who bring small quantities with them when they return home for visits, especially products like emergency contraception that are sold over the counter in other European countries.[43]

Keeping Polish activists reliably stocked with MA requires a detailed knowledge of the regulatory structures for mifepristone around the world. Misoprostol is available over the counter in many places, but stricter regulations on mifepristone mean it is rarely sold without prescription. An activist working in central Europe who frequently sends pills to Poland described the routes that she uses, sourcing pills through sympathetic doctors in her network and from a handful of countries in South America, eastern Europe, and south Asia where mifepristone is either legally available without prescription or is informally sold over the counter. She explains, "We have regular access . . . whenever people travel, they just buy pills."[44] Because abortion pill activists are publicly visible as providers of information on self-managed abortion, they are also sources of support for people who obtain pills through less reliable Internet suppliers.

POLISH PILL VENDORS

People who can afford to shop around for a private gynecologist may be able to find someone who will perform an abortion or refer them to a clinic abroad. Knowledge about how to obtain a clandestine abortion is widespread among women in Poland, who share details through family and social networks.[45] For some younger Poles, the line between private and illegal gynecological services is blurry because they know that abortion is available to those with wealth.[46] There is another reason it can be so difficult for people to determine who they can trust to provide MA, a referral, or information: illicit pill vendors masquerading as medical institutions are flourishing online.

Online pill vendors make claims to legitimacy in two main ways. First, they use stock images of doctors, nurses, and sparkling clinics to convey their medical credentials and trustworthiness. The stock images of photogenic doctors from medical website templates are identified with a Polish name ("Dr. Jarosław," "Dr. Barbara," "Dr. Maciej"). Second, several of these sites present themselves as the web presence for brick-and-mortar clinics in the Netherlands. Some Polish pill vendors list the actual street address of the Vrelinghuis clinic in Utrecht. The Polish pill vendors use this fake Dutch address to lend authenticity to the products they sell. One site (wrongly) claims that is permitted to sell genuine mifepristone and misoprostol to Poles because it is a clinic operating in the Netherlands, where such medications are legally obtained. Another site, which also lists its contact address as that of the Vrelinghuis clinic, offers Poles the option to read about "our friendly clinic in the Netherlands" and links to a legitimate news story about abortion travel to Utrecht. The Vrelinghuis clinic has itself posted a disclaimer disavowing these Polish sites.[47] Another Polish pill vendor site identifies itself as a Dutch organization called "Women on Earth" that ships pills from the Netherlands, presumably to attract people who have heard about Women on Web or Women Help Women.

The lack of abortion care in the formal health system, the widespread demand for abortion, and the lack of public knowledge about medication abortion combine to create profitable opportunities for illicit pill vendors. A number of online pill vendors exist just to serve the Polish market. They advertise abortion pill kits like those discussed in chapter 1. A typical MA combi-pack kit contains five pills: one pill of mifepristone (200 mg) and four pills of misoprostol (200 mcg each). This is the standard protocol for a first

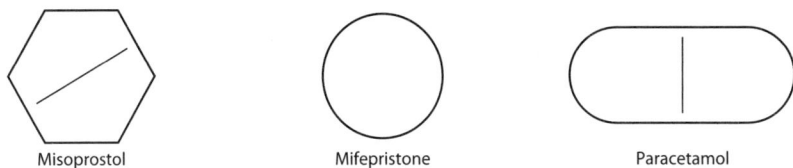

FIGURE 3. Shapes of misoprostol, mifepristone, and paracetamol. Credit: Illustration by Stew Wright.

trimester abortion with mifepristone and misoprostol. A misoprostol-only regime calls for twelve misoprostol pills (200 mcg each, taken four at a time at intervals of three hours).[48]

By contrast, Polish pill vendors online frequently advertise a third regime, known as the 1+12 set, consisting of one mifepristone pill and twelve misoprostol pills. This product advertised by Polish vendors purportedly combines the dosage for mifepristone plus misoprostol and misoprostol-only regimes, in a way that is not used anywhere in the world. The explanation for this novelty is simple: these vendors often do not sell mifepristone. They sell misoprostol, which is available in Poland, with a doctor's prescription. Vendors who sell the 1+12 set tell pill users to take the mifepristone pill, then wait twenty-four hours and proceed with the misoprostol: four misoprostol pills every three hours for a total of twelve misoprostol pills.[49]

The pill sets sold online vary in content. Customers usually know to expect two distinct types of pills, so vendors who sell fraudulent pills are known to package several labeled blister packs of misoprostol—twelve pills in total— with a thirteenth, unlabeled pill cut from a separate blister pack, which is passed off as mifepristone. This thirteenth pill often has a different shape. Sometimes it is another misoprostol, but often it is only paracetamol or acetaminophen. In some cases, customers receive thirteen paracetamol pills, mislabeled as misoprostol.[50]

To the uninitiated, all these pills look relatively similar. For activists, however, they are easily distinguishable by their shape and markings (fig. 3). People who have received pills online sometimes send a photo to activists who can check the packaging and verify whether the pills are genuine before they are used. Other people call afterward, when they have used the pills but have not had a successful abortion. An activist describes her exchanges with callers in this situation:

[The caller says,] "I took mifepristone!"

[And I say,] "What did it look like? OK, you didn't take mifepristone." . . .

Sometimes we have this after we warn people, saying, "Look, these are the webpages that are just sending misoprostol. It's just misoprostol and not mifepristone, but it's not poison."[51]

These Polish pill vendors present a dilemma for people engaged in the work of destigmatizing abortion. One of the most significant cultural trends around abortion (in Poland and elsewhere) is its "awfulization": the depiction of abortion as "an exceptional, morally dubious procedure" that harms women and, by extension, the nation.[52] Activists and clinic workers who support Poles traveling abroad report that they often encounter abortion seekers who assume abortion is highly dangerous, performed only by incompetent profiteers, and likely to leave them injured or infertile.[53] Similar stigma attaches to abortion pills, which are frequently discussed in the media as dangerous or low-quality medicines that will cause grave harm to women who use them. Activists who support people who buy pills online feel conflicted, to some extent, about the medications that online pill vendors send out. Mislabeled abortion pill packages—passing misoprostol off as mifepristone—are clearly problematic because the different pills require different dosages and protocols. Nonetheless, misoprostol can be safely used to manage an abortion. A Polish activist explains, "It's better than nothing."[54]

A misoprostol-only regime is less effective than mifepristone plus misoprostol, but if used correctly it is likely that twelve misoprostol will be effective in ending a pregnancy. According to a 2019 meta-analysis, taking at least three doses of 800 mcg misoprostol (twelve 200 mcg misoprostol pills) over a forty-eight-hour period has an 87 percent likelihood of terminating a pregnancy in the first trimester.[55] However, without knowing whether your pills are mifepristone plus misoprostol or misoprostol only, correct administration of the medications and successful abortion are less likely. Activists see both outcomes: for some people, the misoprostol by itself is effective; for others, who do not know how to use it, it does not work.[56] The reason the Polish online vendors sell misoprostol as mifepristone is cost: mifepristone fetches a far higher price than misoprostol online. For example, one Polish site that is known to send out mislabeled misoprostol advertises pill products (labeled as a 1+12 set of mifepristone and misoprostol) priced at between 440zł and 550zł ($100–$125). Assuming that, based on users' and activists' reports, these sets contain misoprostol only, these vendors sell each misoprostol pill at dozens of times the average retail price.

People trying to buy pills from these online vendors find themselves wading through various forms of misinformation and obfuscation. Those who are aware of activist support groups can rely on them for information, but others who attempt to obtain medications and self-manage abortion without support can be vulnerable to fraud by pill vendors and intimidation by police. Stigma, confusion, and misinformation compound each other in this context: suppliers of misoprostol may provide quality products that could be used to safely self-manage abortion, but when those products are labeled as something else, or their origin is obscured, pill users can struggle to find reliable information about how to use them and how to seek medical care (if necessary). The possibility of criminalization adds to their isolation.

ABORTION CRIMINALIZATION

Ending your own pregnancy with pills is not a crime in Poland, but that does not mean it is free from legal risk. The ambiguous status of self-managed abortion with pills is evident in the way that abortion in Poland has been criminalized. Police efforts to crack down on abortion happen, although overall numbers of investigations, prosecutions, and convictions are low. While the Polish government does not record annual estimates of clandestine abortions, it does record the number of crimes identified under the 1993 law each year. Between 1999 and 2019, an average of 125 violations of article 152 (terminating the pregnancy with the woman's consent) were identified, and criminal proceedings were initiated in an average of 86 cases annually.[57] The outcomes of these cases and their details are difficult to determine as government reports provide different levels of data each year.[58] The Polish Ministry of Justice says that neither it nor the State Prosecution Service collects data on how many investigations are initiated against people who help others seek an abortion outside of the law.[59] There is no centralized recording mechanism for these data because cases of violations of the abortion law are usually brought by prosecutors in local district courts, of which there are several hundred. Lawyers and advocates in the field are only able to track these cases through media reporting or when they are approached directly by parties in the case for legal advice.[60]

Convictions for illegal abortions are low, given the estimates of between 80,000 and 200,000 clandestine abortions that take place each year. As I explained above, these clandestine abortions cannot necessarily be assumed to be illegal. Nonetheless, criminalization of abortion-related activities is relatively rare. The legal scholar Atina Krajewska finds that many more cases are registered than end in prosecution: 90 percent of cases registered for crimes against a pregnant woman and/or fetus never proceed to a formal prosecution.[61] Even where prosecutions result, government data do not disclose the number of convictions for abortion-related crimes. Most cases that are registered are later discontinued because of lack of evidence. Unless residue from MA is found on or inside the pregnant person's body, it is impossible to determine whether the pregnancy termination was a spontaneous miscarriage or an abortion.[62]

As pills entered Poland and became a viable option for an abortion—at roughly 10 percent of the price of a clandestine surgical abortion—reports of prosecutions for medication abortion began to surface. Despite the limitations on available data from the state, analysis of media and court documents on prosecutions for illegal abortion demonstrates some notable trends: first, prosecutions before 2009 mostly involved gynecologists, anesthetists, and others who helped directly in surgical abortions in clandestine settings; second, abortion pill prosecutions began to comprise a significant number of abortion prosecutions from 2009 on; and third, prosecutions for involvement in clandestine self-managed abortion are most often against those who helped an abortion seeker get pills: a partner, a parent, a doctor who provided pills, or others who sell pills if they are working in Poland.

Since 2015 when the hard-line anti-abortion Law and Justice party took power, investigations and registered cases of abortion-related crimes have increased.[63] Between 2001 and 2014, there were an average of 13 convictions per year for assisting illegal abortion.[64] In 2018, there were 32 convictions for terminating a pregnancy with the woman's consent.[65] In 2021, a man was sentenced to six months in prison for buying MA for his partner; this punishment was unusually severe: a conviction of this nature would ordinarily result in a suspended sentence without prison time. His purchase of MA came to police attention after his partner sought postabortion care and was reported to police by her doctors.[66] Although most cases are eventually dropped or result in acquittals, they nonetheless have chilling effects.[67] Investigations and prosecutions of online pill vendors have also increased in recent years. It is not unusual for parents, partners, or other close relatives to be targeted in such cases when they pay for abortion pills that are used by another person.

The Polish anti-abortion movement is engaged in efforts to increase prosecutions of abortion-related crimes. Recognizing the apparent loophole for self-managed abortion, they offer alternative interpretations of the law that would criminalize elements of self-managed abortion. In 2017, the anti-abortion group Ordo Iuris drafted a legal memo that urged prosecutors to make better use of the criminal penalties in the 1993 law. Ordo Iuris suggested to prosecutors that the crime of "assisting" an abortion should be more widely interpreted, to include "providing a tool, means of transport, advice or information," including for abortion travel abroad. They went further, suggesting "assistance" should also extend to cover those people who make it easier for another to obtain an illegal abortion "by omission."[68] The head of the Office of the State Prosecutor shared this memo with all appellate prosecutors and instructed them to "make use of it" by circulating it to all their subordinate prosecutors.[69] Interpretations of what constitutes "assistance" to abortion vary depending on the views of the local prosecutor, so such a memo has the potential to influence powerful decision makers.[70]

Although nominally distinct from PiS, Ordo Iuris has an influential network of allies within the PiS government and is relied on to provide the party with legal expertise and social support.[71] As an extreme anti-abortion organization and source of expertise on "legal culture" with close ties to PiS, Ordo Iuris has pushed for an interpretation of the criminal code that creates opportunities for more abortion criminalization.[72] The group was also permitted to join the prosecution of Justyna Wydrzyńska. In some cases, Polish courts allow for private "social organizations" to join public prosecutions to represent the public interest. Ordo Iuris joined her prosecution in order to advocate for "human rights, including the right to life from conception."[73] Wydrzyńska's prosecution, aided by Ordo Iuris, may signal a change in attitudes among Polish law enforcement bodies regarding abortion criminalization. The 2020 Constitutional Tribunal ruling confirmed the PiS's control of the courts and its ability to accomplish through the courts what it struggles to achieve in the legislature.

POLAND AND UKRAINE

The Russian invasion of Ukraine in 2022 has altered Poland's abortion geography once again. Ukraine has long been a destination country for Poles traveling outside the country for an abortion. Ukraine permits abortion on request up to 12 weeks and up to 28 weeks for a variety of medical reasons.[74] Data on precise numbers of Polish abortion seekers in Ukraine are not available because of the structure of abortion care there. Ukrainians can access abortion in public hospitals, but nonresidents cannot, so Polish abortion seekers rely on private clinics in Ukraine that do not publish statistics on the nationality of their service users. Nonetheless, investigations by journalists have regularly documented the Poland-Ukraine abortion pathway, and Poles have even been sentenced for providing information and assistance to people accessing Ukrainian clinics.[75] Although studies of Polish abortion travel pathways show that Poles with financial means preferred to travel west to Germany, Austria, and the Netherlands (or south to Slovakia and the Czech Republic), Ukraine has consistently been a destination state for Polish abortion seekers.[76]

When Russia invaded Ukraine and millions of Ukrainians were displaced, Poland received the largest number of refugees of any European country.[77] Ukrainians who fled to Poland found themselves living in a country with a de facto total abortion ban. The need for abortion among Ukrainian refugees attracted worldwide media attention during the refugee crisis for two reasons: because of the stark difference in abortion laws between the country Ukrainians fled and the country where they arrived; and because Ukrainian refugees who were victims of rape by Russian troops had no recourse to abortion in Poland. Officially, Poland's law allows for abortion in cases of rape, but in practice it is not available because it falls to prosecutors to investigate the rape allegation before deciding whether an abortion can proceed. Refugees who survive sexual violence in a war zone find it almost impossible to satisfy the Polish abortion law's requirements to obtain a legal abortion.[78] These requirements can barely be satisfied by Poles in peacetime. As previously discussed, legal abortion on the grounds of rape in Poland is vanishingly rare, in part because reports of rape are scarce and dismissal rates of rape allegations by prosecutors are high.[79]

Abortion access for Ukrainians in Poland reflects the broader activist infrastructure developed by Polish and pan-European groups: through a system of medication abortion and abortion travel, Ukrainians in Poland now obtain abortions using the same pathways that Poles do. MA activists and abortion funds have introduced Ukrainian-language resources on self-managed abortion with pills and travel abroad, sometimes with dedicated funding for Ukrainians. Just over six weeks into the Russian invasion, Polish activists reported that 158 Ukrainians in Poland had sought their help to use MA.[80]

Ukrainian refugees in Poland also encounter the same anti-abortion obstacles that Poles face. The Życie i Rodzina (Life and Family) Foundation has distributed Ukrainian-language leaflets informing refugees that abortion is "the worst crime" and "the greatest threat to peace."[81] They distributed these leaflets at transport hubs across Poland to reach newly arriving refugees. Ordo Iuris has also launched an "auditing" process in which it calls Polish hospitals to request data about abortions carried out since the Russian invasion of Ukraine. Its audit specifically requests data on abortions provided in cases of rape for noncitizens because it claims (without evidence) that Polish hospitals are providing abortions in violation of the law.[82]

The same obstacles that obstruct Polish abortion seekers now have an impact on Ukrainian refugees, who fled a country that once served as a destination for Poles seeking out legal abortion. They also face a hostile legal climate for abortion seekers and activists who assist them. At the same time, Poland's willingness to accommodate more Ukrainian refugees than any other European country, and the Russian invasion's impact on the geopolitical situation in eastern Europe, has softened attitudes in the EU to the Polish government. The PiS government had fallen out of favor with the EU after its political interventions in the judiciary, efforts to curtail press freedom, and policies on abortion and LGBTQ+ rights. In the wake of the Russian invasion of Ukraine, this posture changed toward Poland and the EU unlocked funds it had previously withheld. The wider geopolitical context matters for abortion in Poland: before the Russian invasion, western Europe might have seen Poland as less strategically important from a security standpoint and may have put greater resources into sanctioning Poland for violations of human rights and democratic norms. After the Russian invasion of Ukraine, when Poland is viewed as a crucial security partner, its abortion restrictions attract less international opprobrium. It is a familiar story: in times of political crisis, gender justice and sexual and reproductive freedoms are the first to be compromised.

———

Abortion restrictions in Poland, combined with the persistent need for safe abortion, have effectively transformed the landscape of clandestine abortion there. Secretive surgical abortion providers have been replaced by abortion pill providers of various stripes: activists working in transnational networks, doctors working as clandestine suppliers, and online pill vendors selling a variety of products. The ambiguous status of self-managed abortion—an unintended outcome of the 1993 law that criminalized abortion providers who carry out abortions outside the law—means that elements of self-managed abortion cannot be charged as crimes, but various acts of assistance with self-managed abortion can. In practice, MA has become much more widely available in recent years, and its availability has come to public attention through patterns of government crackdown and public backlash. As laws tighten further and efforts continue to erode any remaining legal basis for abortion, tens of thousands of Poles undergo self-managed abortions with pills in their homes. These abortions are not illegal, but they are often stigmatized and clandestine.

Poland's transnational system for self-managed abortion illustrates what the beginning of social decriminalization might look like, in practice, in the absence of legal reform. A hostile anti-abortion political and legal climate can coexist with a growing clandestine system for self-managed abortion that draws on transnational information and supply networks. Abortion pills can slip—metaphorically—between legal categories to scramble ideas about what abortion is and who does it, while they can also slip—physically—across territorial borders in quantities large enough to supply a mass movement. The kinds of systems developed in Poland over the past ten to fifteen years have allowed clandestine abortion to flourish even while new restrictions are added to an already highly restrictive abortion law.

CHAPTER 6

Irish Abortions by Plane or Pill

Ireland's tiny, so everyone's a friend of a friend. There'd be someone coming down on the Belfast bus to Dublin and you'd arrange for someone to meet them on the Quays, hand over a set of abortion pills, and then off they go.

— Irish activist

On May 25, 2018, voters in the Republic of Ireland chose to repeal the country's constitutional abortion ban. The outcome of the abortion referendum had been foretold in public opinion polls in the years leading up to 2018: the Irish public wanted more liberal abortion laws and repeatedly said so.[1] In exit polling, 72 percent of voters said they had made up their minds on the abortion question at least five years earlier and had not changed their views during the campaign.[2] If the outcome of the referendum was foreseeable, then perhaps the more important question is this: How did the Irish government get to the point where it chose to hold such a referendum? Medication abortion is essential to answering this question.

Medication abortion fundamentally disrupted the status quo of the abortion ban in Ireland. This disruption forced a reluctant Irish political class to acknowledge that the abortion ban could not continue. In this chapter I discuss the abortion geography of the island of Ireland, first showing how the patterns of abortion access abroad were shaped by constitutional amendments throughout the 1980s and 1990s and then illustrating how the emergence of abortion pill routes during the first decade of the 2000s disrupted these access patterns. Activists' success in developing pill networks and government agencies' inability to halt the influx of pills not only reduced the number of people who relied on travel abroad to obtain an abortion but also began to change the social, political, and legal cultures surrounding MA. By the eve of the 2018 referendum, self-managed abortion with pills had fundamentally changed public and political perceptions of Ireland's abortion ban. Chapters 6, 7 and 8 look at the impact of medication abortion in the politics of the Republic of Ireland and Northern Ireland, respectively.[3]

IRELAND'S 8TH AMENDMENT

Ireland's de facto abortion ban was the product of a constitutional amendment—the 8th Amendment—which had been added to the Irish constitution by referendum in 1983. It accorded the fetus and pregnant person equal "right to life," and it committed the country to "vindicate the right to life of the unborn."[4] While 1983 represents a milestone in Ireland's history of abortion restriction, it is not the starting point. Abortion was already illegal in Ireland in 1983 and had been illegal since the foundation of the state in 1922, when Ireland inherited the abortion laws of its former colonizer, the United Kingdom. Although abortion was illegal, backstreet surgical abortions were rare. Traveling to an abortion provider in England or using abortifacient "herbs, purgatives, or pills" were the most common methods for Irish abortion seekers.[5] Thousands of pregnant women took "the boat to England," as the euphemism went, seeking abortions (or hoping to escape the social stigma of wanted but out-of-wedlock pregnancies).[6] Even before the United Kingdom legalized abortion, illegal abortion was easier to obtain there than in Ireland. The legalization of abortion in England in 1967 formalized this abortion travel route and saw the establishment of more organized support groups that helped women from across Europe travel to England for abortions. Groups supporting people from Ireland emerged from within the Irish diaspora in England.[7]

Ireland's 1983 referendum came about as the result of domestic political debates and the looming shadow of US abortion politics. Anti-abortion activists in Ireland looked on in horror as the US Supreme Court established the constitutional right to abortion on privacy grounds in the *Roe v. Wade* decision of 1973.[8] Their fears were bolstered by US anti-abortion advocates who warned Ireland that it should act to enshrine its ban in the constitution before legal abortion was introduced through the courts in a repeat of the "tragic American experience."[9] One year after *Roe v. Wade* was decided in the United States, the Irish courts reversed a ban on contraception for married couples, finding that they had the right to make private decisions on family planning. This decision provoked outrage among social conservatives.[10] Opponents of abortion in Ireland worried that their courts were on the pathway to permitting abortion, so they sought a constitutional fix and won political support for a referendum. The Pro-Life Amendment Campaign lobbied for the 8th Amendment with direct and vociferous support from the Catholic Church.[11] In contrast, the Anti-Amendment Campaign found itself with limited resources, up against the institutional power of the church and struggling to fight the perception that it was "the Dublin crowd" coming to impose its views on the rest of Ireland.[12] The 1983 referendum passed with 66.9 percent of the vote, albeit with a turnout of just over 50 percent.[13] The 8th Amendment instituted a constitutional abortion ban in a country where abortion was already illegal.

Judicial rulings, legislative efforts, and constitutional referendums all combined to project the fiction of Ireland as a supposedly abortion-free country. Nearly ten years after the 8th Amendment had been adopted, Ireland held three more referendums on abortion—on the proposed 12th, 13th, and 14th Amendments to the constitution.[14] A 1992 court ruling (known as the "X" case) established that abortion could be obtained in Ireland where there was a "real and substantial" risk to the life of the pregnant woman, including risk to her life by suicide. Anti-abortion conservatives objected to this ground for legal abortion and proposed a new amendment (the 12th) that would explicitly remove risk of suicide as a basis for legal abortion. Voters rejected the 12th Amendment. At the same time, two other amendments passed by referendum: the 13th Amendment established that the state "shall not limit the freedom to travel between the State and another state." Although this amendment is sometimes glossed as the "right" to travel, no such right was established: it meant only that the state could not restrict someone's freedom to travel for purposes of going abroad for an abortion. The 14th Amendment established that the Irish constitution's abortion ban did not limit freedom of information on legal abortion services available in other countries.[15] In the referendums on the 12th, 13th, and 14th Amendments, the Irish electorate voted against further restrictions. The legal effect was to institutionalize abortion-travel pathways out of Ireland, but in political terms the referendums demonstrated the growing public dissatisfaction with the 8th Amendment abortion ban.

Feminist scholars have shown how, across the world, women are held up as the embodiment of "the moral-legal boundary of the nation-state."[16] In Ireland, this moral-legal boundary was brought to life by the outsourcing of abortion onto foreign soil. Its abortion ban was a function of a deeply ingrained system of gender inequality that constructed Irish identity in opposition to its former colonizer. Post-independence Ireland was heavily reliant on ideas about Irish women's moral and sexual purity, taken to symbolize Ireland's superiority over Britain. Women who transgressed gender norms were institutionalized in facilities run by religious orders and the state, for example, the Magdalene Laundries, Industrial Schools, and Mother and Baby institutions. These institutions were notorious sites of state abuse, where women were effectively incarcerated and put into forced labor, as well as separated from their babies in involuntary and secretive adoption processes.[17] Clara Fischer argues that such institutions created a "politics of place that forcibly excised women in order to keep intact this fiction of a morally and sexually pure Ireland."[18] This dynamic extended abroad as well. The perceived deviance from dominant moral codes of women with unwanted pregnancies, as well as LGBTQ+ people, interracial and cross-religious couples, and victims of sexual abuse, was "solved" by emigration, whether voluntary or forced by social pressure.[19]

The distinctive moral geography that emerged in post-independence Ireland also encompasses abortion. Anti-abortion politics in Ireland have long been connected to an anticolonial and pro-natalist nationalism, which draws a distinction between Irishness (Catholic, pro-life) and Britishness/Europeanness (secular, pro-choice).[20] During the twentieth century, the issues of abortion and abortion travel to England became especially important sites where ideas about Irish women's moral purity could be defended and enforced. Abortion travel came to symbolize the antithesis of the Irish Catholic identity, a cherished source of Irish distinctiveness. This was not only because it violated Catholic teachings about sexuality, family, and procreation but also because it was seen as foreign corruption of Irish women who were traveling to "obtain abortions on the foreign territory of the colonial oppressor."[21] The 2018 abortion referendum campaign reproduced these ideas about the moral geography of Ireland. Anti-abortion groups relied heavily on messages that portrayed England's abortion regime as Ireland's dark future. Posters with British abortion statistics warned Irish voters, "Don't bring this to Ireland."[22] Others evoked dire historical comparisons: "British authorities killing Irish children: THEN with famine, NOW with abortion."[23]

The geographic separation between Ireland and Britain was portrayed, by anti-abortion forces, as symbolic of the moral gulf between them. This distinction was compounded by the fact that Northern Ireland's abortion laws more closely mirrored those in the Irish Republic than those in Britain. The Irish anti-abortion movement continued to deliberately cultivate the notion of Ireland as an abortion-free island until shortly before the 2018 referendum. This narrative signaled a conservative attitude to abortion, but it also made a broader claim about Ireland's status in Europe. Anti-abortion conservatives in Ireland promoted the idea that Catholic Ireland stood as a "last bastion" of moral conservatism in Europe.[24] (Anti-abortion forces in Poland make similar arguments about Polish Catholicism and the perils of European integration.)

ABORTION TRAVEL PATHWAYS

The notion of the abortion-free island was of course a political fiction. Clandestine self-managed abortion with "traditional methods" had long taken place in Ireland.[25] Irish women obtained abortions, mostly outside of Ireland, from the early twentieth century on. Since the 1967 legalization of abortion in Britain, thousands of people had left Ireland every year to access abortion abroad (primarily in England but also in the Netherlands since its law changed in 1984).[26] Between January 1980 and December 2017, at least 173,308 people traveled from the Republic of Ireland to access abortion services in another country (fig. 4). Of that group, almost all went to the United Kingdom.[27] It is important to note that these figures almost certainly underestimate the true total: government health departments in the United Kingdom and the Netherlands count nonresident abortion seekers based on the home address they give at the clinic, but the stigma surrounding abortion suggests that some number of people probably gave false addresses. The 173,308 people who obtained abortions abroad are not divided evenly across that period; they peak in 2001 at 18 people per day and then decline to roughly 9 people per day by 2017, for reasons I discuss later.

The combination of laws, regulations, and informal practices create "conditional pathways to abortion." Within these pathways, many different figures—institutional, familial, community, public, voluntary, and private—shape what Ruth Fletcher calls the "landscape of care."[28] This landscape of care for Irish abortion seekers has evolved over time according to their needs, the technologies available to them, the infrastructure that they navigate on their journeys, and the support groups that mobilize to help. When information about abortion was scarce in Ireland, activists based in England educated themselves on the procedure, monitored clinic complaints and patient

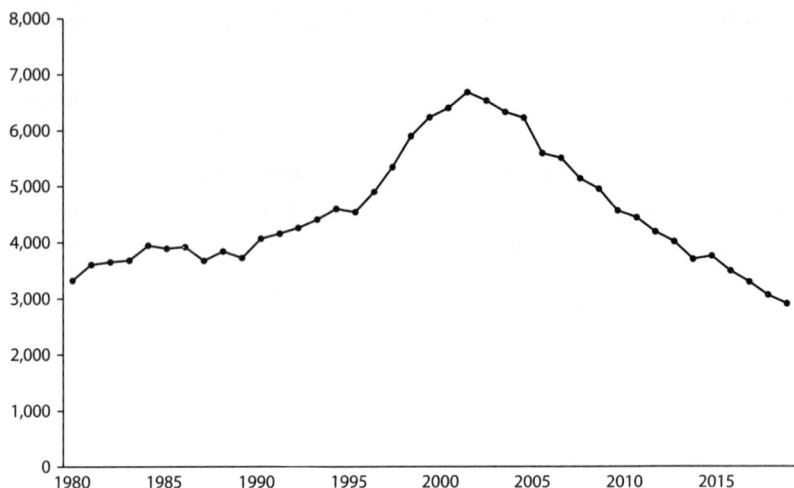

FIGURE 4. Irish residents obtaining abortion in England, Wales, and the Netherlands, 1980–2018. Source: Compiled by the author from UK Ministry of Health and Dutch Ministry of Health reports. Dutch government data collection on nonresident abortion seekers began in 2006.

experiences, negotiated price agreements with clinics, and disseminated information by posting ads in Irish women's magazines and pasting stickers on the walls of public toilets in Ireland.[29] As technology and transportation changed, activists' work did too: cheaper flights, easier access to information, and the internet meant support was needed by fewer people. Support groups operating during the 1990s tended to provide practical support for travel and host abortion seekers overnight.[30] When overnight stays became less common, support groups shifted to financial support for the procedure and associated travel.[31] The landscape of care has been shaped by these support services, all of which differ based on the complex needs of abortion seekers.

The Irish constitution guaranteed the freedom to travel abroad for abortion. After accounting for the obstacles that faced abortion seekers on these journeys, however, this guarantee looked more like a national abdication of responsibility for care. The government established institutions to sustain its "reliance on extra-territorial abortion services."[32] The state used its resources to facilitate abortion journeys abroad. For example, the government agency tasked with reducing crisis pregnancies collected annual UK Department of Health information on Irish abortion seekers in the United Kingdom. It publicly reported these statistics, thereby normalizing the Irish use of foreign services and "normalizing non-Irish provision."[33] Government agencies officially sanctioned and facilitated extraterritorial abortions by producing campaigns and leaflets for people who had already decided to go to the United Kingdom for an abortion, providing them with information on abortion and travel in an effort to lessen the stress of their experience.[34]

For decades, the myth of abortion-free Ireland was sustained by private individuals engaging in abortion travel (with the support of family or activist organizations). The freedom to travel for abortion amounted to little more than an "escape hatch" in Ireland's law.[35] Privatizing the burden of abortion care served to stave off political pressure on the government to liberalize its laws, avoid major public health effects on maternal health, shore up nationalist discourses about the moral distinctiveness of Catholic Ireland, and sustain the social stigma of abortion by geographically displacing its practice. The arrival of medication abortion disrupted this status quo.

ABORTION PILLS ARRIVE IN IRELAND

In 2001, the feminist activist organization Women on Waves, led by the physician Rebecca Gomperts, set sail for Ireland. On board was a shipping container with a reproductive health clinic inside it. Women on Waves' strategy, which they would later implement in other countries, was to bring abortion seekers on board, then sail outside of Irish territorial waters and into international waters. There doctors could legally carry out abortions for passengers of any nationality on their Dutch-flagged ship as long as they complied with Dutch abortion laws. The organization intended to visit multiple ports in Ireland, carry out twenty abortions per day on board the ship, and operate five days per week.[36] Before the ship reached Ireland, however, several obstacles presented themselves: Dutch authorities suggested that the organization had voided its inspection certificates and might be prosecuted on its return, the Irish port authorities imposed restrictions on the ship's ability to pick up passengers in Ireland, and the calls from Irish women seeking abortion pills far outstripped the ship's supply.[37] As a result, Women on Waves did not provide any abortions during their 2001 campaign in Ireland, but they did provide counseling, ultrasounds, and contraception and took calls from three hundred people seeking abortions.[38]

Although they were unable to provide MA, Women on Waves saw the Irish campaign as an important catalyst of the pro-choice movement there. The Dutch organization had been invited by a few Irish pro-choice organizations and mobilized its own team of Irish volunteers.[39] However, activists aboard the ship saw the Irish pro-choice movement as highly skeptical of their tactics: "The women's groups said, 'Oh, great, yes you can come, but by the way no woman in her right mind will go to have an abortion on the boat because they can easily travel to the UK.' . . . Then hundreds of women called, they came to the ship, they asked us, 'Can we get the pills? Because we can't go to the UK.'"[40] Irish activists contradict this account: they expected the ship to provide abortions until it docked in Dublin, and they expressed anger at the Dutch activists for reducing "a real challenge to government" to "a publicity stunt."[41] The Ireland campaign was the first of Women on Waves' ship campaigns that sought to conduct abortions in international waters. It was the first—but not the last—of such campaigns to be prevented from carrying out abortions at sea, instead serving a primarily symbolic function.[42] Although it did not provide abortions, the 2001 ship campaign raised the profile of the Dutch group and drew attention to the possibility for transnational abortion activism with pills.

MA began to enter Ireland through the post in 2006, through Women on Web, Gomperts's newly established sister organization of Women on Waves.[43] In this initial stage, Ireland-based pro-choice organizations were not collectively involved in obtaining or distributing pills, although individual activists did undertake this work. The number of people distributing pills in Ireland was low at this time as there was little public knowledge about MA and the demand tended to be small.[44] One activist involved in pill distribution across the island estimated only one hundred people ordered pills in 2008.[45] However, by 2009, pills were coming through the post in large enough numbers that the Irish customs agency began to seize them.[46] Customs agency seizures of the pills sent by Women on Web also coincided with a court challenge brought against Gomperts in Austria, apparently instigated at Ireland's request, which sought to prohibit her from prescribing MA to patients in Ireland. The Austrian courts initially ruled against Gomperts, finding that her practice did not comply with laws that required doctors to "treat patients personally and directly," but she won on appeal in 2012.[47] In the meantime, customs seizures in Ireland disrupted WoW's service to the extent that it developed alternative routes to move pills into the country. I explore these routes in detail later.

ACCOUNTING FOR ABORTION PILLS

The availability of MA in Ireland fundamentally disrupted the geography of the 8th Amendment abortion ban, which had institutionalized abortion travel abroad through private journeys, informal activist networks, and formal state initiatives. Abortion travel numbers peaked at the turn of the new millennium, with the highest totals recorded between 1999 and 2004. At its peak in 2001, eighteen people from Ireland obtained abortions in English clinics every day (see fig. 4). From 2001, daily travel numbers declined by 2 to 10 percent annually.[48] By 2016, daily travel numbers had fallen by half, to nine people per day (3,265 per year).[49] The growing availability of MA contributed to this decline.

People living in Ireland who wanted to end a pregnancy with pills faced few options. Misoprostol was licensed for the treatment of ulcers, but it was not available without a prescription and was not licensed for any reproductive uses. Like most countries with very restrictive abortion laws, mifepristone was banned entirely in Ireland.[50] Feminists in the pro-choice movement were involved in sourcing pills for individuals, and feminist networks like WoW (and later Women Help Women) mailed pills through the postal system, although these were often confiscated by customs.[51] Purchasing pills from online pharmacies was possible in theory but difficult in practice: Irish law prohibits ordering any prescription-only medications online, and the Irish customs agency intercepts all such products.[52] Growing interference by Irish customs eventually prompted the feminist networks to reorganize their system for moving pills into Ireland.

It is difficult to say exactly how many people in Ireland used MA in the years leading up to the 8th Amendment referendum. There are a few reasons for this difficulty. The first is perhaps the most obvious: people who obtained pills to end their pregnancies almost always did so in secret because of anti-abortion stigma and fears of criminalization. Until 2013, self-managing an abortion was criminalized under the Offences Against the Person Act (1861), which criminalized the use of any "poison or noxious thing" used to "procure [a] miscarriage."[53] In 2013, parts of this older law were replaced after the passage of the Protection of Life During Pregnancy Act, which imposed a possible fourteen-year prison sentence on anyone who sought to "intentionally destroy unborn life."[54] This provision was widely interpreted as criminalizing self-managed abortion. However, the 2013 law was never used to prosecute anyone who purchased medication abortion to end their pregnancy during the five years it was in force.

The second reason for the lack of clarity on abortion pill numbers is the multiple sources for these pills. Women on Web (and later Women Help Women) established infrastructures for getting MA into Ireland and later reported their data on the requests for pills there.[55] Their services were not the only source of pills, however. Online pharmacies like those highlighted in chapter 1 were available to individuals if the pills could get through customs. In addition, local groups were known to source pills from abroad, especially among migrant or refugee communities with close ties to countries where misoprostol could be obtained over the counter and brought back into Ireland in a suitcase.[56] Irish activists whose work mostly took place among white Irish abortion seekers became aware of these independent networks of abortion pills within migrant communities, but these migrant networks effectively ran parallel to feminist activist groups without much interaction between their pill supplies. As further evidence of pill suppliers operating in migrant networks, it is notable that the only prosecution for importing mifepristone into Ireland was brought against Fang Huang, a Chinese citizen residing in Ireland who imported mifepristone from China and sold it in a Dublin pharmacy; she was fined €5,550.[57]

How, then, can we measure the quantity of MA that entered the country and understand whether the growing availability of pills reduced the number of people who traveled for an abortion? We might look first to the feminist networks distributing pills through the post. Part of the campaign strategy of groups like Women on Web is to show the demand for MA within a given country in order to contradict claims by anti-abortion groups that there is no need for these products.[58] Irish anti-abortion conservatives, like the Polish groups discussed in chapters 4 and 5, refuted the idea that abortion pills were used in large numbers inside the country. Women on Web, operating since 2006, and Women Help Women, operating since 2014, both supplied pills to Ireland, although they took different approaches to publicizing the extent of the demand for pills there. Women on Web partnered with Irish politicians from 2014 to stage highly public campaigns spreading information about how to get and use MA. They also partnered with public health researchers who used their data for peer-reviewed publications in medical journals.[59] Women Help Women has been more reticent to share its data by directly publicizing the number of pill requests it receives in particular countries because of the potential for backlash or police interest.[60] Nonetheless, Women Help Women did publish some data before the 2018 referendum in Ireland to demonstrate the scale of the use of MA there.[61] Taken together, the data published by Women on Web and Women Help Women provide the most complete (although still partial) picture of demand for, and access to, MA in Ireland.[62]

Second, we might look to the Irish customs agency and its seizures of medication abortion, which it often publicized in the national media. The Irish customs and drug agencies chose to treat imported MA as part of the trade in online pharmaceuticals. All goods from overseas pharmacies and prescription-only goods from Irish online retailers were prohibited.[63] This means that the products were considered illegal and seized, but the individual consumers who purchased them were not usually subject to criminal sanctions. This is still the case in Ireland today.[64] The decision to treat MA in this way represents a notable act of categorization by the state. Importing abortifacients was a violation of the Family Planning Act of 1979, and intentionally ending one's own pregnancy was a criminal offense under the Offences Against the Person Act (1861) and the Protection of Life During Pregnancy Act (2013). Despite this criminalization, Irish customs treated MA as analogous to other pharmaceutical products whose importation from foreign online pharmacies was illegal because of concerns over quality and safety.[65] The Irish medicines agency indicated it would only prosecute the commercial importation and sale of MA, as in the conviction of the woman importing mifepristone from China for resale.[66]

The Irish customs agency was able to intercept medication abortion by looking out for markings on the packaging that indicated pharmaceutical products within.[67] Women on Web placed orders for MA with a pharmaceutical distributor in India that shipped pills directly to the recipient.[68] With this export system, the pills were sent from India in their pharmaceutical packaging and were not repackaged or disguised by Women on Web. This meant, however, that when they entered Ireland through customs hubs, the packages could be visually identified and intercepted, along with other pharmaceuticals that were considered contraband.[69] When customs intercepted a package of pills, according to the Irish medicines agency, the intended recipient of the package received a standard letter that told them their package had been detained. The recipient was then given the "opportunity to explain why the products should be released to them under Irish law" but warned that prosecutions could result.[70]

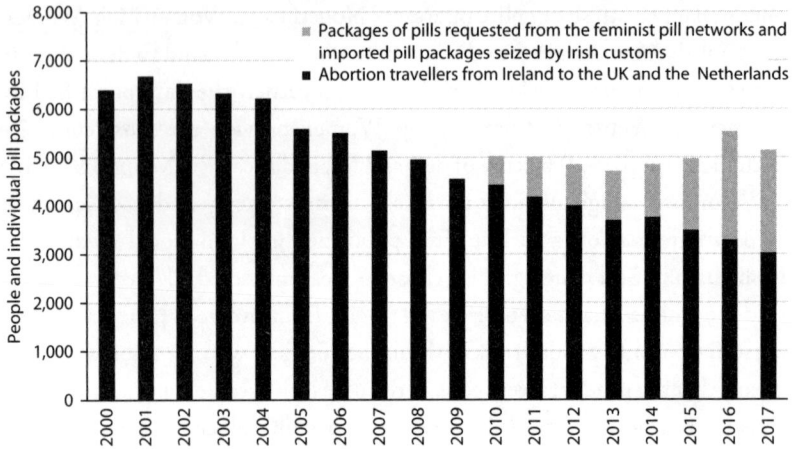

FIGURE 5. Abortion travelers from Ireland and abortion pills requested/ imported into Ireland, 2000–2017. Source: Compiled by the author from UK Department of Health, Dutch Ministry of Health, Women on Web, Women Help Women, and Irish Medicines and Healthcare Regulatory Authority data.

After it began seizing pills in substantial quantities at customs hubs around the country, the Irish medicines agency published periodic reports about its interventions, spoke to journalists about the number of shipments seized, and released figures of annual MA interceptions.[71] As part of a coordinated annual international police action, Irish customs seized thousands of shipments of illegal medicines each year and held press conferences at which seized MA was displayed alongside steroids, diet pills, and sedatives.[72] The Irish customs and medicines agencies first released data on abortion pill interceptions in 2008, echoing activist reports that pills were not intercepted in the early years but that interceptions escalated over time.[73] In 2009, Women on Web stopped shipping pills directly into Ireland through the post because of these interceptions; Women Help Women never shipped directly to Ireland. That customs seizures of MA continued from 2009 indicates the demand for pills through channels other than feminist networks, like online pharmacies.

Taken together, we have three sources of data to compare to understand the relationship between abortion travel and abortion pills (fig. 5).[74] Each of these is an estimate that likely reflects the lower bounds of the real number; there are many different incentives for people to hide their nationality at the clinic, to obtain MA through clandestine and informal routes, or to disguise packages to move them through customs more discreetly. All of these tactics would make the abortions disappear from data. Nonetheless, these data can tell us something significant: they show that abortion travel numbers from Ireland declined steadily while numbers of people attempting to obtain MA in Ireland grew.

MAPPING ALTERNATIVE PILL ROUTES

With Irish customs seizing pill packages from around 2009 on, feminist activists were forced to develop alternative routes to move pills into the country. They did so by playing with the idiosyncratic boundaries that shape the flows of goods and people within the United Kingdom and on the island of Ireland. To understand the pill routes that took shape from 2009 on, it is essential to detour into the political geography of Ireland.

The political and economic border across the island of Ireland, separating the Republic of Ireland from Northern Ireland, was established by treaty in the early 1920s. South of the border, an independent Irish state was established, while north of the border, Northern Ireland remained a part of the United Kingdom, although its status was fiercely contested. In later decades, especially during the 1970s through the 1990s, the Irish border became a heavily militarized site of political violence.[75] Today the historical significance of the border has been "diminished" and "overtaken," in practical terms, by a set of legal and political agreements: the Common Travel Area, European Union rules, and the Belfast/Good Friday Agreement. The Common Travel Area, which has existed almost since the partition of Ireland, enables Irish and British citizens to move freely in a zone that comprises Ireland, the United Kingdom, the Channel Islands, and the Isle of Man. Membership in the European Union allows Irish and EU citizens free movement across member states. The Belfast/Good Friday Agreement allows people born in Northern Ireland to hold Irish and thereby EU citizenship.[76] In effect, these agreements allow free movement across a "soft land border between Northern Ireland and the Republic of Ireland."[77] The agreements diminished the practical impact of the Irish border on the daily lives of people on the island of Ireland, at least until a resurgence of debate about the future of the border in the context of the United Kingdom's decision to exit the European Union in 2016.

Although they are different legal jurisdictions, Northern Ireland and the Republic of Ireland both had very restrictive abortion laws until 2018 that created similar demands for clandestine self-managed abortion. They also had active domestic pro-choice networks that engaged in cross-border cooperation to create an islandwide system for distributing MA. These systems for moving MA into Northern Ireland and on into the Republic were structured to take advantage of the island's political geography. Customs agencies in the two countries treated MA differently, although this was the result of policy differences on imported medications rather than policy differences on abortion. Medications ordered online fell under a blanket ban on importing prescription pharmaceuticals into the Republic of Ireland, with a corresponding effort by customs to intercept all such products.[78] By contrast, in the United Kingdom, there is no such ban on medication purchased online and no corresponding policy of consistently intercepting medications at customs hubs.[79] Activists in Northern Ireland saw this discrepancy as an opportunity. As one activist told me:

> Because we're part of the UK, we actually benefit in this regard. The pills in the south of Ireland all get seized, or nearly all get seized, because everything is seized. They seize aspirin in the south, they seize everything. But here, all the customs, everything for Northern Ireland, goes through the British customs hubs . . . and there are only periodic customs raids on those hubs, when they're looking for diet pills or that. So the pills get stopped occasionally in those places but all the time in the south.[80]

People in Northern Ireland who ordered pills from the feminist MA services could generally get the packages mailed to their homes.[81] By contrast, people in the Republic of Ireland could not order the pills directly, so activists developed a system for moving pills. It ranged from the very informal—giving a friend some boxes of pills before she got on the bus south—to the more complex—using cross-border postal systems to move pills. People in Ireland who could travel across the border to collect their parcels might order it sent to Northern Ireland by providing a UK shipping address like a P.O. box or the *poste restante* holding service at a Northern Irish post office.[82] Alternatively, people in Ireland could use Parcel Motel, a service through which Irish customers could get a "virtual address" in Northern Ireland, to save on shipping costs for online purchases. Such a service also offered a workaround for those seeking abortion pills. Activists in the north developed systems for sending pills south when people could not collect or redirect the goods themselves.[83] This usually meant changing the packaging to disguise its contents, as a Northern Irish activist explains: "In order to get them into the south, quite a lot, we'd repackage them, so they didn't look like medicine. Because they'd come from other countries where they would have posted on the package—because they were doing it legally—'This contains prescribed medicine.'"[84]

Repackaged and disguised medications could be sent south to the recipient's home address, avoiding customs scrutiny. Activists in the north and south kept small stockpiles in their homes to fill gaps in the supply.[85] When parcels were delayed or abortion seekers were very close to the time limit for using pills, activists would supply them with the medications from their domestic reserves. When that abortion seeker's parcel eventually arrived, they would send it back to the activists, who would add it to the reserve. Not all pills came in through Northern Ireland: activists replenished this supply through shipments from other European countries where large shipments of pills could be ordered from suppliers without being confiscated. The pills would be repackaged, disguised, and shipped on to the Irish Republic.[86] Occasionally, replenishment of Irish activists' stockpiles also came in the form of foreign visitors simply carrying whatever medications they could fit inside their suitcases.[87] State officials could close off one source of pills by intercepting marked pharmaceuticals at customs ports, but as soon as these interceptions began to bite, activists developed alternative routes that could not be so easily interrupted. Ireland's political geography was key to the continued flow of MA: situated in a complex web of island-based and regional travel agreements and trade flows, activists were able to maintain reliable pill supplies for abortion seekers there.

THE STATE'S RESPONSE

The Irish state's response to the growing use of MA for self-managed abortion was slow and fragmented. Irish customs sought to intercept all pills at customs ports, but their efforts did not end pill flows. When MA continued to enter the country after the 2009 customs crackdown, other arms of the state interacted with pills and pill users. Criminal justice authorities largely feigned ignorance of the issue, declining to prosecute individual pill users and only pursuing one case against a distributor.[88] As self-managed abortion with pills became more prevalent, it became an issue for the health service. Although they took years to acknowledge the extent of self-managed abortion, health authorities eventually came to treat abortion pill use as a public health problem to be managed with information to minimize harm. Health authorities discouraged self-managed abortion, instead promoting abortion travel to

England, but they also downplayed the criminal aspects of self-managed abortion by encouraging pill users to seek medical care. As it was integrated into public health messaging on abortion, MA underwent what Máiréad Enright and Emilie Cloatre call "transformative illegality." This is a socio-legal process made possible over time by "relentless illegal activism" to demonstrate the incoherence of laws, and it results in new legal meanings being attached to illegal objects.[89] Enright and Cloatre show that the legal status of an object is not a fixed property but something that can change during heightened periods of action or the slow buildup of daily activities.[90] The illegality of medication abortion in Ireland was contested in both ways. The influx of pills, though illegal, became so substantial and regular that state authorities were forced to acknowledge it and formulate their response in a way that would reassure the public that using pills designated illegal would not trigger criminal prosecutions of individuals.

The health service's Crisis Pregnancy Agency (CPA) was the main vehicle for public health action on medication abortion in the Republic of Ireland.[91] The CPA was established as part of a government strategy to use domestic governance tools to reduce the number of Irish abortion seekers abroad.[92] To this end, the CPA monitored UK Department of Health data on Irish residents obtaining abortions there and reported on those numbers in annual statements. Noting the steady fall in Irish abortions abroad, the CPA initially assumed that the decline could be equated with a straightforward reduction in abortions. To explain the apparent reduction in abortion travel, the health service offered several explanations. It assumed that fewer abortion travelers meant fewer unwanted pregnancies and thus fewer abortions. It pointed to its success in providing greater support for women with unwanted pregnancies, greater uptake of contraception among young people, and state-funded counseling services that "provide women with the space and time to consider their options."[93]

Although pill interceptions by customs continued and had increased since 2009, the health service was slow to consider the role of self-managed abortion in changing patterns of access. The Irish health service first publicly acknowledged the domestic use of abortion pills in 2015, noting that abortion pills "are not legally available in Ireland and it is not legal to supply or receive 'prescription-only' medicine through online sources." It further cautioned that the medicines agency, customs agency, and national police force "monitor and investigate instances of illegal supply of medicinal products in physical sales and via the internet and actively enforces against suspected breaches of the law."[94] In 2016, the health service cited data from the national medicines agency to concede that "some women may be ordering the abortion pill online" but to discourage this practice: "If a woman makes the decision to have an abortion, it is safer for her to attend an abortion clinic in the UK or other country where abortion is legally available, than ordering the abortion pill online or from other sources and taking it at home alone."[95] The health service's statement mentions the legal availability of abortion abroad, but it foregrounds safety when it explains why Irish women should seek abortion abroad rather than with pills at home. From 2016, these statements emphasized the extent of the demand for MA inside Ireland and pointed abortion seekers to aftercare services provided by the state. In subsequent statements, the agency's tone changed, and its recognition of domestic MA use came to the forefront. The health service's 2017 press release was headlined, "Increase in Number of Women Consulting with Online Abortion Pill Service," and it went on to cite published data from Women on Web.[96] Women on Web's data would become important in the legislative hearings and debates; information about abortion pills in Ireland was extensively cited in decision making on the 2018 referendum.

The state funded sites like AbortionAftercare.ie to provide information about the side effects of medication abortion and when to seek medical care. It reassured visitors that people who had taken MA could visit their doctor without fear of being reported to the police. A doctor, it explained, is "not required to report to the Gardai [police] that a woman has taken an abortion pill" and may only breach patient confidentiality if ordered by a court or for safeguarding reasons. Public-facing statements and resources produced by the Irish health service encouraged pill users to seek aftercare without fear that they would be turned over to the police. Similarly, the state prosecutor expressed the view that pill users would not be reported to the police because they would be protected by doctor-patient confidentiality.[97] However, this protection was subject to interpretation. The Irish Medical Council guidelines stated that doctors were justified in breaching confidentiality when the disclosure is "in the public interest."[98] Furthermore, studies of Irish doctors suggested that a significant proportion (12–26 percent) might be prepared to report an illegal abortion to police.[99] Criminal cases against pill users in Northern Ireland, where patients were reported to police by their doctors, also served as a signal that it was risky to assume that doctors would treat disclosures about self-managed abortion with confidentiality.

Together, Irish state agencies had created the "general understanding" that for women who had abortions at home in Ireland with MA they obtained online, the law would "remain unenforced." This understanding was built up, over time, through the repeated actions (and inaction) of various state agencies and authorities. Government agencies displayed what the legal scholar Sally Sheldon calls "choreographed ignorance" about the extent of clandestine self-managed abortion (as well as the safety of the pills and reliability of the providers).[100] The health agency encouraged abortion travel abroad, provided free pre- and post-abortion counseling, and discouraged the use of MA at home with messages about risk and safety rather than illegality. The state prosecutor's office did not pursue any prosecutions against pill users but only pursued a single prosecution against someone who imported mifepristone for commercial resale. The prosecutor's public statements assured individuals that they should not expect their doctors to report them to police if they sought aftercare, nor would police arrest them for ordering pills.[101] The customs and medicines agencies intercepted and confiscated most of the abortion pill packages coming through the post, but they did not take action against the people who ordered the pills except to send them notices that their packages had been seized.[102] Media reports about the seizure of abortion pills carried official warnings about their use that emphasized health risks and uncertainty about the quality of medications ordered online, not the criminal penalties that self-managed abortion carried under Irish law.[103]

Official responses to MA by the Irish state echo the pattern of "limited, uneven, ambivalent interruptions" in the 1970s and 1980s against violations of the state's ban on contraceptives. The ban on contraceptives was continuously, creatively, and dramatically flouted by activist groups that undermined the official policy so completely that it was reformed. Cloatre and Enright's study of cross-border contraceptive activism illustrates some important parallels with abortion pills. As with medication abortion, Ireland's official condom prohibition "coexisted with an elaborate organized distribution network" that operated in full view of state authorities.[104] The Irish state response to illegal contraceptives was characterized, like medication abortion, by state knowledge of flows, partial interruption of cross-border flows, and deliberate inaction when confronted with activist displays of illicit products. The fragmented state responses to condoms and abortion pills contradict the idea that the state is a unified entity: instead there are "complex layers of micro-interactions" comprised by encounters and negotiations with individual agents.[105] The absence of a unitary state with a perfectly coordinated and uniform response to illegality also suggests that illegal practices can open up spaces for new and experimental forms of action.[106] Persistently challenging the "illegal" label of a product or practice can contribute to changing its status over time, as social decriminalization models of medication abortion activism demonstrate. Furthermore, by choosing the path of strategic ignorance about medication abortion, the Irish state was able to diffuse some of the tensions that resulted from its unworkable abortion laws.[107] The limits of this ignorance became apparent as pro-choice activists and campaigners for reform mobilized in the mid-2010s.

By this time, the following situation had crystallized in Ireland. The numbers traveling abroad for abortion had fallen by half in fifteen years. Abortion pills were being seized by customs officials at ports of entry, but pills continued to enter the country in increasing numbers through routes that state agencies could not close down. Feminist networks that supplied MA were reporting growing demand by people in Ireland, and well-coordinated networks across the island were moving pills across borders by a variety of methods. Self-managed abortion with pills, which officially carried a maximum fourteen-year jail sentence, was a method being used by several thousand people each year. Obtaining and using MA, although logistically difficult and socially stigmatized, was becoming easier and more widespread. Despite claims by the Irish anti-abortion movement that the 8th Amendment successfully kept Ireland "abortion-free," the island was in fact a laboratory of experimentation by the political movement for self-managed abortion. Next, I address the question of medication abortion in law and politics at the time of the 2018 referendum.

CHAPTER 7

Abortion Pills and Ireland's 8th Amendment Referendum

Well, if they go to England, it's not on our soil. It's over there, but it's still in a clinic, where they maybe have a nurse or a doctor. But if it's pills coming into the country—do you really want girls coming in with complications because they're sitting in their bedroom taking pills?

—Irish politician

By the time of the 2018 referendum, medication abortion had been in clandestine use in the Republic of Ireland for more than ten years. Estimates from pill providers put the demand at three to five people per day.[1] Abortion pills entered the country in growing numbers and had a substantial impact on reducing the number of Irish people who traveled to England in search of an abortion. While authorities in other countries (e.g., Northern Ireland and Poland) had shown a willingness to criminalize individual pill users and the people assisting them, authorities in the Irish Republic never adopted this approach. Irish state agencies were slow to grapple with the significance of pills and confronted their impact in different ways. Abortion pills remained marginal to mainstream political conversations until 2016–17, when they became a focus of legislative committee debates.

This chapter explores the political life of abortion pills in the Republic of Ireland from the mid-2010s. Medication abortion was essential to changing the consensus among Irish politicians, who came to endorse reform in part based on their understanding of how easily available and widely used MA was in Ireland. Political conversations about pills centered on the idea that abortion pill use was dangerous and pill users were vulnerable, both of which became important in the referendum campaign and the abortion law that followed the referendum.

A TRAGIC DEATH AND A NEW LAW

For nearly twenty years after the 1992 referendums, the issue of abortion was frozen in Irish politics. A few critical events—most notably, a tragic and preventable death—changed the political context of abortion reform in Ireland. After a 2010 European Court judgment that found Ireland's abortion ban violated human rights, the government began to explore its options for implementation of this decision.[2] This political process coincided with the 2012 death of Savita Halappanavar. Halappanavar died in a Galway hospital after being denied a life-saving abortion. At seventeen weeks of pregnancy, her water broke and she began to miscarry but did not expel the fetus. Her doctors refused to intervene because the fetal heart could still be heard. She experienced sepsis and died of a heart attack seven days after her miscarriage began.[3] During the miscarriage, the Indian-born Halppanavar told her midwife that in the Hindu faith, and under Indian law, a termination would be possible; her midwife responded, now infamously, that termination was not possible because Ireland is a "Catholic country."[4] Halappanavar's death provoked public anger and mobilized the pro-choice movement, sparking mass protests in the streets of Dublin. Meanwhile, the climate of anti-abortion stigma in Ireland was shifting as personal stories about experiences of abortion travel became more common in public discourse.[5]

The public demanded abortion reform, but the political response was only to tinker at the edges of the constitutional abortion ban. Public pressure after Savita Halappanavar's death, compounded by European court rulings against Ireland, pushed the government to introduce abortion legislation.[6] Until that point, abortion law had been the product of constitutional referendums and court judgments, not legislation. In 2013, the legislature passed the Protection of Life During Pregnancy Act (PLDPA), which clarified the circumstances under which abortion could be obtained legally. Abortion would be legal, it established, only where two doctors certified that there was "real and substantial risk of loss of the woman's life" from physical illness, emergency illness, or suicide and that the risk could only be averted by abortion.[7] It also introduced a potential fourteen-year criminal penalty for anyone who "intentionally destroy[s] unborn human life." While the constitutional ban had existed since 1983, the 2013 legislation marked the first time a regulatory framework for abortion was introduced in Irish law.[8]

Although it was only in force for five years, the PLDPA is an important milestone for a study of medication abortion in Ireland because it represents the first moment when the Irish legislature—the Oireachtas—publicly confronted the issue of clandestine self-managed abortion with pills. The PLDPA primarily dealt with the narrow legal grounds for abortion in hospitals. However, the issue of self-managed abortion with pills was present in the debates from the committee stage to the passage of the bill. The PLDPA introduced criminal penalties that were interpreted as targeting pill users at a moment when self-managed abortion with pills was attracting increased attention in the Irish press.

Testimony by members of a pro-choice campaign group before a 2013 parliamentary committee first made legislators aware of the growing number of women in Ireland accessing medication abortion. At this early stage, even pro-choice activists tended to frame MA as a dangerous alternative to legal abortion provided by doctors, although the danger could be eliminated with proper regulation.[9] As the PLDPA took shape and came before the legislature, MA became central to debates about its criminal penalties. Section 22, which criminalized intentional destruction of "unborn human life" with a maximum fourteen years in prison, was especially significant because it raised concerns that pill users themselves could face prison time.[10] The government insisted that criminal penalties for violating the PLDPA would be enforced against rogue abortion providers only. However, increased media coverage of self-managed abortion undermined the government's account of who would be likely to violate the abortion law and who might be criminalized by it.

In legislative debates, the health minister, James Reilly, supported the fourteen-year prison penalty for illegal abortion and defended it as a modern, proportional measure. In response, a Teachta Dála (TD; member of the lower house of the Oireachtas) called on the minister to explain whether criminal penalties like prison time could fall upon a hypothetical fourteen-year-old who used "abortifacient tablets" bought online. The health minister replied:

> The Director of Public Prosecutions will use his or her discretion and the wisdom of the office in deciding whether to refer a case. The courts will also have discretion. None of us would want to see a 14-year-old in the situation described by TD Kelleher. I cannot imagine how it would happen but equally I cannot give a cast-iron guarantee that it will not happen.[11]

Minister Reilly's ambivalence about criminalization reflects a broader public discourse at the time. Even the anti-abortion activists who opposed the PLDPA as too permissive (because it provided several grounds for legal abortion) publicly disputed the idea that criminal penalties should be applied to women who ended their own pregnancies. Anti-abortion campaigners like the Iona Institute argued that the PLDPA would not be used to criminalize doctors who acted in "good faith." Proponents of criminal penalties in the law instead invoked the threat of an imagined backstreet abortion provider who could only be deterred by the possibility of prison.[12]

In response to another question about women buying MA online, Minister Reilly countered that the bill's criminal penalties existed to deter a "backstreet operator," a "recidivist" who performs "dangerous procedures on vulnerable people."[13] These debates illustrate a mismatch between the mythical criminal abortionist and the reality of self-managed abortion with pills. Since abortion had become legally available in England, reports of so-called backstreet (i.e., illegal surgical) abortions in Ireland had been vanishingly rare.[14] Nonetheless, what the historian Ricki Solinger calls the "spectral icon" of the backstreet provider continues to shape political arguments about clandestine abortion and its criminalization.[15] Pills came to be known in Irish politics, to the extent that they were discussed on the periphery of the 2013 PLDPA, through legislators' narratives of self-managed abortion as the last resort of "isolated and vulnerable" "young girls."[16] This framing would remain resonant in the abortion debate, and it would play an important part in the public conversations on MA that took place during the 8th Amendment referendum process.

THE CITIZENS' ASSEMBLY AND THE JOINT OIREACHTAS COMMITTEE

The 2013 Protection of Life During Pregnancy Act was a reluctant government response to a human rights court judgment and the outcry after the death of Savita Halappanavar. It proved too little, too late. It introduced the first regulatory framework for legal abortion in Ireland, but its limitations highlighted the need for larger constitutional change and helped build momentum for the campaign to repeal the 8th Amendment. Because it was inserted in the constitution by referendum, the 8th Amendment could only be removed by referendum. By 2016, mounting public pressure for abortion reform became a central issue in the general election. Several political parties made explicit commitments to hold a referendum on the 8th Amendment and civil society organizations lobbied candidates to endorse its immediate repeal.[17] In what was seen as a stalling tactic at the time, the center-right political party Fine Gael did not commit to a referendum but promised to hold a "convention or assembly" on the 8th Amendment.[18] Upon forming a minority government in 2016, it passed a resolution to convene a Citizens' Assembly that would deliver a nonbinding recommendation to legislators.

The Citizens' Assembly on the 8th Amendment was an "exercise in delib-erative democracy": over five weekends, it assembled ninety-nine registered voters, chosen for their representativeness of the electorate.[19] Members heard testimony from experts and advocates, as well as submissions from the general public, on topics such as the history of the 8th Amendment, the current state of abortion access in Ireland, and abortion laws around the world. Abortion pills were not included on its agenda. At the time, the Citizens' Assembly was viewed with skepticism by pro-choice groups in Ireland, which saw it as a cynical maneuver by the socially conservative government to avoid a referen-dum. Feminists were critical of the Assembly's structure and program, as the legal scholar Fiona de Londras explains:

> The Assembly was designed with a literal adherence to a notion of balance that meant any lawyers who had expertise in abortion rights were not invited to address it; instead, "general" constitutional lawyers played that role. Furthermore, "bal-ance" was interpreted to ensure that anti-choice speakers received equal time to pro-choice speakers, even when their presentations were based on abortion myths or made by representatives of discredited organizations.[20]

Despite these flaws, when it came to final ballots and its report, the Citizens' Assembly surprised its critics by going "far beyond what anyone had really expected."[21] In its recommendations to the legislature, 87 percent of Assembly members wanted the 8th Amendment to be removed or reformed. Nearly half (48 percent) recommended that abortion should be legal on request up to twelve weeks of gestation. Furthermore, majorities supported legal abortion on mental health grounds (78 percent), on the grounds of serious fetal anom-aly (80 percent), and on socioeconomic grounds (72 percent).[22] If the Citizens' Assembly had been Fine Gael's attempt to "kick the can down the road," as observers had speculated, the outcome was not what they had anticipated.[23] It showed that the 8th Amendment abortion ban—and the Protection of Life

During Pregnancy Act, passed only four years earlier—were decidedly at odds with public opinion on the matter of abortion.

The Citizens' Assembly's recommendations were brought to members of both legislative chambers in the Joint Oireachtas Committee (JOC) for examination. At the first meeting of the committee, Justice Mary Laffoy, chair of the Citizens' Assembly, singled out medication abortion as the main issue that the Assembly had not covered sufficiently. She cited recent statements from health authorities that indicated "increasing numbers of women from the island of Ireland are making contact with online abortion pill providers."[24] These statements marked a shift in the state's attitude to medication abortion: health authorities were increasingly forced to acknowledge that the reduction in abortion-travel numbers was the result of medication abortion bought online. When Catherine Noone, chair of the JOC, was interviewed after the committee adjourned, she admitted to a "high level of ignorance" about MA on her part and among other colleagues on the committee.[25] At that point, abortion pills had been entering Ireland for at least a decade.

Although many members of the legislature and the parliamentary committee on the 8th Amendment claimed ignorance of MA, its membership included two legislators who were closely affiliated with abortion pill activism: TD Ruth Coppinger, who consumed abortion pills in front of TV cameras as part of the 2014 Abortion Pill Train (see chap. 8), and TD Bríd Smith, who brought a package of MA into the legislative chamber in 2016 and explained how to order them. She held aloft a package of A-Kare, manufactured by DKT India, obtained through Women on Web.[26] She challenged her colleagues: "You could arrest me for having it . . . but you know that if you dare to implement [the law] you would bring hell-fire and brimstone down on top of this house, and in wider society, because we have moved on."[27] TDs Coppinger and Smith were by no means the only advocates for repealing the abortion ban in the Oireachtas, but they were the most visible political spokespeople for abortion pill users in Ireland. Within the Irish political system, they nonetheless sat on the fringes in the Solidarity–People Before Profit party, which held very few seats in the Oireachtas. Nonetheless, the TDs' position on the Joint Oireachtas Committee, their affiliation with pro-choice feminist activists, and their partnership with Women on Web all contributed to elevate the position of MA in the committee's deliberations.[28]

Abortion pills became known to the Irish political class largely through published research from Women on Web when it was presented to the Joint

Oireachtas Committee by Dr. Abigail Aiken and later when Aiken's evidence was discussed in 2018 Oireachtas debates. In the words of a Fine Gael senator on the committee, the data Aiken presented on MA were "a game changer."[29] Aiken's collaboration with Women on Web had begun some years earlier, and their first peer-reviewed study was published in 2016. This collaboration was built around a concerted strategy to study and publish Women on Web data in top medical journals, whose institutional infrastructure would showcase the "quality and reliability" of their data and help inform public conversations on MA, which had so far lacked data.[30] Their first joint publication on Ireland, which formed the basis for Aiken's testimony to the JOC, analyzed consultations and questionnaires of 5,650 people in the Irish Republic and Northern Ireland who had obtained pills from Women on Web between 2010 and 2015. It found that the vast majority (98 percent) had positive experiences with telemedical abortion. Aiken showed data indicating that abortion travel from Ireland had declined as abortion pill access in Ireland had grown.[31]

Aiken's testimony was referenced throughout the remainder of the JOC's term and in the subsequent legislative debates, where politicians used her research to make the case that reform was urgently needed.[32] Other advocacy groups saw that politicians were more willing to engage with the findings of Aiken's peer-reviewed research than they had been with anecdotal evidence from Irish counseling and support services, which had also reported growing numbers of clients using MA obtained online.[33] The prominence of Aiken's evidence in Irish debates reflects Women on Web's strategy of publishing its data in scientific and medical outlets to push for legal change. WoW faced criticism from other groups that saw a potential contradiction between ensuring the safety of pill distribution networks and publicizing the extent of the demand for pills.[34] Given that abortion pill use had been publicized in media coverage well before the committee, Aiken herself was surprised that many politicians in the room had no knowledge about medication abortion. Aiken saw the impact of her testimony as generating interest in reform—not enforcement—of the existing laws:

> Many of the politicians had never heard of this and were really unfamiliar with it. . . . It could have easily been "Oh my gosh, all these thousands of women a year using the pills, why aren't we prosecuting them? Why aren't we bringing the long arm of the law down on them?" That was not the reaction of anyone, not even the most anti-abortion person in the room. Instead their reaction was a lot more: "Wow, this is happening! Tell us about this. Who is affected by this, and what do we need to do to change things?"[35]

When the JOC released its final report, it recommended that abortion be made available up to twelve weeks with no restriction as to reason, delivered through a GP-led service.[36] In making this recommendation, the committee reported that it could not "ignore the extent to which Ireland has an underlying rate of terminations, the majority of which are carried out either in medical clinics in the United Kingdom, or in Ireland through unsupervised use of abortion pills procured through the internet."[37] Its report also recommended the repeal of the Protection of Life During Pregnancy Act because its criminal penalties created a chilling effect without any impact on "the overall incidence of abortions." The place of abortion pill use, and the presumed vulnerability of abortion pill users, was at the center of the committee's response. A Fine Gael senator who sat on the committee described the change in attitude in the following terms:

> [The committee hearings] shone a light on the availability, the lack of regulation, the lack of quality control, the frequency at which the tablets were being used, the fact that they could land at your doorstep via a courier or An Post [the Irish postal service]. I think that changed the debate, in that people recognized and realized it wasn't about going—like you see in America—going to a Planned Parenthood, a facility or to an 'abortion clinic' in inverted commas. It was available at your doorstep and there were women taking these tablets or pills … unsupervised, unregulated, and they had the potential to be dangerous and cause harm and, in some cases, death. That created huge awareness and that was, I think, a turning point.[38]

The committee's report set the tone for much of the pill-related debate that would take place over the next few months, which would also be typified by shock at the prevalence of pills in Ireland, anxiety about the potential danger of unsupervised use, and acknowledgment of the unworkable nature of the 8th Amendment ban.

ABORTION PILLS IN THE OIREACHTAS

From the committee process to legislative debates about repealing the 8th Amendment and then to the referendum campaign itself, medication abortion entered public discourse in a new way. Previously, pills had been marginal to the abortion debate in Ireland, mainly coming to public attention through campaigning by activist groups or media reports about pill seizures by customs. As a consequence, the Oireachtas debates of 2018 show how politicians worked to understand and interpret the scientific, moral, and political significance of the pills for the Republic of Ireland and its abortion laws. I argue here that MA took on a sociopolitical life in two ways: first, through a set of technological and temporal frames that were used to interpret the social impact of pills in Ireland; and second, through the abortion seekers conjured in Oireachtas debates and campaign material.

Opponents of reform were almost entirely absent from discussions about MA. This is notable because anti-abortion legislators in other contexts have seized on MA to promulgate restrictions that prevent their uptake in abortion care (see chap. 2). In Ireland, opponents of abortion scarcely engaged with the topic of pills in the 2018 debates. When they did, it was for two reasons. The first was to contest the evidence presented about the widespread use of pills. Because this evidence undermined the narrative of the "abortion-free" island, anti-abortion legislators like Ronán Mullen argued that abortion pills were used in Ireland in very small numbers, so they were just a red herring in the abortion debate. Anti-abortion campaigners like Mullen maintained that Ireland still had a far lower abortion rate than neighboring countries because its ban reduced the number of people who wanted to end their pregnancies in the first place.[39] The second reason that anti-abortion legislators discussed the inflow of MA was to accuse the state of failing to properly enforce its abortion laws. Some defenders of the 8th Amendment argued that the state's tolerance of illicit MA amounted to an unlawful concession to global criminal forces. They drew parallels between MA and other illegal drugs to argue against the widely held view that the state should respond to the growth in self-managed abortion by reducing or removing the criminal penalties attached to it.[40] Others analogized MA to social harms of the internet. For example, TD Kevin O'Keefe, of the Fianna Fáil party, argued, "People being able to access abortion pills online is a manifestation of global interference in our society. Similar issues such as cyber-bullying and the age of consent in regard to accessing mobile phones and so on have recently arisen. . . . It worries me that we would acquiesce to such a problem."[41] Grasping for metaphors or analogous flows to understand MA, many legislators seized on the online dimension of abortion pill purchases to equate online pills with the internet more generally. For opponents of abortion, this meant that abortion pills were best understood as a by-product of external online forces that caused concrete harms in Irish society.

For advocates of reform, and for the large group of politicians who expressed ambivalence about abortion, MA purchased online took on a different meaning.

For this group, equating MA with the internet served to demonstrate that the 8th Amendment was an outdated pre-internet relic that was incompatible with contemporary Irish society where life was increasingly—and irreversibly—entwined with online culture and commerce. Many politicians presented themselves as reluctant supporters of reform, motivated by pragmatism rather than pro-choice or feminist political commitments. Among this large group, abortion pills were commonly used to demonstrate the impracticality of the 8th Amendment abortion ban. Advocates of reform in 2018, especially those who presented themselves as ambivalent about abortion itself, often drew technological analogies between MA and internet technology.

> If we want to become hardline on it, we can say we will ban the Internet, or ban abortion on the Internet, but reality is reality. (TD Bernard Durkan, Fine Gael)[42]

> In the absence of shutting down the Internet, we will never be able to stop women in crisis pregnancies—women who are desperate, alone and afraid—from taking [pills]. (TD Hildegarde Naughton, Fine Gael)[43]

> Now we have the Internet which did not exist thirty years ago. Kids and young people can go online and purchase abortion pills, unregulated and unethically, which they can use without medical supervision. (Sen. Martin Conway, Fine Gael)[44]

Here abortion pills are used to advance a narrative about contemporary Ireland, which is at odds with the Ireland of 1983 when the constitutional ban was introduced. These legislators use technological change as a way to illustrate social change, drawing a parallel between the two to argue that access to abortion pills can no more be reversed than the technological integration of the internet into modern life can be rolled back. There is a temporal comparison at the core of these claims: the "old" Ireland of 1983 and the "new" Ireland of 2018 are different places. Máiréad Enright identifies this as part of the Irish state's "common sense" narrative of its own history, "neatly divided into religious past and secular present." In this narrative, abuses like those carried out by religious institutions are designated as "leftovers from a different time."[45] Much of the 2018 political discourse on the 8th Amendment reflects this temporal split: the 8th Amendment is framed as an unwelcome hangover from the religious past. Abortion pills feature in these narratives as evidence of the distinction between the pre-pill era and the current era of frequent pill use:

> Irish women have abortions every day. With the advent of the abortion pill we cannot even say, as we did years ago, that they have abortions every day, but they

> just do not have them here. They do have them here, every day, and we cannot
> deny that. To continue to deny that is to continue to perpetuate the kind of place
> Ireland was in 1983 and we have moved on. (TD Louise O'Reilly, Sinn Féin)[46]

TD O'Reilly draws a line between the "kind of place" Ireland was in 1983 and
the Ireland of 2018 when abortion routinely happens in clandestine, self-
managed settings. Times have changed, but so too has geography: abortions
happen "here" in Ireland, not just abroad. Her words illustrate another important feature of the political discourse on pills, asking her colleagues to consider
that pills were already in frequent use as politicians were debating their existence. In their speeches, legislators frequently evoked the idea that "this eve-
ning," "as we speak," someone was in the process of ending their own pregnancy
with pills.[47] Politicians spoke in vivid and emotive terms about the abortion
pill usage that was taking place alongside political debates. The ideas and
images they employed to understand the pill users themselves merit closer
scrutiny, because a particular type of pill user became a notable feature of
politicians' messages and the campaign that would follow. As in the 2013 abortion debates, abortion pill users came to be known through well-worn tropes
about youth, vulnerability, and protection. The idealized young pill user was
not representative of people self-managing abortions in Ireland, but her image
nonetheless captured the political imagination.

KNOWING ABORTION PILLS THROUGH THEIR USERS

Reproductive technologies come to be understood through ideas about their
users, and their users are simultaneously framed through ideas about the
technologies that they employ. A technology and its users are socially coproduced, so the same technology can be subject to different interpretations
depending on context-specific ideas about the device, its users, and users'
bodies.[48] Reproductive technologies are differently understood depending on
the geographic location, socioeconomic status, and racialization of their users,
all of which shape ideas about the meaning of fertility and its control. Using
these feminist frames to examine the MA debates in Ireland, we can see that
this technology came to be understood through the repetition of particular
narratives about abortion pill users: the young and vulnerable pill user who
needed medical support, contrasted to the demanding, irresponsible pill user
whose conduct required state regulation.

The first group's characteristics were imagined through tropes of the isolated places where they used MA. In the 2018 debates, legislators evoked pill users in the following ways (emphasis below is my own):

> The *young women* who seek to terminate a pregnancy by obtaining pills over the Internet which will bring on a miscarriage do so in *lonely bedrooms or sheds* dotted around the country. (TD Timmy Dooley, Fianna Fáil)[49]

> Since the technology of the abortion pill was introduced, girls have been taking it, whether in *toilets in colleges or in their own bedrooms*. (TD Joan Burton, Labour)[50]

> We have abortion in Ireland. . . . We have it in *lonely bedrooms* with pills bought on the Internet by approximately three women every day. (TD Jan O'Sullivan, Labour)[51]

The language used to discuss abortion pill users stressed their age and marginality, through references to "girls" in their "lonely bedrooms" or "toilets in colleges." These assumptions were at odds with available data on Irish abortion pill users presented in the Joint Oireachtas Committee, which showed that only 7.9 percent of people who obtained pills through Women on Web from 2010 to 2012 were under 25 years of age. The greatest share of demand for pills came from people ages 30 to 34.[52] Nonetheless, the imagined abortion pill user who came to animate Oireachtas debates about MA was the familiar figure of the isolated young woman, who had also appeared in 2013 debates about criminalizing vulnerable pill users. Tropes of the abortion-seeking woman as a "helpless victim" with "culturally potent" reasons for abortion— like youth, poverty, or family pressure—have long been used to attract support for legal abortion, because they frame women's reasons for seeking abortion in ways that comport with gendered expectations and moralism about female sexuality.[53] As a rationale for reform, narratives like this often lead to bad policy because they continue to see abortion seekers as victims in need of protection, not rights holders or decision makers.[54]

These frames resonated with conservative Irish politicians who, according to an advocate working in reproductive health policy, "responded empathetically" to the framing of "a vulnerable teenage girl alone in her bedroom." The power of this image even motivated some conservatives to extend their support for abortion beyond the circumstances of risk to life or in the case of rape.[55] As earlier debates had shown, tropes about predatory backstreet abortion providers fit poorly with the model of self-managed abortion supported online, because abortion seekers end their pregnancies by swallowing pills themselves, at the time and place of their choosing. In the absence of this abortion-provider figure, the idea about vulnerability and victimhood of abortion seekers continues, albeit through the figure of young women facing isolation, social pressure, and stigma.

Compounding the vulnerability of pill users in these accounts were the criminal prohibitions on self-managed abortion that forced pill users to act secretly. Many politicians stressed the feelings of anxiety, uncertainty, isolation, shame, and fear that abortion pill users would feel because they were unable to seek out medical care. People who order pills from services like Women on Web or Women Help Women have consultations beforehand and communicate with trained help desk staff during the process of self-managing abortion.[56] However, "telemedicine" was never mentioned in the Oireachtas debates, nor was the remote medical supervision provided for pill users. Instead, politicians characterized self-managed abortion with pills as the total absence of supervision. If abortion pills signified the idea that abortion was happening *in Ireland*, where no medical or clinical infrastructure was established for abortion provision, they also indicated to Irish politicians that this new method for abortion would proceed whether or not it was available in the formal medical system. A pro-choice senator and member of the Joint Oireachtas Committee suggested that the perceived absence of "supervision and control" was the key difference that motivated politicians to act on abortion pills when they had been complacent about the informal system of abortion travel.[57] This claim is illustrated by a speech by TD Micheál Martin, an antiabortion legislator who had served as health minister in 2002 when the government again tried to pass a constitutional amendment to remove the risk of suicide as legal grounds for abortion.[58] In 2018, Martin changed his position to support abortion reform: "It is clear that the reality of the abortion pill means we are no longer talking about a procedure that involves the broader medical system during the early stages of pregnancy. We must have a system which actively encourages women to seek support from medical professionals as soon as possible."[59]

Among Irish politicians who called for reforms in order to bring self-managed abortion into the formal healthcare system, and under medical supervision, the perceived danger of MA was a common theme. Many TDs and senators advocated for liberalization of Irish abortion law on the grounds that abortion pill users should be entitled to seek medical care before, during, and after an abortion without fear of criminalization. Proponents of reform who relied on pragmatic arguments about pill use often worked to frame the debate in medical terms. This is a familiar feature of abortion debates in other countries: advocates of abortion reform try to lower the temperature by framing the issue as a matter of healthcare, not a religious or moral question.[60] Politicians in the Oireachtas debates, including the health minister, and later the Taoiseach (prime minister) on the campaign trail, warned that without swift action, an Irish woman taking MA "in the not-too-distant future will rupture her uterus and die."[61] The perceived danger of clandestine self-managed abortion was a common message among pro-choice spokespeople on the campaign trail, and it provoked serious disagreement among pro-repeal activists.

DEMAND, REGULATION, AND CONTROL

While the figure of the young, vulnerable pill user evoked paternalistic sentiments of protection and concern, a second type of pill user was conjured during abortion debates to project an alternative relationship between abortion seekers, doctors, and the state after repealing the 8th Amendment. This second figure—the demanding, irresponsible pill user—was evoked to frame the concern over the unregulated nature of the online abortion pill supply. Opponents of reform sometimes downplayed the number of self-managed abortions taking place in Ireland. By contrast, some proponents of abortion reform countered that the 8th Amendment regime in the Irish Republic had inadvertently created a system of unregulated abortion with pills. This was partly a pragmatic argument about the extent of pill use and partly a democratic argument about the need for the legislature to determine if, how, and when abortion would be available. If the 8th Amendment were repealed, a legislator argued of pills, "we could make a decision to ban them, regulate them, or limit their availability to medical practitioners."[62]

Legalization as a path to regulation, restriction, and medical supervision became a prominent theme in the discussion of MA. This narrative about regulation configured the abortion pill user in a distinct way. TD Lisa Chambers, Fianna Fáil, stated:

> We do not suggest one should be able to walk into one's local convenience store and purchase an abortion pill as one would a box of Panadol [acetaminophen]. What is being proposed is highly restricted and regulated and will be carried out in conjunction with the medical profession. Women buy abortion pills online and self-administer them without medical supervision. *That* is unrestricted.[63]

This is a familiar feature of debates about medication abortion around the world: the idea of an easier, more convenient, and less invasive abortion outraged anti-abortion activists and motivated campaigns against the introduction of MA during the 1980s and 1990s. Opponents of medication abortion have routinely objected to the technology on the basis that it makes abortion too easy—a "social convenience abortion," as it was described in Australian debates on mifepristone. This characterization of MA as easy, convenient, and trivial also suggests characteristics of the abortion seeker, of course. For example, opponents of abortion use the phrase "abortion on demand" to signal their disapproval and malign the behavior of "demanding" women.[64]

Abortion debates often turn on the question of how limits can be imposed and who can verify that abortions are being obtained for the "right" reasons. Doctors are usually tasked with this gatekeeping role, interpreting the law and its restrictions before deciding whether or not the abortion request is legal. This was a feature of Irish abortion debates well before the 2018 referendum: in 2013, then Taoiseach Enda Kenny argued that doctors who could make judgments about genuine medical grounds for abortion were the "only line of defense" against abortion "on demand."[65] The emergence of self-managed abortion with pills cast doubt on the idea that doctors could reliably continue to play that role. This anxiety was apparent in the 2017–18 Oireachtas debates and the referendum campaign itself: "demanding" women who felt entitled to abortion might expect to be able to buy MA in the same way they buy other medications.[66] Many of the politicians who called for pragmatic liberalizing reforms did so while offering reassurances that abortion legislation would impose medical supervision and limitations.

Taoiseach Leo Varadkar—a physician who opposed abortion when he served as minister of health from 2014 to 2016—became one of the most prominent political supporters of the repeal of the 8th Amendment, along with the health minister, Simon Harris. Varadkar was a vocal advocate of the idea that MA posed an imminent danger to Irish people, repeatedly telling the media and the public that it was "only a matter of time before somebody hemorrhages or bleeds to death or dies as a result of using these pills unregulated."[67] Varadkar's messages on the campaign trail amplified two narratives that had emerged prominently in the Oireachtas debates: first, abortion pills were dangerous because they were unregulated; and second, any law to regulate abortion after repeal would impose suitable restrictions and regulations. The demanding abortion pill user also appeared in his campaign messages as a cautionary tale about how the state would regulate pills after repealing the constitutional ban: "No woman who is experiencing crisis pregnancy will be able to go into the pharmacy and bang the table and demand abortion pills. Not that I think anyone would ever do that."[68]

A persistent anxiety about pills is visible in Irish political discourse around this time: if clandestine self-managed abortion was already widespread in Ireland under a constitutional abortion ban, would legislation be able to impose a system to regulate who can end a pregnancy and when? Or would women flout the law by using pills regardless? This points to a tension at the heart of the referendum campaign: because the referendum dealt only with the question of repealing the 8th Amendment and allowing the legislature to regulate abortion, it raised questions about what kind of abortion law and gestational age limits would follow. For instance, a campaign poster from the anti-abortion group LoveBoth implored voters, "If killing an unborn baby at six months bothers you, vote no."[69] The resonance of this messaging affected the pro-choice side as well. Advocates of repeal, particularly those in the political establishment who had only recently become public supporters of abortion reform, took pains to emphasize the message that legislation following repeal of the 8th Amendment would impose limits on abortion.[70]

ABORTION PILLS IN THE PRO-REPEAL CAMPAIGN

The referendum on the 8th Amendment offered an up or down vote on the constitutional abortion ban, but it did not determine the specific abortion law that would govern after repeal. Together for Yes (TFY), the pro-repeal civil society campaign, recognized this as a problem early on, noting a nervousness on the "degree of choice" and an aversion to "unlimited choice" among likely voters.[71] Based on public opinion research, TFY oriented its campaign around a three-pronged strategy: first, set an "informative, reasoned, calm, and non-confrontational" tone; second, position abortion as a necessary part of healthcare; and third, shift the emphasis of the abortion debate "from 'choice' to 'needs', from 'rights' to 'healthcare', and from judgement to empathy and compassion."[72] Together for Yes was a coalition of seventy civil society organizations composed of groups with different political strategies and stances on abortion, everyone from "establishment figures to anarcho-feminists."[73] Such a coalition had its own internal respectability politics. As they had in 1983 fighting the 8th Amendment, some parts of the 2018 pro-choice campaign felt maligned in the national press (and more conservative segments of the Irish women's movement) as "blue-haired feminists in their Repeal jumpers" who would alienate undecided voters.[74]

At times, the professional gloss of the organization, which developed messaging based on market research, polling, and focus groups, was alienating to veteran activists who were used to working in more grassroots ways. Some found themselves reluctant to share TFY's messaging about "the conditions, the regulations, the limitations" on abortion that would follow repeal.[75] There was also division among campaigners about their overall stance on abortion: necessary but unfortunate reality or basic right to be demanded without apology? As feminist analyses of the campaign have suggested, Together for Yes's campaign messages positioned abortion seekers as "vulnerable recipients of love, compassion and decent medical care," as opposed to "political agents"; this decision had broader ramifications for the referendum outcome and future abortion politics in the Irish Republic.[76]

Among the groups in the TFY coalition, there was disagreement over how MA should be discussed, and the campaign's messaging changed over time.[77] Its pre-referendum messaging research had showed that a campaign for abortion reform should emphasize that delays to reform would result in further deaths, in keeping with its emphasis on abortion as essential healthcare.[78] This message resonated with public anger over the death of Savita Halappanavar six years earlier. During the 2018 campaign, the message about the preventable deaths caused by the 8th Amendment came to focus, in part, on the purported health threat of self-managed abortion. The campaign's focus on so-called middle-ground voters resulted in a discourse on self-managed abortion that presented it as "dangerous and risky."[79] Together for Yes spokespeople appeared at press conferences with doctors, to emphasize that repeal was "required to regulate the use of abortion pills," along with parents, who discussed the dangers of "unregulated access" to abortion pills.[80] This approach divided activists and generated pushback from groups who were directly involved in providing pills. They found TFY's language on pills "stigmatizing" and pushed it to change its language to describe MA as "safe but illegal" when discussing medicines supplied by feminist networks like Women on Web and Women Help Women.[81] Nonetheless, Together for Yes campaign material continued to equate unregulated pill use with unsafe abortion in its literature, as in this quote from a campaign leaflet:

Every day at least two women take an abortion pill at home alone with no medical support. Most are already mothers. Vote YES to ensure women who need an abortion will have the support of their doctor. Voting NO means unsafe and unregulated abortions will continue to happen all over Ireland every day.[82]

This kind of messaging divided activists and campaigners because they perceived it as "instrumentalizing" the issue, emphasizing negative aspects of self-managed abortion and diminishing the autonomy of pill users.[83] Moreover, some activists saw the message as short-sighted. Because the pills being framed as dangerous during the campaign would be the same ones dispensed by doctors under the government's proposed scheme for abortion provision after repeal, a message that associated MA with danger had the potential to undermine public confidence in any future abortion service.[84] This confusion was compounded by the Together for Yes briefing material, which used "medical abortion" as a synonym for self-managed abortion. In one campaign briefing, TFY concluded that while "the option of medical abortion is generally safe and effective, it cannot be considered acceptable healthcare as it does not reflect an active preference, but the lack of safe options and alternatives."[85]

Disagreements among pro-repeal groups over the framing of self-managed abortion during the campaign speak to larger strategic questions that activists and campaigners faced. Critics of TFY thought it too cautious, middle class, and concerned with the perceptions of "middle-ground" voters who wanted limited reform. Its messaging, workshopped over several years and carefully designed to frame abortion reform as a medically necessary change, was at odds with the vision that MA activists had developed in the years leading up to repeal. Similar debates have emerged elsewhere, dividing pro-choice advocates over the extent to which self-managed abortion should be framed as a regrettable practice that is the last resort of desperate women—little better than the coat hanger of the past—or as a safe and acceptable method of abortion, which requires decriminalization but not necessarily the introduction of tight medical controls over it.

When the referendum vote was held, 66.4 percent voted to repeal the 8th Amendment. It was a resounding victory for the TFY coalition and activist groups that preceded it.[86] Repeal won in every county (except Donegal) and among all age groups (except those over sixty-five). Asked when they had made their decision on the 8th Amendment, 75 percent of voters in the exit poll said they "always knew" how they would vote and only 12 percent said they had made their decision during the campaign. Of the Joint Oireachtas Committee and the Citizens' Assembly, only 2 percent said they had made their decision after these bodies published their recommendations. The exit poll also asked about the factors that most influenced voters' choice: of those who supported repeal, 84 percent cited the right to choose as a leading factor in their decision.[87] The risk to health and life, pregnancy as the result of rape, and serious fetal anomaly were the next three most-cited factors in the exit poll. The prominence of health messaging suggests that the pro-repeal campaign's decision to emphasize abortion as healthcare was highly effective, but the overwhelming support for the idea of choice suggests that TFY might have been overly cautious with its messaging about compassion and care rather than choice and bodily autonomy. Self-managed abortion was not among the factors that the exit poll explored.

PILLS IN THE REPUBLIC OF IRELAND AFTER REPEAL

In discussing the committees, legislative debates, and campaign in the lead-up to the repeal of the 8th Amendment, I have argued that themes of danger, risk, and regulation were the most important frames used to interpret the impact of clandestine self-managed abortion. These frames matter enormously for what came after the referendum, when it became clear that promising regulation of self-managed abortion was not just a rhetorical stance of politicians who wanted to advocate for a middle-ground compromise on abortion. MA came to be understood in 2017–18 as a risky and unregulated technology whose unfettered movement was a threat to public health and state control over reproduction. For procedural and political reasons, this framing not only defined the messaging around pills during the campaign, but it also shaped their position in the system of legal abortion that was introduced after the constitutional ban had been removed.

After the referendum, the legislature debated and passed the Health (Regulation of Termination of Pregnancy) Bill to introduce regulations for legal abortion in the Irish Republic's healthcare system by early 2019. Much of this bill reflected the political process that had taken place prior to the referendum, when the government had released a draft bill as an indication of what a post-repeal law would look like. However, after the referendum passed, the bill introduced to the legislature showed significant additions that contradicted the recommendations of the Citizens' Assembly and Joint

Oireachtas Committee. One such feature, directly at odds with the recommendations of those bodies, was the bill's proposal to retain criminal penalties for self-managed abortion outside of approved medical settings. The bill contained provisions for decriminalizing the pregnant person while criminalizing people who assisted self-managed abortion; it also maintained a maximum fourteen-year prison sentence. The bill added new language targeting MA, which had not been present in pre-referendum drafts:

> It shall be an offence for a person to prescribe, administer, supply or procure any drug, substance, instrument, apparatus or other thing knowing that it is intended to be used or employed with intent to end the life of a fetus, or being reckless as to whether it is intended to be so used or employed, otherwise than in accordance with the provisions of this Act.[88]

During the debates over this bill in late 2018, months after the referendum result, legislators debated criminalization as a proxy for the meaning of the entire referendum. Legislators who defended the continued criminalization of self-managed abortion argued that the threat of criminal penalties was necessary to encourage people to obtain abortions within the formal healthcare system only. Health Minister Simon Harris justified retaining criminal sanctions in these terms:

> Helping a pregnant woman to end her pregnancy outside the provisions of the Bill is not in her best interests and may put her health or life at risk. One of the primary purposes of this legislation and repealing the eighth amendment was to ensure we could eliminate the risks that women face in consuming abortion pills sourced online or seeking an illegal abortion.[89]

TD Stephen Donnelly, for example, endorsed the criminal penalties in the bill by citing his experiences during the campaign: Donnelly argued that his constituents "who intended to vote 'Yes' were doing so in the clear knowledge that this section existed" in the law that would follow repeal.[90] Pro-choice legislators attempted to remove the criminal penalties in the bill at the committee stage but were unsuccessful.[91] Just as pills animated much of the pre-referendum debate about the dangerous realities of the 8th Amendment, they appeared in post-referendum debates as a threat to the integrity of any system for legal abortion.

The bill passed with criminal sanctions intact, albeit with the exemption for the "pregnant woman in respect of her own pregnancy."[92] The Irish medicines regulator approved mifepristone for termination of pregnancy on

November 30, 2018, in anticipation of the new abortion service opening at the beginning of 2019.[93] The Republic of Ireland's new abortion law permits abortion on request, without regard to reason, up to twelve weeks of pregnancy and after that point for limited reasons, including threat to health and life or serious fetal anomaly. The service for abortion before twelve weeks is almost exclusively managed with medication abortion provided by general practitioners and sexual health clinics, with surgical abortions only available in hospitals in limited cases. In the first full year of provision, Irish government data showed 6,666 abortions had been obtained in the country, while there were 375 abortions in England and Wales for Irish residents.[94] The new abortion law, immeasurably better than the 8th Amendment regime, still contains unnecessary barriers like a three-day waiting period, and service provision is still characterized by obstacles for people who are poor or live in rural areas.[95] As a result, some people still self-manage abortion with pills. The customs and medicines agencies continue to seize abortion pills at the border, as they did before the referendum. Figures published in 2020 by the medicines regulator indicate that abortion pill seizures are falling year on year.[96] As before, pill seizures continue, but there have been no prosecutions under the new law against people who attempt to help someone else end a pregnancy.

———

In countries where surgical abortion was already legal when MA became available, MA came to attention as one method among others. In the Republic of Ireland, where all abortion was effectively banned, MA came into the country as a clandestine mode of self-managed abortion in the absence of any domestic alternatives. It reshaped the geography of Irish abortion, giving people a choice to end a pregnancy at home, without traveling abroad. By extension, it brought abortion into a country that had previously thought itself free from abortion. MA entered the public debate in a distinctive way: debating abortion pills in Ireland was tantamount to debating the presence of any abortion—legal or illegal—inside the country. Political conversations on medication abortion therefore started from the question of how it upended the 8th Amendment abortion ban.

When Ireland had criminal penalties in place for self-managed abortion—against the person having the abortion and people who help them—the state did not pursue any prosecutions against individual pill users or their close supporters. It stopped pills coming in through the post by seizing them at customs. Across the border in Northern Ireland, the authorities took a very different approach to MA. Northern Irish authorities pursued investigations and prosecutions of individual pill users and the people who supported them, despite the public unpopularity of such prosecutions. At the same time, Northern Ireland served as the supply route for pills used by people across the entire island of Ireland because activists coordinated across the two jurisdictions. Next I turn to Northern Ireland, exploring the contradictions that made it both a hub for MA and a dangerous place for pill users.

CHAPTER 8

From Criminalization to Decriminalization in Northern Ireland

Changing a law isn't necessarily that feminist. It doesn't always put the means to access abortion back in women's hands. . . . So, our main concern wasn't necessarily changing the law, it was showing people they could get pills easily, cheaply, safely, and were unlikely to be prosecuted.

—Northern Irish activist

The geography of self-managed abortion on the island of Ireland was shaped by cross-border cooperation. Activists overcame obstacles to moving pills through the Irish postal system by shipping pills to Northern Ireland and transporting them across the land border. The fact that medication abortion could be reliably mailed to Northern Ireland might seem to signal a less restrictive environment for self-managed abortion than in the Republic of Ireland, but the opposite is true.[1] The enforcement climate in the Republic of Ireland was far more lax, with customs interception of MA but little police or prosecutorial action. By contrast, Northern Ireland was the source for most of the pills that made their way into the Republic, but it was the only one of the two jurisdictions that actively investigated MA stored in homes and workplaces, pursued investigations against individuals who ordered pills online, and brought charges against pill users and the people who helped them procure pills.

This chapter explores the abortion geography of Northern Ireland, explaining its position as both a source of pills and a site of criminalization of pill users. I begin with the unique political culture and institutions of Northern Ireland, where opposition to abortion has been historically framed as an issue that unites communities in conflict. The uneasy postconflict political settlement in Northern Ireland, and its position in the United Kingdom, shaped how abortion pills moved around the island of Ireland, how authorities treated pill users, and how abortion reform was eventually achieved.

THE POLITICAL CONTEXT OF NORTHERN IRELAND

Abortion has been legally available in England, Scotland, and Wales since 1967. Not so in Northern Ireland: although it is part of the United Kingdom, Northern Ireland has a devolved government, different political parties, and a distinct political culture that set it apart on many issues, including abortion. Until 2019 when it was decriminalized, abortion in Northern Ireland was governed by the 1861 Offences Against the Person Act. This is the same law that was inherited by the Republic of Ireland on its independence, criminalizing someone who procures the miscarriage of another, as well as a person who procures their own miscarriage. It banned the use of "any poison," any "noxious thing," or "any instrument" to procure a miscarriage.[2] Elsewhere in the United Kingdom, abortion became legally available under the 1967 Abortion Act, which maintains the criminal status of abortion but effectively created an exception for abortions carried out on certain grounds and with medical approval. The 1967 act applies in England, Scotland, and Wales but has never applied to Northern Ireland, where the 1861 law governed. Beyond the 1861 law, Northern Ireland's legal standard for abortion was shaped by court judgments that held abortion was only lawful if continuing the pregnancy posed a "serious and long-term" risk to physical health.[3] The vagueness of this standard led to "wide variation in implementation," driven partly by uncertainty among doctors who feared prosecution.[4]

The ambiguous legal standard for abortion, the reluctance of Northern Irish doctors to act within the law to provide abortion, and the proximity to abortion services on the UK mainland meant that large numbers of abortion-seekers left Northern Ireland to obtain care in other parts of the country.[5] Government data show that over 60,000 women traveled from Northern Ireland to England for abortions between 1968 and 2020. These numbers rose sharply in the 1970s, hovering between 1,400 and 1,800 per year during the 1980s and 1990s, then declining in the 2000s as emergency contraception became available and, later, as MA became more widely used.[6] Abortion travel from Northern Ireland, like abortion travel from the Republic of Ireland, has generally declined over the past twenty years (fig. 6).[7]

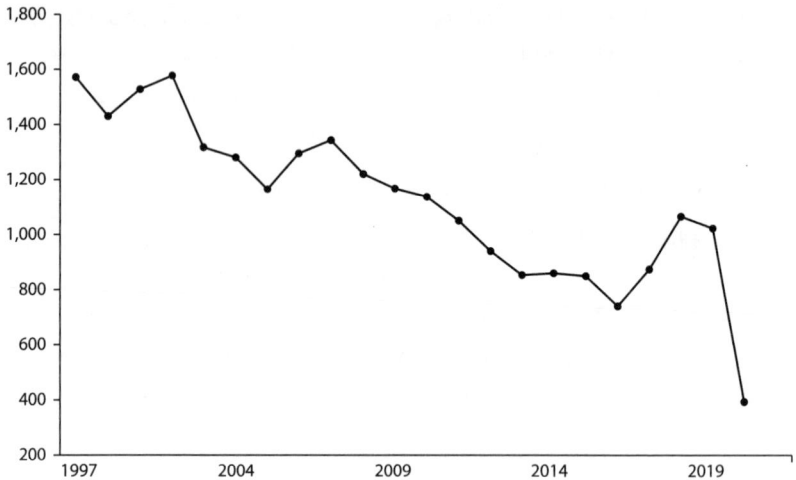

FIGURE 6. Northern Irish residents obtaining abortion in England, Wales, and the Netherlands, 1997–2020. Source: Compiled by the author from UK Department of Health reports.

The issue of abortion occupies a peculiar place in Northern Irish society and politics. Northern Ireland is a postconflict society with persistent sectarian divisions that have been politically institutionalized since the end of the period of political violence known as "the Troubles." During this conflict, paramilitaries and state forces fought over the question of whether Northern Ireland would remain part of the United Kingdom or reunify with the Republic of Ireland. The government established by the 1998 Belfast/Good Friday peace agreement was based on a system of power sharing between Catholics/Republicans/Nationalists and Protestants/Loyalists/Unionists. These political positions generally map onto religious identities, but the conflict is territorial and not theological. Broadly, Republicans/Nationalists want political reunification with the Republic of Ireland, while Unionists/Loyalists oppose Irish reunification and support the existing political union with the United Kingdom.

Although the political violence of the Troubles was concentrated in the 1970s and a peace agreement has been in force since 1998, sectarian divisions continue to shape the political landscape of Northern Ireland. The majority of Northern Irish Catholics continue to identify as Nationalists (59 percent), while a larger majority of Protestants continue to identify as Unionists (67 percent). The main parties draw their votes from distinct identity communities, and as such, there is little convergence in voters.[8] In practice, Northern Irish politics functions as an "ethnic dual-party system" where elections are divided into "two simultaneous but largely separate contests."[9] These two contests take place among Catholics/Republicans/Nationalists, who mainly vote for Sinn Féin or the Social Democratic and Labour Party, and among Protestants/Unionists/ Loyalists, who mainly vote for the Democratic Unionist Party or the Ulster Unionist Party.

While politics has become largely peaceful and power sharing between communities more entrenched, sectarian divisions continue to shape the political landscape of Northern Ireland. Dominant culture war issues related to identity and belief—like flags, marches, and language rights—still divide communities along Nationalist and Unionist lines. However, opinion on sexual and reproductive freedoms is not divided evenly along identity or party lines.[10] Social conservatives in both communities still maintain shared opposition to abortion and same-sex marriage. The importance of sectarian politics means that voters' preferences are usually determined by the community they represent rather than the party's position on abortion or same-sex marriage.

In Northern Ireland, conservatism on sexual and reproductive freedom is often identified as a "distinctive cultural value" that unites communities who are usually at odds.[11] Anti-abortion sentiment has sometimes been celebrated as a point of commonality by political parties that represent different communities in Northern Ireland (and as a value shared with Catholic conservatives in the Republic of Ireland). This is best illustrated in the words of a conservative Unionist politician speaking in 2013 in support of an abortion restriction:

> Across the island of Ireland, we share a common bond in seeking to protect and provide the best care for mothers and unborn children. . . . People ask what a shared future looks like, and I point to this moment of [one Nationalist legislator and two Unionist legislators] bringing forward proposed legislation related to the most basic of human rights: the right to life.[12]

Social conservatives advanced a related argument to warn the central government in London against trying to impose reforms: in Northern Ireland, moral conservatism and opposition to abortion were portrayed as the glue that held together warring communities. Any liberalizing reforms, the argument followed, would prompt a return to conflict.[13] On the contrary, opinion polling since the 1990s shows growing support for abortion reform among the general public and doctors, with substantial support for abortion in cases of risk to health and life, rape and incest, and fatal fetal anomaly; opinion polls on abortion also demonstrate a significant gulf between the views of voters and those of Northern Irish political parties.[14]

Anti-abortion attitudes among the political class lead feminist critics of Northern Ireland's power-sharing model to argue that it perpetuates the conflict by preserving the power of ethno-national elites. This model incentivizes voting along sectarian lines and thereby dampens pressure for parties to change their position on social issues that do not divide evenly across community lines. Within each of the power blocs, women are sidelined, and feminist issues are often viewed as irrelevant (or even dangerous) to the community's political agenda.[15] With Northern Irish political parties largely unsupportive of abortion reform but receiving their support from voters on the basis of other issues, feminists have seen little scope for achieving change through the devolved Northern Ireland Assembly. The local parties that make up the Northern Ireland Assembly are different from the dominant political parties in the UK Parliament in London, so feminists have also faced significant challenges lobbying representatives in the central government. While they are in theory doubly represented by the Northern Ireland Assembly and the UK Parliament, in practice Northern Irish pro-choice activists have found themselves sidelined by both institutions, which pass responsibility for abortion back and forth.[16] Because Northern Irish abortion restrictions have been rooted in statute, reform was a matter for the legislature, and there was no possibility of mobilizing for a referendum as in the Republic of Ireland. Political obstacles, including institutional structures, political parties, and the political culture of Northern Ireland, essentially prevented abortion reform for decades. Feminists in the region were eventually able to trigger reforms by seizing "contingent, and often unexpected," opportunities.[17] Medication abortion activism proved essential in their efforts.

IRISH ABORTION PILL GEOGRAPHIES

As in the Republic of Ireland, medication abortion started arriving in Northern Ireland in 2006, when Women on Web first launched its online pill service. Demand was low in the early years because there was little public knowledge about the pills. The availability of MA in Northern Ireland came to public attention through media coverage in 2008, when a journalist on the BBC investigative show *Spotlight* ordered pills from four websites, had the pills chemically analyzed, and then revealed on air that only one site—Women on Web—provided the correct pills with a doctor's consultation. Activists were glad for the publicity. As one campaigner in the NGO Alliance for Choice put it, "From then on women in Northern Ireland especially, but increasingly in the south, knew about these pills—and it was the BBC that did it!"[18]

When customs authorities in the Republic of Ireland began to intercept pills in large quantities in 2008 and 2009, activists changed their shipping routes to send most pills to Northern Ireland and distribute them across the border. Northern Ireland and the Republic of Ireland are separate legal and political jurisdictions, but they are separated by a soft border across which people and goods can move with relative ease. Authorities in these countries also take different approaches to imported medication. While any packages that could be identified as abortion pills were impounded by customs agents in the Republic of Ireland, abortion pills entering the United Kingdom were only sporadically seized.[19] As shipments of pills increased, they came to the attention of the UK National Crime Agency, which passed information about pill shipments to police in Northern Ireland and encouraged them to investigate further.[20]

For the most part, abortion pills ordered to be sent to Northern Ireland arrived at their intended destinations. Data released by the UK medicines agency shows that between 2013 and 2016 it only seized six packages of pills: one of those shipments contained five combi-packs, but the other shipments contained between 25 and 375 combi-packs.[21] This indicates that the state made an effort to intercept bulk orders but little effort to intercept individual orders. These seizures all came during Operation Pangea, a coordinated campaign led by the international police organization Interpol. During this annual weeklong operation, national medicines regulators and customs agencies work with Interpol to target "counterfeit and illicit medicines."[22] Periodic interceptions disrupted the supply to Northern Ireland but, compared to the blanket policy of seizing all MA in the Republic of Ireland, sporadic seizures in the north presented a more manageable disruption for activists.

The majority of people seeking pills online for delivery to Northern Ireland could order directly from feminist networks like Women on Web and Women Help Women. By stockpiling to fill supply gaps during customs crackdowns, activists were able to develop workable systems for distributing pills across the island.[23] Local activists in Northern Ireland served as intermediaries to offer information—and in some cases, the pills themselves—to people who needed them. For those who could not receive a package at home, or who could not wait a few weeks while the package was shipped, activists kept a supply of pills for immediate use. For pills moving south, packages were ordered to Northern Ireland and collected by individuals or repackaged and sent south through the post. Because of the Republic of Ireland's prohibition on ordering any prescribed medicine online, this repackaging effort involved disguising the pills as something other than medicines, for example, by gift wrapping them.[24]

"AROUND, ABOVE, AND BEYOND" THE LAW

Activists' confrontations with the state over abortion criminalization esca-lated in 2013, after the pro-choice movement across the island was galvanized by the death of Savita Halappanavar. In the preceding years, Northern Irish activists had noticed a large increase in the demand for MA from Women on Web. These pills arrived at their intended destination consistently but irreg-ularly. Activists began to strategize about a legal challenge that could clarify the status of MA or at the very least test the state's position on actually enforc-ing its laws against MA. Furthermore, they saw an urgent need to dispel fears about MA as the public tended to assume that illegal abortion pills were poor quality or dangerous.[25]

In 2013, one hundred people signed an open letter, organized by Alliance for Choice, stating that they had "either taken the abortion pill or helped women to procure the abortion pill in order to cause an abortion here in Northern Ireland."[26] Founded in 1996, Alliance for Choice is generally recog-nized as the main abortion lobbying group in Northern Ireland. Its original aim was to extend the 1967 Abortion Act to Northern Ireland, though its position evolved over time to support "free, safe, legal, local" abortion and eventually full decriminalization.[27] Alliance for Choice worked to facilitate access to pills, supplying information on how to order pills across the island and coordinating a clandestine supply system to fill gaps in supply (north and south) when customs seizures blocked the flow of medications.

Groups that were engaged with abortion pill activism in Northern Ireland and the Republic of Ireland trod a fine line between raising awareness and drawing scrutiny. Courting public, police, and media attention could bring pills into the lives of more abortion seekers, but it could also make it difficult for the state to turn a blind eye to clandestine pill use. MA activists believed that the Northern Ireland Assembly was unlikely to enact meaningful legal reform that would benefit abortion seekers in the region. They engaged in simultaneous forms of activism that undermined the law, exposed its limitations, and irreverently disobeyed it. Emma Campbell of Alliance for Choice gave a pithy summary of this strategy: "The law is an ass, so we'll do whatever we can around, above, and beyond it."[28] This meant coordinated clandestine activities, public spectacles, and some strategic crossover between the two.

The 2013 open letter represented the "first public outing" for activists challenging the state over MA. Activists subsequently escalated their confrontations with the state. Alliance for Choice organized another open letter in 2015, signed by more than two hundred people and "inviting prosecution" for their work providing MA.[29] They tried to tempt the state into prosecuting them in order to challenge the abortion law in court. In May 2016, three members of Alliance for Choice turned themselves in at a police station in Derry, where they submitted a statement saying they had taken delivery of abortion pills for others who were too scared to receive pills at their own homes.[30] Despite repeated public admissions that they had broken Northern Ireland's abortion laws, activists in Alliance for Choice were not arrested. As one activist explained:

> We've been on the radio saying, "We don't understand why we haven't been arrested, we've helped so many women to get these pills, we've had pills delivered to our houses, we've sat with women as they've miscarried." We've said that so often. And we've never had so much as a visit from the cops! It's not like they don't know where we live! . . . So all of that really does lead you to think that the last thing they want is any kind of political trial.[31]

Ultimately, public displays of defiance by MA activists exposed the limits of authorities' willingness to enforce abortion laws. Pill actions served to test the law, revealing what activists saw as its "hidden limits" and "hypocrisies."[32] Alliance for Choice undertook these kinds of activities, but so too did ROSA, a socialist feminist group based in the Republic of Ireland and closely associated with the People Before Profit political party there. From 2014, ROSA collaborated with Women on Web/Women on Waves to stage abortion pill actions that attracted international media attention. Alliance for Choice and ROSA both favored an irreverent approach that emphasized public defiance of the abortion law. ROSA similarly designed MA actions with the aim of provoking a state response; they believed that a police crackdown would trigger a public backlash against the state and mobilize opposition to abortion criminalization.[33]

ROSA carried out pill actions beginning in 2014 with the Abortion Pill Train that paid homage to the Contraceptive Train, a well-known 1971 protest action staged by the Irish Women's Liberation Movement to protest the Republic's contraception ban.[34] During their 2014 action, ROSA activists, including TD Ruth Coppinger, who sat on the Joint Oireachtas Committee on the 8th Amendment, traveled by train to Belfast where they collected abortion pills shipped by Women on Web to ROSA activists in the north. They returned to Dublin with the pills in hand. When they disembarked, the group carried a banner advertising Women on Web, as well as packages of pills. TD Coppinger and nine other activists swallowed pills in front of supporters, journalists, and police gathered at the station. Anxious that the police would seize the pills or the banner, activists had split up the pill packages between them and stashed a spare copy of the banner; the police stood by without intervening.[35]

After the Abortion Pill Train, ROSA and WoW continued to pursue joint actions across the Irish border. With WoW's characteristic affinity for designing protests that attract media attention, the group carried out symbolic border crossings of MA by drone (in which pills were moved from the Republic of Ireland into Northern Ireland) and by robot (in which a wheeled robot remotely controlled from the Netherlands attempted to deliver pills to activists waiting outside Belfast City Hall).[36] Like the Women on Waves ship campaign, these acts were largely symbolic: they attracted a great deal of media attention but did not facilitate a significant number of abortions (if any).

Among the Northern Irish abortion activist groups, there was intense disagreement about strategies and tactics. ROSA drew criticism for its public-facing actions, which were perceived as triggering police crackdowns on pill supplies by groups like Alliance for Choice and Abortion Rights Campaign in the Republic of Ireland. They accused ROSA of jeopardizing pill networks by engaging in public actions that led to a total customs shutdown for weeks across the island. Furthermore, ROSA's critics argued that the Bus for Repeal in March 2017 and the surrounding publicity was the direct cause of authorities in Northern Ireland undertaking pill raids in homes and workplaces.[37] For ROSA's part, it responded that the news media had already widely publicized abortion pill routes so no customs crackdowns could be directly attributed to their actions and that the group had planned for possible crackdowns by stockpiling pills ahead of every action. ROSA sourced pills through its partnership with Women on Web and referred pill requests to them.[38] ROSA and its political allies strategized that it was more important, in the long run, to raise awareness of medication abortion, without which political change would not occur.

Activists routinely disagree, and feminist activists are no different. Disputes about abortion pill activism are important because they demonstrate how groups grappled with two competing imperatives: how to make more people aware of medication abortion and facilitate the process of social decriminalization of self-managed abortion without jeopardizing the networks they had built to supply pills. Provoking the state could catalyze reform, just as it could trigger a police or customs crackdown. On the other hand, clandestine systems for providing illegal abortion had the potential to help the state maintain unjust laws by quietly managing the demand for abortion.[39] Scholarship on institutional ignorance highlights this bind: protecting clandestine self-managed abortion from public attention makes it easier for states to strategically ignore the issue and choose not to criminalize pill users. Equally, strategic ignorance about clandestine self-managed abortion relieves pressure on states to undertake reforms and provide services for safe, legal, and local abortion when there is widespread disobedience of unjust abortion laws.

Ultimately, these disagreements center on the question of how best to balance competing goals: distributing pills to people who need them, sustaining pill networks by avoiding customs clampdowns, confronting the state to demonstrate the extent of demand for pills, and campaigning for legal reform on abortion. When abortion activists adopt a deliberate strategy of public disobedience, running parallel to clandestine abortion provision, their efforts to expose law's hypocrisies can also expose fragile systems of illegal abortion. This tension is a familiar feature of feminist abortion politics. A similar debate was present in the 1960s–1970s underground abortion movement in the United States between the Los Angeles Feminist Women's Health Center and the Jane Collective. Both groups promoted lay abortions, but the Los Angeles group "sought publicity (including getting arrested) and Jane relied upon secrecy."[40] The groups were wary of each other's strategies: the Los Angeles group viewed arrest as a way to "test the laws," while the Jane Collective preferred to avoid a confrontation with the police so that they could keep providing abortions in secret.[41] In 1970s France, activists decided to stop providing illegal abortions when they realized their work meant that "doctors and hospitals could conveniently go on ignoring the problem, while militants provided a much-needed service."[42] Decades later and thousands of miles away, Northern Irish groups confronted the same dilemma.

ROSA activists in the Republic of Ireland felt certain that the Irish political establishment was so fearful of a public backlash that pill actions would not provoke arrests of individuals.[43] They were right in this regard: the criminalization of individual pill users never materialized in the Republic of Ireland. Nonetheless, the debate over ROSA's actions highlights one of the key features of abortion pill activism in Ireland. As political and legal jurisdictions, the Republic of Ireland and Northern Ireland are distinct entities. But much of the pro-choice movement in these countries operated on an all-island basis, as did the pill networks, by virtue of the customs and border infrastructures on the island. Activist efforts to publicize the availability of pills in the Republic of Ireland could therefore trigger a crackdown or criminal penalties for people in the north without provoking any police reaction in the south. The smooth functioning of pill networks across the island depended on customs officials in the United Kingdom deciding not to intercept packages of pills, as well as police and prosecutors in the Republic of Ireland deciding not to pursue criminal sanctions against pill users. By contrast, Northern Irish authorities did crack down on pills: the state chose to raid private residences in search of MA, investigate reports of illegal MA use, and prosecute MA users.

PROSECUTING ABORTION PILL USERS

Public displays of disobedience, where activists admitted to supplying abortion pills or even swallowed abortion pills in front of police, did not lead to arrests or prosecutions, but the Northern Irish state did investigate and prosecute individual pill users during this period. Their targets were not activists. Instead, the targets were vulnerable abortion seekers and the people who assisted them.

Between April 2007 and April 2015, no woman in Northern Ireland was convicted of illegal abortion under the 1861 Offences Against the Person Act.[44] The law had been used to prosecute some men who committed acts of domestic violence that resulted in miscarriages, but it had not been used to prosecute any women who deliberately ended their own pregnancies in many years.[45] However, between 2013 and 2015, Northern Irish prosecutors' attitudes and practices regarding abortion criminalization changed. During this period, the Northern Irish state pursued cases against four people who procured their own abortions or helped others end their pregnancies: the first was a young woman reported to police by her flatmates, the second was a mother who procured MA for her daughter, and the third was a young couple (he supplied the pills; she consumed them). These three cases are worth examining in detail because they illustrate the mechanisms through which pill users came to the attention of authorities and the government's selective enforcement of the law.

In 2013, a Northern Irish mother bought MA for her fifteen-year-old daughter who became pregnant while in an abusive relationship. The teenager went to her doctor to seek counseling because of the abusive relationship, and at that point she disclosed that she had self-managed an abortion with pills. Neither she nor her mother thought they had committed a crime when she disclosed the abortion to the doctor. Two months later, someone at the medical practice reported the girl and her mother to the police, who seized the girl's medical records. When she was interviewed, without a lawyer, unaware she had committed a crime, the mother disclosed everything to police.[46] The mother was charged with "procuring and supplying poison with the intent to cause a miscarriage" under the 1861 act. Her trial was set to take place in June 2015, but it was delayed when her lawyers challenged her prosecution and obtained a judicial review of the decision to prosecute.[47] (Later, after abortion was decriminalized in 2019, she was formally acquitted.)

The first conviction of an abortion pill user in Northern Ireland occurred in April 2016. A young woman had ordered MA online and used it to end a pregnancy at ten to twelve weeks' gestation. She had tried to have a legal abortion in England but had been unable to raise the money to travel. The woman, who was nineteen years old at the time of the abortion, came under police scrutiny after she self-managed her abortion and left remnants of the abortion "in a plastic bag in a household bin." Her flatmates reported her to police and later told a newspaper that they had gone to police in part because of her attitude to the abortion: "We tried so hard to support her when she told us about the pregnancy, but it made me so angry when she kept calling it 'the pest.' Then, after the abortion, she showed no remorse."[48] The woman was convicted and sentenced to three months in prison, but the sentence was suspended, meaning she did not serve prison time.[49]

In another case, in 2015–16, a young couple was charged with crimes under the 1861 act: the woman, with "administering noxious substances" (mifepristone and misoprostol) to end her pregnancy; and the man, with "supplying a poison with the intent to procure a miscarriage."[50] In early 2017, the charges against the couple were withdrawn, and they accepted a formal caution, meaning they admitted to the crime but the prosecutor declined to prosecute. Prosecutors issued the caution, in part, because it was determined that her mental health was fragile and would be harmed by a prosecution and the ensuing media coverage.[51] Information on how her use of MA came to police attention has not been made public.

The criminalization of medication abortion also proceeded through police actions that stopped short of prosecution but nonetheless provoked intense anxiety among abortion seekers. During winter and spring 2017, between fifteen and twenty women who ordered pills in Northern Ireland had their pills seized at customs, and police visited each of the delivery addresses. The police invited people who ordered pills to be interviewed under caution, meaning they were suspected of having committed a crime. Of the fifteen to twenty people summoned by police, only four were interviewed before the investigations were halted, although authorities waited one year before giving notice that they would not be charged.[52]

Because activists who tried to attract prosecution for a test case did not succeed in challenging the abortion law in court, they instead intervened in the cases of individual pill users, contacting their lawyers and advising on strategies for challenging the police.[53] When the 2017 spate of pill seizures and police visits took place, Alliance for Choice activists advised women who were to be interviewed on defenses available to them:

> You have to say: "I didn't believe it was a crime because I was dealing with a doctor. Under the EU, this is an e-service under EU commercial law, how could that be illegal? The law says you shan't get any poison or noxious substance, but these aren't poisons. They're on the WHO Essential Medicines List!" ... It was only once [the lawyer's] clients put forward these defenses, all of a sudden [police] stopped interviewing everybody.[54]

In March 2017, around the time that police were visiting the homes of people who had ordered MA, police also conducted raids on the homes and workplaces of a few activists affiliated with Alliance for Choice. Police searched a man's workplace, seizing his laptop and phone. On International Women's Day, while the celebrated feminist Angela Davis addressed a rally at Belfast City Hall, police raided a woman's art studio with a warrant to search for "drugs or instruments which cause abortion." The police seized her laptop, mobile phone, and bank documents. Neither person whose property was raided was charged with a crime.[55] Nonetheless, police sent activists across the country scrambling to get rid of pills they had stockpiled, as they feared further raids were coming.[56]

Activist efforts in 2013, 2014, and 2015 to "test" the law by staging public acts of defiance had led to some scrutiny of activists and interception of pills, but no charges had been brought against any activists. By contrast, the authorities only chose to bring charges against people who had been turned in "by members of the public and medical staff."[57] Law enforcement actions against abortion pill users proved to be an important turning point in Northern Ireland, because they brought greater public attention to the legal framework for abortion. Investigations and prosecutions of pill users commenced a few years before they became public knowledge, but once these cases came to public attention, they provoked a public backlash.

THE POLITICS OF ABORTION CRIMINALIZATION

MA rapidly transformed the geography of abortion in the Republic of Ireland and Northern Ireland from 2006 on. Authorities in the Irish Republic reacted with choreographed ignorance and declined to criminalize any pill users.[58] Even staunch anti-abortion figures in the Irish Republic defended laws with harsh criminal penalties by promising that those penalties would not be applied, in practice, to any individual women seeking abortions. By contrast, authorities in Northern Ireland carried out raids, investigations, and prosecutions and instituted other policies designed to criminalize and stigmatize abortion. For all the mythology about the shared values on the "abortion-free" island of Ireland, the two countries on that island took very different approaches to abortion criminalization and paths to abortion reform. What prompted Northern Irish law enforcement authorities to actively pursue abortion pill users?

A few important factors shaped the political context in which the crackdown on pill users took place. First, the process of devolution from the government in London to Belfast gave the Northern Ireland Assembly powers over justice and policing in 2010, in addition to the powers it already held over health. At that point, abortion policy was a "transferred matter" under control of the devolved Assembly, and any reform imposed from London would be considered a violation of the devolved power arrangement.[59] There was little prospect of abortion reform through the Assembly, because key authorities in the Northern Ireland government were vociferous opponents of abortion.

The second and third factors shaping criminalization during this period were the men in charge of important government bodies: the attorney general and the health minister. John Larkin, attorney general between 2010 and 2020, was known as a fervent anti-abortion campaigner. In a radio debate, Larkin expressed the view that abortion was the same as "putting a bullet in the back of the head of the child two days after it's born."[60] In his official capacity, Larkin was seen by activists working in Northern Ireland as the main driver of efforts to enforce abortion criminalization.[61] Larkin was perceived by stakeholders as having "a key influence" on legal guidance that required doctors to report suspected abortions by their patients.[62] The public prosecution service, which makes decisions about whether to bring charges, is an independent body that is not overseen by the attorney general. Nonetheless, a lawyer working on these issues cited Larkin's fervent anti-abortion stance as part of a "push for change [in] the wider legal system" that likely shaped the decision to pursue the prosecution of the mother who supplied pills to her daughter.[63] The anti-abortion advocacy of Larkin took place amid growing awareness of abortion pill use and political shifts in other parts of government.

Shortly after Larkin assumed the role of attorney general, Edwin Poots of the Democratic Unionist Party became the health minister. Poots took control of the department in the middle of a years-long process to draft guidelines that would clarify Northern Ireland's abortion law for doctors. When Poots took office, the guidelines were nearly agreed on, but he withdrew them and issued a new draft in 2013. It bore little resemblance to the previous guidelines. The new draft guidelines sought to involve doctors more directly in the identification and criminalization of abortion pill users. It threatened healthcare providers with up to ten years in prison if they failed to report unlawful medical procedures.[64] It read:

> Health and social care professionals have a legal duty to refuse to participate in, and must report, any procedure that would not be lawful in Northern Ireland. A person who has knowledge of the carrying out of a procedure which is not lawful in Northern Ireland and who has information which is likely to be of material assistance in securing the apprehension, prosecution, or conviction of any person in relation to that lawful [sic] procedure is under a duty to give that information, within a reasonable time, to the police.[65]

The proposed requirement for doctors to report illegal medical procedures was partly the result of the increase in the number of abortion pills entering Northern Ireland at the time. Earlier iterations of the guidelines, before pills came into the country in large numbers, had no such requirements for health-care providers to report on illegal procedures.[66] The specter of criminal penalties for doctors who knew about abortion pill use illustrated the state's new willingness to ramp up criminalization. In fact, the new draft guidelines issued by the Department of Health were such a "game changer" that human rights bodies in Northern Ireland intervened in the abortion debate for the first time.[67]

The 2013 draft guidelines never came into formal effect but nonetheless had a significant chilling effect on medical practice, making doctors reluctant to perform abortions that they might previously have considered legal. The small number of legal abortions carried out in Northern Ireland fell as a result: while fifty-one legal abortions were performed in 2012–13, only sixteen were performed in 2014–15.[68] The Royal College of Midwives advised its members to take a "don't ask, don't tell" approach to MA, because they feared that members could face criminal penalties if they did not report knowledge about pill users to the police.[69] Activists also observed doctors' reluctance to pre-scribe misoprostol in post-miscarriage care. Because of its association with elective abortion, misoprostol was "kept under lock and key." Women who needed misoprostol to complete a spontaneous miscarriage reported that they were only able to access it if they knew to ask directly.[70] These activists' obser-vations resonate with studies of misoprostol use in other contexts: as miso-prostol is a drug used for miscarriage management *and* induced abortion, anti-abortion stigma has been known to reduce doctor's willingness to use it for any purpose, including a legally approved purpose.[71]

These events took place in the broader context of significant and growing support for abortion liberalization in Northern Ireland. The public reaction to the criminalization of abortion pill users was overwhelmingly negative at the time and helped shift opinion in favor of abortion liberalization. In 2014, before the criminal cases became public knowledge, polling by Amnesty International found that 69 percent of voters in Northern Ireland wanted abortion to be available in the case of rape and 60 percent in the case of fatal fetal anomaly. Nonetheless, public opposition to abortion on demand remained substantial: in 2016, 60 percent said they did not believe abortion should be legal where a woman simply did not want to have children.[72] Before 2015–16, the criminalization of pill users had been hidden from the public for the most part as the people interviewed by police about MA had quietly accepted cautions. The prosecution of the mother who obtained pills for her teenage daughter was especially powerful as an illustration of the true impact of abortion criminalization. It was the "small details" that "absolutely horrified" the public when they came to light, like the fact that police had taken the teenage girl from her school classroom for questioning.[73] Information about the criminalization of pill users provoked public opposition and further contributed to liberalizing attitudes. In a 2016 poll, 71 percent of respondents said that a woman should never go to prison for having an abortion. By 2018, this number had risen to 89 percent.[74]

Activists saw public distaste for criminalizing self-managed abortion as an opportunity to change views on the question of abortion more broadly. Before the criminal cases came to light, the Northern Irish abortion debate was limited by its focus on the so-called hard cases like fatal fetal anomaly and pregnancies resulting from rape. Activists who advocated for self-managed abortion felt pushed to the margins of these debates, cast as "the scary strident super-feminists" by groups like the Royal College of Midwives.[75] This changed when clear public opposition to the criminalization of pill users demonstrated the growing gulf between public attitudes and the views of elected representatives. Politicians who were unaccustomed to being challenged on their position on abortion found themselves confronted much more directly on this issue. Political discourse began to change, reflecting a softening of attitudes. Politicians who had previously expressed extreme anti-abortion views moderated their approach, advocating "mercy" and "compassion" for people in these circumstances.[76] A further political change on abortion came in 2017, when Sinn Féin (the all-island Irish republican party) modified its position to support abortion in limited circumstances, and again in 2018, when Sinn Féin politicians prominently campaigned for repeal in the 2018 referendum in the Republic of Ireland.[77] Committed to a unified policy platform across the island, Sinn Féin's position on the 8th Amendment referendum in the Republic of Ireland meant it adopted a pro-reform position in Northern Ireland.

Opposition to criminalization of pill users helped change the tone of public discourse on abortion and, to some extent, discourse among political elites.[78] Nonetheless, because political party preference in Northern Ireland is mainly determined by community affiliation, not the party position on issues like abortion, parties that take an unpopular stance on abortion are still unlikely to lose votes on this basis.[79] Changing public attitudes on abortion did not make the Northern Ireland Assembly any more hospitable to abortion reform in the short term. The Assembly was barely able to agree to a new commission on abortion in cases of fatal fetal anomaly, let alone pass legislation for broader reforms.[80] Meanwhile, in London, the prosecution of the mother for supplying pills to her teenage daughter had "set off alarm bells" among politicians who anticipated a national public outcry across the United Kingdom if the prosecution were to proceed.[81] After the 2017 general election, the Conservative Party formed a minority government and relied on the Northern Irish Democratic Unionist Party to vote through its policies; this arrangement brought a new level of UK-wide public scrutiny to that party's positions and activities in Northern Ireland.[82] An intervention by an international human rights body also increased pressure on the central government to take action. For these reasons, abortion reform advocates looked to other institutions outside of Northern Ireland where they could pursue change.

DECRIMINALIZATION WITHOUT ABORTION SERVICES

The referendum to repeal the 8th Amendment in the Republic of Ireland generated momentum for action in the north. However, in Northern Ireland there was no option for a referendum on the abortion issue. Instead, the power to legislate for abortion was in the hands of an unwilling devolved legislature that was both divided along sectarian lines and united around opposition to abortion. Abortion reform came as the result of feminist activist efforts that seized opportunities across institutions: short-term actions to take advantage of political opportunities, long-term legal work, lobbying in national legislative bodies, and engagement with international human rights treaty bodies.

Abortion was considered a devolved issue by the UK government in London, which carefully avoided intervening in the issue on the grounds that it would pose an unspecified threat to the peace process. The Northern Ireland Assembly was unwilling and unable to use its legislative powers to pass reforms. In the face of this deadlock, a coalition of feminist civil society organizations in Northern Ireland filed a complaint with the United Nations Convention on the Elimination of All Forms of Discrimination Against Women (CEDAW), an international human rights treaty.[83] In three previous reports, CEDAW had challenged the UK government on Northern Ireland's restrictive abortion access regime, but each time it declined to take action.

Because CEDAW allows civil society groups to bring complaints directly, in 2010, Northern Irish feminists submitted a request for an inquiry into "grave and systemic human rights violations" by Northern Ireland's abortion law.[84] Abortion pills and their criminalization played a significant role in the report's findings and recommendations. Although the CEDAW application was filed in 2010, CEDAW's monitoring committee carried out a visit in 2016 at the height of the controversy over criminalization of pill users.[85]

When CEDAW released its findings in 2018, the verdict was damning. The report concluded that the UK government violated women's human rights in Northern Ireland through its abortion laws. It found that the United Kingdom was "perpetrating acts of gender-based violence against women through its deliberate maintenance of criminal laws disproportionately affecting women and girls."[86] CEDAW therefore recommended, among other things, "a moratorium on the application of criminal laws concerning abortion and to cease all related arrests, investigations and criminal prosecutions."[87] The call for a moratorium was significant because there was still an ongoing prosecution for MA: in the case of the mother who bought pills for her teenage daughter, the decision to prosecute her was under judicial review, but no decision had been made and a conviction was still possible.

The use of CEDAW's human rights framing was crucial for breaking the deadlock of devolved institutions that passed responsibility back and forth. London and Belfast both considered abortion a "transferred issue" because health, justice, and policing powers were devolved. By contrast, CEDAW's findings were directed at the UK government, not the devolved government of Northern Ireland, thus putting the responsibility on London to act.[88] The civil society groups who applied for CEDAW's review saw this as one of the main advantages: health is a devolved issue, but human rights is not, so CEDAW's conclusion that human rights violations were taking place challenged London's usual response that abortion was an issue for the devolved Northern Ireland Assembly. The United Kingdom was not blocked from taking action on abortion in Northern Ireland but in fact had an international human rights obligation to do so.[89] Despite CEDAW's limited enforcement mechanisms, Northern Irish feminists hoped that the findings could "shame" the UK government into action.[90]

CEDAW's findings, targeted at the UK government, provided the basis for Northern Irish feminist campaigners to lobby for reforms in London. In an indirect way, sectarian politics in Northern Ireland played an important role in the accomplishment of abortion reform. The Northern Ireland Assembly, which was unable to agree on any abortion legislation, had collapsed because of a corruption scandal and was unable to reconvene for three years because parties could not agree on the terms of a power-sharing arrangement.[91] With the collapse of the Northern Ireland Assembly, abortion campaigners saw an opportunity. In the political vacuum, feminists in Northern Ireland looked to the central government in London to implement the human rights obligations that an international treaty body required. MP Stella Creasy, a prominent voice for abortion rights in Parliament, proposed a measure that would require the UK government to act to decriminalize abortion in Northern Ireland if the Northern Ireland Assembly did not reconvene by a deadline. Creasy's measure passed in the House of Commons, and when no executive had been formed in the Northern Ireland Assembly by October 21, 2019, it became law.[92]

The measure passed, in part, because abortion attitudes among MPs from England, Scotland, and Wales tend to be more liberal than those in Northern Ireland. The possibility of a criminal conviction for the mother who supplied pills to her daughter also helped push reluctant MPs to support the reforms, because it showed them that abortion reform without decriminalization in Northern Ireland would not be enough. A lawyer who lobbied politicians on the vote explains how the prosecution persuaded MPs:

> [Some MPs] supported the notion of reform, but they weren't sure about decriminalization. That case brought it to life. Ultimately, when the negotiations were going back and forth with the government, around the final details and the need for the moratorium, that was done with the mother's case in mind. There was no other way to save her. That's ultimately what it boiled down to. It wouldn't be enough for MPs to say, "We legislated to overturn this 160-year-old ban," if you still had this situation with the mother. So it had to be [the UK central government in] Westminster, and it had to be at that moment.[93]

By implementing the CEDAW recommendations, the amendment did a few things: it repealed the sections of the Offences Against the Person Act of 1861 that criminalized abortion; it prohibited future investigations and prosecutions under those sections and discontinued any ongoing ones; and it required the secretary of state to introduce regulations for the provision of abortion in Northern Ireland.[94] When Creasy's measure came into force, abortion was decriminalized (in Northern Ireland only) and all pending prosecutions were dismissed. Alliance for Choice saw a direct link between this achievement, the prosecutions of abortion pill users, and the medication abortion activism that surrounded it. Alliance for Choice cochair Emma Campbell explained:

> Because they used CEDAW in making the law in the UK parliament, and they included that moratorium, then those pills and those arrests were directly responsible for the decriminalization that we have now. . . . Using the CEDAW framework was so helpful, because you can't argue with the minimum human rights standard.[95]

CEDAW, an international human rights treaty, lacks clear enforcement mechanisms, so while it offered a stark condemnation of Northern Ireland's abortion laws, the route to implementing its recommendations was unclear. London's consistent position on devolution to Northern Ireland had meant decades of inaction by the central government, out of deference to the supposedly special status of abortion in postconflict Northern Ireland. In the absence of the devolved assembly, pro-choice legislators seized an opportunity to pass abortion reform through the legislature in London. Furthermore, because they used the CEDAW findings as a basis for the reforms, they achieved change on a scale that would have been impossible in the Northern Ireland Assembly. Bypassing the regional assembly, legislating at the national parliament, and drawing on the findings of an international human rights treaty body, feminists were able to achieve a staggering transformation in abortion law. After parts of the 1861 Offences Against the Person Act were repealed and abortion was decriminalized, Northern Ireland was left with a less restrictive legal framework than England, Scotland, and Wales. The 1861 act still prohibits abortion in the rest of the United Kingdom, but the 1967 Abortion Act sets out a few circumstances under which legal abortion can be obtained.[96] Abortion is still a criminal offense everywhere in the United Kingdom except Northern Ireland, and, as of August 2022, there are two women awaiting trial in England for abortion-related offenses.[97]

––––––––

The legal reforms that decriminalized abortion in Northern Ireland did not mark the "end of a struggle" but the beginning of a new phase.[98] While abortion was decriminalized in 2019, as of 2023 it is still not widely available past twelve weeks. It is provided in some places, and under some circumstances, but many Northern Irish residents continue to travel to England because they cannot obtain abortions at home. Anti-abortion parties, politicians, and institutions act as obstacles to implementing the new law because they refuse to commission health services to provide abortion care. Having decriminalized abortion via London, the devolved government in Belfast still retains responsibility for establishing an abortion service. But the Department of Health has refused to do this because it claims that such a "contentious issue" as abortion requires approval from the executive, which lacks a mandate for this decision. As a result, services are provided on an ad hoc basis only. The Northern Ireland Assembly, meanwhile, has already attempted to pass legislation that would narrow the scope of the reforms achieved and outlaw some abortions.[99]

Northern Ireland's partial abortion service is an urgent reminder that removing laws that criminalize abortion is not the same as creating services that give people local and affordable access. Without functioning abortion services that create access to supported, local care—with medication abortion or surgical abortion options where needed—abortion reform in Northern Ireland is unfinished. People can order medication abortion online, without fear of criminalization, but they cannot reliably access abortion services in their home region and are frequently required to travel elsewhere in the United Kingdom for care.

This ambivalent ending suggests that we should be cautious about any straightforward, triumphalist narrative that argues self-managed abortion paves the way for free, safe, legal, local abortion. As it became widely used and discussed in Northern Ireland, medication abortion helped catalyze reform. Its social decriminalization (evident in widespread opposition to imprisonment of abortion pill users and highly visible abortion pill activism) proceeded even as political elites maintained their support for unpopular anti-abortion policies. Prosecutions of people who bought and used abortion pills met with opposition from the public and lawmakers in the central government, both of which were leveraged by activists who turned to international institutions for support. When the Northern Ireland Assembly was suspended, the central government merely removed abortion's criminal penalties rather than impose any kind of new regulations on it. The achievement of decriminalization of abortion in Northern Ireland is remarkable, moving it from the most to the least legally restrictive part of the United Kingdom. But the ongoing opposition to abortion in the regional government means that, in practice, people in Northern Ireland who want abortion continue to confront reproductive injustices every day.

CHAPTER 9

The Future of Reproductive Freedom

The *Dobbs* decision overturning *Roe v. Wade* is a momentous loss in the struggle for abortion access. In the months after the decision, the legal ground is rapidly shifting. Some states are passing laws to ban abortion inside their state and for their residents who travel elsewhere, while other states are passing laws to shield their abortion providers from lawsuits. The federal government is issuing some limited executive orders and agency decisions to protect abortion where it has jurisdiction. Post-*Dobbs* abortion bans in the states show a new level of extremism in the anti-abortion movement, lacking even the exceptions for rape and incest that used to be commonplace.[1] Downstream from these new anti-abortion laws, we have seen an immediate chilling effect in medical practice. Within weeks of the *Dobbs* decision, horrifying stories emerged of women denied medical care until they were on the brink of serious injury or death because their doctors were uncertain about the law or afraid of legal repercussions.[2] There will certainly be preventable deaths caused by state abortion bans in the United States, just as there are in every country with restrictive abortion laws. These deaths will not be caused by a lack of resources, training, knowledge, or technology but by political choices made in courts and legislatures.

In this concluding chapter, I reflect on the possibilities and limitations of medication abortion in the United States after *Dobbs*, in the short and the long term. In the short term, self-managed abortion with pills will be a lifeline for Americans because it is relatively difficult for governments to block, and, as we have seen in chapter 3, self-managed abortion with pills is already widespread in the United States. As elsewhere in the world, US activists are engaged in cross-border work that moves people and pills into spaces where abortion is unavailable. Drawing on this extant cross-border work, in the longer term, we should use self-managed abortion with pills to rethink our systems of abortion provision. The models for self-managed abortion that have been developed in restrictive countries have important innovations that can help us imagine better ways to provide abortion to everyone who needs it.

MEDICATION ABORTION AS A LIFELINE

State-level abortion bans are coming into force across the United States. At least twenty-six states are likely to ban abortion in the wake of the *Dobbs* decision.[3] State by state, abortion laws will be a stark patchwork of total abortion bans, progressive abortion protections, and something in between. As it does across the world, such a patchwork of laws will create and expand travel pathways between different jurisdictions—such as those from Ireland to England and Poland to Germany (see chaps. 4 and 6). Abortion travel across state lines in the United States, of course, predates the *Dobbs* decision, but we can expect to see a smaller number of clinics serving a much greater number of abortion travelers in its aftermath. However, many people cannot travel to another state because of the financial, social, and logistical challenges involved.

Self-managed abortion with pills will be a lifeline for Americans whose states ban abortion. It has already become a lifeline for Americans living in states with very restrictive laws or those living in states with liberal laws who are nonetheless unable to afford in-clinic care. Abortion laws have generally regulated abortion providers (and mainly physicians), but self-managed abortion with pills means laws governing the conduct of abortion providers will be less able to determine if, where, and when abortion happens. Self-managed abortion makes the abortion seeker their own abortion provider. In recognition of this change, and in an effort to crack down on newer abortion methods, some anti-abortion authorities in the United States are taking deliberate steps to criminalize self-managed abortion. In some cases, they do this by relying on archaic laws from the nineteenth century that criminalize "procuring" miscarriage through abortifacients, expanding the interpretation of recent laws to grant fetuses the status of born children, or creating new laws with the express purpose of criminalizing self-managed abortion.[4] Nonetheless, as I have shown throughout the book, self-managed abortion with pills is very difficult for governments to prevent or eliminate, even when they try to do so; abortion pills are cheap to obtain, easy to move, hard to intercept, and nearly impossible to detect.

Abortion pills are inexpensive to produce. Treatment activists who organize buyer's clubs for other medications—like Sofosbuvir for hepatitis C or Truvada for HIV—come up against pharmaceutical interests and intellectual property protections that work to keep drug costs high and limit their availability.[5] Not so with medication abortion. It is off-patent and cheaply produced in generic form across the world. In pharmaceutical hubs like India, dozens of brands compete against each other for domestic and international markets (see chap. 1). The emergence of online markets in generic pharmaceuticals means that these products can be bought and shipped abroad with relative ease and, in many cases, without violating national pharmaceutical laws. Vendors like Organic Lifestyle Guru and GetAbortionPillsNow.com buy MA online in bulk, import it to the United States, and resell it to Americans, but they struggle to keep up with the demand. The status of a medicine changes numerous times as it crosses borders, picking up labels like "falsified" and "counterfeit," but these designations do not necessarily mean that the medicine is of poor quality. MA activism depends on a range of chemically equivalent generic products—substituting Mifegest or Mifepro for Mifeprex—because so many brands are manufactured across the world. The abortion pills that circulate in clandestine abortion networks and online pharmacies are, according to the best available evidence, simply generics of good quality.[6]

Manufacturing hubs for medication abortion are mainly countries where abortion is legal. To reach abortion seekers in countries with very restrictive laws, the pills need to move. It is difficult for state authorities to intercept medication abortion shipped from abroad. Even when they are motivated to block incoming shipments, the sheer volume of international mail makes it impossible to verify the contents of all packages at customs points. Where a package is labeled "prescribed medicine" and it is illegal to import prescribed medicine, customs agents can block a significant volume of incoming pills (see chap. 6). But when activist intermediaries in a different country repackage the medications, wrapping them as birthday gifts or hiding them inside packages of personal goods, they can pass through domestic and international mail with ease (see chap. 8). Online pharmacies use similar tactics, sometimes disguising abortion pills inside packages with other goods that make the medications harder to detect (see chap. 1). In this way, abortion medications move inside the enormous volumes of global cargo that cross borders each day.

Small and portable medications can be easily smuggled by people crossing borders. Pills move in this way in quantities large and small. Whether this is one person taking a short bus trip over the border to pick up their own MA or a friendly doctor crossing the border with a suitcase stuffed with combipacks (see chap. 6), pills move when people do. Activist networks collaborating across borders have developed sophisticated assessments of the medical regulations in different countries, and they use this information to keep stocks of medications at regular levels. Some countries permit mifepristone and misoprostol to be sold over the counter, so these become important travel stopovers where supplies can be replenished (see chap. 5). Studies on the extent of self-managed abortion in the United States, and the methods used to self-manage abortion there, demonstrate that many US residents already engage in cross-border travel for abortion pills.[7]

Abortion pills are not only difficult to detect as they cross borders, but they are also difficult to detect inside the human body. An abortion induced with medication is (almost always) indistinguishable from a spontaneous miscarriage. Mifepristone and misoprostol are difficult to detect in blood tests after an abortion. Misoprostol sometimes leaves a residue, so medication abortion activists tell people to take misoprostol by mouth rather than insert it in the vagina, which is the way it is usually administered.[8] If the pills are swallowed, no residue is detectable, whereas if fragments of the pills remain in the vagina, a doctor could find evidence of misoprostol and therefore determine that the abortion was deliberately induced.[9]

Anti-abortion states are largely unable to impede the flow of abortion pills, and anti-abortion doctors are largely unable to detect an abortion induced with pills. People who are criminalized for having an abortion with medication are often identified after they tell doctors what they have taken, when family or friends report the abortion to the police, or when evidence of the abortion (like blood and tissue) is discovered. Medication abortion providers, especially feminist networks, counter this risk by providing information on how to seek post-abortion care and what to say to doctors. They also use secure digital platforms to erase evidence when a person obtains abortion pills, because digital data is a key tool that law enforcement uses to prove a miscarriage was intended rather than spontaneous.[10] One abortion pill service, for example, delivers all email via temporary Web links that erase the message's content after it is read.[11] However, when people are criminalized for self-managed abortion, it is usually those who lacked the support of medication abortion activists, self-managed their abortions in the second trimester, and faced heightened scrutiny from medical staff (see chap. 3). These are a small number of pill users, but they tend to represent the most marginalized groups in society.

Cheap, mass-produced, portable, and largely undetectable: it is difficult for state authorities to stop people from using MA to self-manage abortion. Governments and law enforcement officials who do want to criminalize self-managed abortion can, occasionally, prosecute and convict people who self-managed their abortion or those who help them. But they risk provoking public backlash against a particular prosecution and against the criminalization of pill users in general. Irish politicians sought to maintain the legitimacy of their abortion ban by promising they would not prosecute individual abortion seekers (see chap. 7). Across the border, Northern Irish prosecutions of abortion pill users and the people who helped them met with public protest, increased the public's opposition to abortion criminalization, and galvanized reluctant politicians to take action (see chap. 8). The April 2022 arrest of a Texas woman, Lizelle Herrera, for an alleged self-induced abortion illustrates this dynamic in the United States. Murder charges against Herrera were dropped but only after reporting on her arrest made national news and provoked large protests.[12] Opinion polling from March 2022 shows that 50 percent of Americans think the pregnant person should not face penalties for having an illegal abortion; and 47 percent favor penalties of some kind (3 percent are not sure).[13] Very few cases of prosecution for illegal abortion have come to widespread national attention, although it seems likely that more such cases will occur in the years after *Dobbs*. Based on trends in other countries, we might expect to see public opinion shift more strongly against penalties for illegal abortion if more prosecutions take place.

MEDICATION ABORTION IN THE BORDERLANDS

Across a mosaic of different abortion jurisdictions, border zones appear as spaces of opportunity. The Northern Ireland–Republic of Ireland border has been one such space, as has the Polish border. Border zones—physical and digital—are spaces that abortion providers and MA activists have used to build the infrastructure to support self-managed abortion. They engage in border work, mapping a state's abortion laws, customs procedures, medicines regulations, border infrastructure, postal systems, cross-border transport links, and regional activist mobilization. From that point, they can construct networks and procedures to move medications between the places where they are easy to obtain and the places where they are needed but hard to obtain. Each jurisdiction requires its own tailor-made pathways. What works varies across all types of borders—by city, county, province, region, or country.

Sometimes this border work is deliberately kept secret so that authorities cannot identify pill pathways. Sometimes it goes unnoticed only because it is mundane: the physical spaces where the state enforces its border are usually bureaucratic and unglamorous. In Poland, a group of activists wanted to stage a protest against customs officials who were illegally withholding and tampering with abortion pill packages coming into the country. As they planned this protest, they realized that the customs building where these decisions were made was "just somewhere in a field, in no man's land!" Not only could they not stage a protest there, because supporters and media would not attend, but they realized that this bland and remote building, where abortion pills were being seized and destroyed, was an important site that reproduced the state's power to oppress abortion seekers. People whose pills were illegally held in this building would be afraid to confront decision makers: "You'd have to go there and argue with some man in a suit who's very important, and is yelling at you, threatening you, using terms you don't know, and you wouldn't know if they are telling the truth or not."[14] States oppress women and pregnant people when they limit their reproductive autonomy, and they do it in ways large and small. Protesters mobilize in city centers and in front of government buildings after these institutions make decisions that restrict abortion, but the quotidian decisions that matter for abortion seekers, like where and when pills get through which customs offices, attract much less attention. We have seen a similar dynamic at play in the United States in recent decades. The *Dobbs* decision that overturned *Roe v. Wade* mobilized enormous protests and intense public anger after the leaked draft decision. But years of smaller, complex, mundane laws that tinkered with the medical regulations governing abortion and effectively eroded access met with much less public anger. Who, besides specialists in the weeds of abortion law and medicine, could really understand them and see their full impact across all fifty states?

Activists engage in cross-border work in secret in some places and in full view of the media in others. Activists often disagree on whether and when to publicize their work: some want to prioritize the work of secretly moving pills to the places they are needed, avoiding police attention at all costs; others see this as a futile, piecemeal effort, instead seeking publicity for abortion pill actions that will expose hypocrisies and catalyze change (see chaps. 5, 6, and 8). These are long-standing disagreements within the activist movement that provides clandestine abortion and advocates for abortion reform. These disagreements have long-term strategic as well as immediate practical importance. If a particular pill pathway is exposed in the media, will law enforcement shut it down? Without media attention to abortion pills, will anyone other than feminist activists realize that they can have a safe, self-managed abortion with pills? Can a public media spectacle give abortion seekers enough information to obtain pills, use them effectively, and avoid scrutiny from police or anti-abortion doctors? If activists try to provoke the state authorities and authorities take the bait, is someone willing to go to prison for the cause?

The relationship between medication abortion activism and legal change is not straightforward. The countries studied in this book show the variety of possible outcomes. Widespread defiance of unjust abortion laws and use of medication abortion for clandestine self-managed abortion can help drive legal change, as it did in Ireland. Legal change is insufficient, as we see in Northern Ireland, where resistance to abortion throughout the political system still means the absence of any functional abortion services in the government-funded health system. In Poland, self-managed abortion occupies a unique legal position: it is not a crime, but assisting it is. Activists in Poland and allies abroad have developed systems to facilitate widespread self-managed abortion with pills there, but the only legal change in abortion in Poland has been to further restrict its abortion law. The emergence of an informal system for self-managed abortion across Poland has not produced progressive political change: instead, the scale of abortion is denied, minimized, and ignored by lawmakers, while a small number of criminal prosecutions creates a chilling effect. Medication abortion and self-managed abortion have upended much of the conventional wisdom, not least because they change the relationship between abortion's legality and safety. But they do not have a predictable, uniform impact on the social and political systems that states use to govern the termination of pregnancy.

Ultimately, the most important point of agreement that unites medication abortion activism across borders and group affiliations is its emphasis on social decriminalization. Changing the availability of medication abortion and public attitudes to it now, activists argue, will contribute to legal reforms and decriminalization. Defying unjust laws now by facilitating practical, immediate access to abortion with pills is the priority. As a consequence of widespread defiance of the law, growing social acceptance of self-managed use of medication abortion will likely precede legal change. This is because widespread change of social attitudes on abortion creates public dissatisfaction with anti-abortion laws and causes these laws to lose legitimacy. Legal scholars call this the "regularization of transgression": breaking the law becomes so routine, so organized, that an alternative system "on the periphery of the legal order" emerges and begins to influence governmental practices.[15] The highly organized system for self-managed abortion that exists on the periphery of the legal order has come to influence that legal order in different places. When anti-abortion laws are widely defied, medication abortion activists argue, they simply cannot be enforced and will be changed. In the face of prosecutions and restrictions, activists and pill users put it plainly: "They can't arrest us all." An informal, activist-driven system for clandestine self-managed abortion on the periphery of the legal order already exists in the United States and will undoubtedly grow. For those who cannot or will not travel across state lines, it will likely become the main way to access abortion.

Abortion border work in the United States takes many forms. Medication abortion crosses national borders, whether from Mexico or India, whether in a suitcase or a labeled parcel from a pharmaceutical distributor. People and pills cross domestic borders, moving across the American mosaic of abortion regulations and bans. Medication abortion access in the coming years will likely be defined by complex patterns of interstate mobility by people and their pills. Digital technologies mean that consultations with doctors and community health providers can happen across long distances, but ultimately the pills need to get into the hands of pregnant people. That will mean mobile clinics just over state borders from which pills can be dispensed. It will mean mail forwarding services through which abortion providers can legally prescribe pills and those pills can be legally delivered within a state that permits medication abortion but then forwarded to another state where those pills could not have been legally obtained. It will mean well-connected cross-border networks of activists who maintain stockpiles of pills and refresh those stockpiles through travel or shipments from elsewhere, as activists in other countries have done. Through these routes, and more that will develop over time, self-managed abortion with pills will certainly become available to more people in the United States who live in abortion-hostile states.

MEDICATION ABORTION AS A PARADIGM SHIFT

In the short term, then, self-managed abortion with pills will be widespread regardless of its legal status in each state, as it is in abortion-restrictive places across the globe. It will not be accessible to everyone, nor will it be medically suitable to everyone. For all its transformation of clandestine abortion and its transgression of the laws and borders that usually govern abortion, medication abortion has its limits. Some people need abortions in medical settings with intervention from doctors. Self-managed abortion cannot ever eliminate the need for medical services that treat people who need later abortions, have medical complications, need medical care to complete a miscarriage, or need to terminate a pregnancy for urgent health reasons, among other things. But in the context of reversals and draconian anti-abortion laws that offer almost no grounds for legal access, it will be a lifeline. It will take long-term committed political mobilization to repeal anti-abortion laws and institute protections for abortion that mean states cannot ban it. The *Dobbs* decision has set abortion access back by decades, and restoring abortion services—even to 2021 levels—will take time. But we should go much further.

Self-managed abortion with pills should not be limited to a stopgap measure in countries with restrictive abortion laws. In the long term, the design and delivery of abortion services should be influenced by models of self-managed abortion with pills that MA activists developed in contexts where there was little or no legal abortion. This requires a shift in the way we think about self-managed abortion. It should not be imagined as a harm reduction measure, taken only to minimize health risks of even less safe abortion methods. For those who imagine abortion care only in terms of in-clinic abortions supervised by doctors, self-managed abortion with pills might seem like an acceptable alternative to a coat hanger abortion but not a long-term model for care. If policy makers see self-managed abortion as a harm reduction measure, activists and lawyers caution, they continue to imagine the conventional clinical setting as the only "desired place of care," and as a result, they fail to reckon with the transformative social change that self-managed abortion with pills can drive. Like earlier generations of activists in the reproductive self-help movement, advocates for self-managed abortion do not want to move abortion back into the medical settings where unequal power relations between doctors and patients are pervasive. Advocates argue that self-managed abortion with pills means a paradigm shift in abortion care. It allows for more autonomy in the decision-making process and procedure of the abortion. It also allows community health workers and lay activists to support abortions as providers, expanding the pool of people who can give care.

By changing the institutional power dynamics and social roles around abortion, demedicalizing abortion would also help to destigmatize it.[16] Expanding the spaces of abortion care to include the home would help normalize abortion as a matter of routine health.[17] Many years of public health study support these arguments. Since its earliest trials, medication abortion has been shown to be safe, acceptable, and even preferred. Evidence shows that people prefer medication to surgical abortion because it allows them to act as their own abortion provider rather than submit to a procedure carried out by another person. People also prefer self-managed abortion with remote support because it is less expensive, they can choose when and where to take the pills, and they can undergo the abortion in the comfort of their home with people there to support them.[18] Abortion with medication is often experienced and conceptualized differently, as more analogous to a menstrual period than a surgical intervention.[19] For Americans especially, having an abortion at home is often preferable because it means they do not have to risk harassment or violence from anti-abortion protesters who gather outside abortion clinics. The advantages of medication abortion show the importance of choice of abortion method, not just the need to replace one method with another. Studies show that when people who are eligible for medication and surgical abortion are given the choice, they choose medication abortion at higher rates, but regardless of the method they choose, satisfaction with the abortion is higher for people who participated in the decision about their abortion method.[20]

Ironically, when they can access safe and supported abortion pills through international feminist networks, people in legally restrictive settings sometimes have more control over their own abortions than they do in settings where abortion is legal but highly regulated.[21] Instituting new legal and regulatory frameworks on abortion can have the effect of disempowering abortion seekers. The discussion of Ireland in chapter 7 illustrates this point: an Irish woman who obtained abortion pills from Women Help Women in 2017 would have been able to obtain those medications in her own home, without having to search for a pro-choice doctor, justifying her reasons to that doctor, or undergoing a mandatory waiting period. The same Irish woman who obtains an abortion in 2023, under the new Irish abortion law, has to find a doctor willing to provide abortion, meet with that doctor in person or by phone, and undergo the three-day waiting period to obtain abortion pills. This comparison is not to suggest that the previous legal regime was preferable, because the woman who self-manages an abortion today does so without fear that she could be criminalized for ending her own pregnancy. Nonetheless, with the extra burdens on abortion that are imposed in the name of regulation and control, it is clear why abortion seekers might prefer some elements of the online system run by feminists who see abortion as a social good. In fact, an Irish NGO reports that some people in Ireland still choose to obtain abortion pills through online feminist networks because of the obstruction and delay they face getting a legal abortion in the Irish health system.[22]

The COVID-19 pandemic also gave weight to the argument that self-managed abortion models developed on the periphery by activists should be studied as models of design and delivery of abortion services. When lockdowns forced people to stay home and pushed medical providers to shift as many services as possible to telemedicine systems, some countries moved their abortion services in this direction. They introduced no-touch telemedicine abortion services, with phone consultation and pills sent by mail, reduced the number of in-person visits required to obtain a medication abortion, and/or expanded the places that medication abortion could be dispensed.[23] Policy makers may have seen telemedicine abortion as a temporary measure adopted in a moment of crisis, but evaluations of the services found them to be safe, effective, and acceptable to service users well beyond the pandemic.

The United Kingdom provides one example: an evaluation of one "pills by post" service initiated there during the COVID-19 pandemic found that the service reduced waiting times and lowered the gestational age at which the abortion was completed. Even a relatively abortion-permissive context like the United Kingdom puts numerous regulations on medication abortion—typical of the exceptionalism that surrounds abortion—and these regulations impose significant barriers to care.[24] People in the United Kingdom regularly look to foreign telemedicine services like Women on Web for abortion care (which is a crime under the UK abortion law). Once the pills by post telemedicine service was introduced during COVID-19, the number of English, Scottish, and Welsh people requesting abortion pills from Women on Web dropped by 88 percent.[25] These findings about the safety and accessibility of telemedicine abortion echo years of work by public health researchers who have studied the international feminist MA services—like Women on Web, Aid Access, and Women Help Women—and determined that those services were not only safe and acceptable, but essential.[26] The pandemic has presented a moment for governments to learn from the experience of medication abortion networks that operate outside the formal medical system (and sometimes outside the law) and to integrate elements of these services into improved models of clinical provision.[27]

By adapting abortion services from the activist models of remotely supported self-managed abortion, these services become more available to people who face barriers to obtaining in-clinic care. Abortion that is more available, more autonomous, less costly, and restricted by fewer gatekeepers is a requirement of Reproductive Justice. Reproductive Justice analysis of abortion pushes us to consider the gap between a legal or constitutional right to an abortion and the resources to practically obtain one.[28] Moving beyond the "right to choose" framework, Reproductive Justice asks us to think about the conditions under which people make choices and the structures that constrain their choices. The gap between rights and resources in the United States is a factor of class, race, and geography, among others.[29] The poorest Americans are disproportionately likely to want access to abortion services.[30] When abortion services are confined to a few clinics, when those services are expensive, and when those services require in-person visits, the poorest and most marginalized groups are the least likely to be able to access it.[31] There is an abundance of evidence—from before the *Dobbs* decision and state-level abortion bans—to show that financial and logistical barriers delay and ultimately prevent people from obtaining a wanted abortion.[32] Being unable to obtain a wanted abortion has damaging consequences for women and pregnant people, their children, their wider networks, and society as a whole.

Simply put, autonomy over reproductive decisions about if, whether, and when to have children is "a requirement for social justice."[33] Medication abortion delivered through remotely supported services advances us toward such a goal. It lowers the financial barriers to abortion, because it costs a fraction of what in-clinic abortion costs. It reduces the logistical burdens of obtaining abortion care, because no-touch models do not require in-person clinic visits.[34] Such a system would also mitigate the geographic barriers to abortion care that make access especially difficult for people living in rural areas, without access to private transportation, or with limited mobility for other reasons. Going one step further, we could imagine more flexible models for distributing medication abortion that would remove barriers that make it costly or cumbersome to access. Abortion pills should, in the future, be sold over the counter in pharmacies. People could purchase them as needed or ahead of time for quicker access. Preliminary studies suggest this change would lower costs and improve the availability of medication abortion.[35] In the United States, even states with liberal abortion laws will be unable to make this change until the FDA removes regulations on medication abortion that severely restrict where it can be sold and by whom (see chap. 2). Regulations on medication abortion were relaxed during the pandemic to allow for no-touch abortion care, but federal restrictions that overly burden mifepristone compared to medications of equivalent safety still remain in force.[36]

In the short term, safe self-managed abortion with pills will be the main way that many Americans can access abortion. Abortion pills, whether bought online from foreign pharmacies, sent through feminist online abortion providers, or smuggled across state borders, will save lives. Many people will still need to travel, with the help of abortion funds and support networks, to obtain an abortion in medical settings where it remains legal. Some will not be able to access abortion at all. In the long term, however, the struggle to restore abortion services across the United States should not treat demedicalized models of self-managed care as substandard and acceptable only in times of dire need. Medication abortion models, developed on the periphery of the law, are potentially transformative for all abortion seekers and all legal contexts.

Writing in 1984 about the development of surgical abortion methods that replaced herbal abortifacients, Rosalind Petchesky cautioned against placing too much stock in new technological developments. Reproductive freedom, she wrote, is "not simply a matter of developing more sophisticated techniques" for performing abortion. The pursuit of reproductive freedom remains a "political, not technological," agenda.[37] Petchesky's words resonate as deeply today as they did in the 1980s, and I conclude with them here as a warning against too much technological optimism about medication abortion. To be sure, medication abortion has been transformative. It has changed the experience of abortion, its availability, its relationship to law, the state's ability to enforce prohibitions against it, and pregnant people's ability to obtain it regardless of where they live. However, medication abortion by itself will not instantly trigger abortion reforms, because these are political, not technological, problems. The systems for safe self-managed abortion flourishing across the world provide us with a glimpse of a future of greater reproductive freedom. And the feminist struggle to realize that future continues.

Appendix

A Note on Interviews and Anonymity

All participants in the project were offered anonymity for their interviews, as a default. Some people specifically asked to be named in publications, while most remain anonymous.

Participants gave informed consent for their interview. Most interviews were recorded and transcribed verbatim. If not, I took written notes during the interview. I carried out all the interviews below except where otherwise noted. Research assistants asked not to be named in association with the interviews they conducted.

In some cases, additional steps to protect the anonymity of participants were required. The field of abortion pill activists is small, and people who are publicly known as campaigners do not always publicly disclose their work providing abortion pills. I have protected the anonymity of some participants by assigning separate interview labels to the same person: one label to cover instances where they spoke about well-known public activities that could be easily identified and another label to refer to clandestine activities that require additional measures to protect identities. The 2022 prosecution of Justyna Wydrzyńska demonstrates the high stakes for activists who do this work.

I refer to interviews cited in the book using the labels below. This is not an exhaustive list of every interview that I conducted for the research, but it reflects the interviews directly quoted or paraphrased in the text.

INTERVIEWS: TRANSNATIONAL

T317	Director of a pan-European abortion travel support group, 2017
T518	Public health researcher working on self-managed abortion, 2018
T618	Former crew member on Women on Waves' Latin American ship campaigns, 2018
T718A	Leader in Women on Web/ Women on Waves, 2018
T718B	Activist working for reproductive rights for refugees in Europe, 2018
T818	Latin American researcher with knowledge of regional pill networks, 2018
T1118	A founder of Women Help Women, 2018
T2019A	Activist working in a transnational European network that facilitates abortion pills and travel, 2019
T2019B	Doctor working with a transnational European pill network, 2019
T2019C	Polish activist involved in clandestine pill supply networks, 2019
T2019D	Polish activist involved in clandestine pill supply networks, 2019
T519A	Director of a pan-European abortion travel support group, 2019
T519B	Director of Safe2Choose, 2019
T719A	Gynecologist who works in a research and advisory capacity with Women on Web, 2019
T719B	Doctor who is a medical supervisor for Women on Web, 2019
T819A	Volunteer on the Women on Web help desk, 2019
T919	Doctor who is a medical supervisor for Women on Web, 2019
T1119	Maltese activist working in transnational abortion solidarity groups, 2019
T1219	Senior executive of the British Pregnancy Advisory Service (BPAS), 2019
T120	Austrian abortion provider and researcher, 2020
T520	Operator of an online pharmacy selling abortion pills, advertised as a Moscow-based company, 2020

INTERVIEWS: NORTHERN IRELAND

NI518A   Activist working with several pro-choice and feminist groups in Belfast, 2018

NI518B   Activist affiliated with Alliance for Choice, working in rural Northern Ireland, 2018

NI518C   Activist working in pro-choice and feminist groups in Belfast, 2018

NI818A   Derry-based activist and campaigner in Alliance for Choice, 2018

NI818B   Activist and campaigner in Alliance for Choice, 2018

NI1018   Activist working in Alliance for Choice, 2018

NI220   Activist involved in pill provision and campaigning, 2020

NI721   Lawyer involved in defending people charged with abortion-related crimes in Northern Ireland, 2021

INTERVIEWS: REPUBLIC OF IRELAND

ROI317A   Leading figure in Irish campaign for abortion reform, 2017

ROI317B   Spokesperson for an Irish support group and campaign group on medical grounds, 2017

ROI317C   Spokesperson for an Irish pro-choice campaign group, 2017

ROI317D   Activist and artist in the Irish pro-choice movement, 2017

ROI518A   Doctor who worked in Dublin sexual health clinics during the 1980s, 2018

ROI518B   Activist who campaigned as part of the Anti-Amendment Campaign in 1983 and for repeal in 2018, 2018

ROI518C   Academic and activist, campaigning for survivors of historical abuses in Ireland, 2018

ROI718A   Pro-choice activist and campaigner who worked on medication abortion provision from the mid-2000s, 2018

ROI718B   Campaigner with London Irish Abortion Rights Campaign, 2018

ROI718C   Spokesperson for Doctors for Choice, working in rural Ireland, 2018

ROI1118A   Activist working with ROSA in Dublin, 2018

ROI1118B Politician who has campaigned on abortion reform and medication abortion, 2018

ROI719 Senator who served on 2013 and 2018 legislative committees on abortion legislation, 2019

ROI819 Activist affiliated with ROSA, based in west of Ireland, 2019

ROI919 Staff member on the policy team of a large Irish reproductive rights NGO, 2019

ROI1219 Senator and member of the Joint Committee on the 8th Amendment, 2019

ROI421 Activist in the west of Ireland, involved in pro-choice campaigning and pill networks, 2021

INTERVIEWS: POLAND

PL518 Polish activist in Dublin working with a transnational solidarity campaign, 2018

PL618A Activist and campaigner leading a local branch of a national women's rights group in a large Polish city, 2019

PL618B Campaigner working on feminism and church-state separation, 2019

PL519A Activist and lawyer working on abortion access, 2019

PL519B Activist and educator working on abortion access, 2019

PL519C Scholar and activist writing and campaigning on reproductive rights, 2019

PL519D Polish activist based in London, working in a transnational solidarity group, 2019

PL519E Staff member of Polish NGO, working on sexual and reproductive rights, 2019

PL719A Doctor and activist working with Doctors for Women, 2019

PL719B German activist leading an abortion fund and travel support group for Polish abortion seekers, 2019

PL819A Feminist intellectual and activist, 2019

PL819B Polish activist living abroad, working with a support group that helps Polish abortion seekers travel, 2019

PL819C   Lawyer and staffer with a large Polish reproductive rights NGO, 2019

PL919   Activist working with a transnational solidarity group for Polish and Irish migrants in Germany, 2019

PL1119A   Sexual health educator and advocate, 2019

PL1119B   Follow-up interview with PL719A, 2019

PL220A   Dutch activist working with a group that helps Polish abortion seekers come to the Netherlands, 2020

PL220B   Polish politician and campaigner, a prominent advocate of abortion rights, 2020

PL220C   Activist living in Sweden, leading an organization to help Polish abortion seekers travel abroad, 2020

PL220D   Research assistant interview with Polish woman who formerly worked as a translator for Polish patients in an Austrian abortion clinic, 2020

PL320   Research assistant interview with Polish woman working as translator and advocate for Polish patients in an Austrian abortion clinic, 2020

INTERVIEWS: INDIA

IN621A   Research assistant interview with operations head of an Indian firm that manufactures MTP kits for the domestic market, based in Punjab state, 2021

IN621B   Research assistant interview with managing partner of an Indian firm that manufactures MTP kits for the domestic market, based in Punjab state, 2021

IN621C   Research assistant interview with employee of an Indian firm that manufactures MTP kits for the domestic market, based in Maharashtra state, 2021

IN621D   Research assistant interview with technical director of an Indian firm that manufactures MTP kits for the domestic market, based in Punjab state, 2021

IN721A   Research assistant interview with president of a local pharmacists' association in Uttar Pradesh state, 2021

IN721B   Research assistant interview with employee of a pharmaceutical wholesale business operating in a market in Uttar Pradesh state, 2021

IN821A   Research assistant interview with enforcement official of the Food and Drug Control Administration of Maharashtra state, 2021

IN821B   Research assistant interview with enforcement official of the Food and Drug Control Administration of Maharashtra state, 2021

IN821C   Research assistant interview with enforcement official of the Food and Drug Control Administration of Maharashtra state, 2021

IN822   Abortion and contraception activist based in the southern state of Tamil Nadu, 2022

INTERVIEWS: UNITED STATES OF AMERICA

US1018   Activist and campaigner working on abortion pill pathways, 2018

US1118   Activist and campaigner working on abortion pill pathways, 2018

US719   Activist working on DIY medical technologies including misoprostol, 2019

USA819   Activist who leads a transnational pill network, 2019

US520A   Person living in a southwestern state who bought abortion pills online for another, 2020

US520B   Person living in a southeastern state who bought abortion pills online and used them to self-manage an abortion, 2020

USA620A   Staff member at an international trade association for reproductive health products manufacturers, 2020

USA620B   Two researchers from international reproductive rights NGOs, working on abortion pill supplies, 2020

US1020   Operator of an online abortion pill business, 2020

US1220A   Public health researcher and advocate for medication abortion provision, 2020

US1220B   Lawyer and advocate against criminalization of pregnant and abortion-seeking people, 2020

USA621   President of US-based international marketer and manufacturer of sexual and reproductive health supplies, 2021

NOTES

INTRODUCTION

1. Rickie Solinger, *Pregnancy and Power: A Short History of Reproductive Politics in America* (New York: New York University Press, 2007), 121.

2. Leslie Reagan, *When Abortion Was a Crime: Women, Medicine, and Law in the United States, 1867–1973* (Berkeley: University of California Press, 1997), 3–4.

3. For all the media debate about language and gender identity in abortion work, I found little disagreement about this issue in the medication abortion movement. The activist groups discussed in this book are inclusive of trans and nonbinary abortion seekers and actively oppose anti-trans elements of the abortion movement. In the text, I alternate between referring to women, people, and pregnant people where appropriate. Where I refer to women, it is usually to a specific woman or a specific group of people identifying as women. For more general discussions, I usually refer to people rather than women.

4. David Cohen, Greer Donley, and Rachel Rebouché, "The New Abortion Battleground," *Columbia Law Review* 123, no. 1 (2023): 2.

5. Guttmacher Institute, *Abortion Worldwide 2017: Unequal Progress and Unequal Access* (Washington, DC: Guttmacher Institute, 2018), 12.

6. Jonathan Bearak et al., "Unintended Pregnancy and Abortion by Income, Region, and the Legal Status of Abortion: Estimates from a Comprehensive Model for 1990–2019," *The Lancet Global Health* 8, no. 9 (2020): e1152–e1161.

7. Guttmacher, *Abortion Worldwide*, 34–35.

8. Heidi Moseson et al., "Self-Managed Abortion: A Systematic Scoping Review," *Best Practice & Research Clinical Obstetrics & Gynecology* 63 (2020): 88.

9. Bela Ganatra et al., "Global, Regional, and Subregional Classification of Abortions by Safety, 2010–14: Estimates from a Bayesian Hierarchical Model," *The Lancet* 390, no. 10110 (2017): 2372–81.

10. Mariana Prandini Assis and Joanna Erdman, "Abortion Rights beyond the Medico-Legal Paradigm," *Global Public Health* 17, no. 10 (2022): 2235.

11. Kinga Jelinska and Susan Yanow, "Putting Abortion Pills into Women's Hands: Realizing the Full Potential of Medical Abortion," *Contraception* 97, no. 2 (2018): 87.

12. Elizabeth Raymond, Margo Harrison, and Mark Weaver, "Efficacy of Misoprostol Alone for First-Trimester Medical Abortion: A Systematic Review," *Obstetrics and Gynecology* 133, no. 1 (2019): 137. The figures quoted here come from this systematic review, but more recent data suggest that misoprostol-only regimes may be up to 99 percent effective.

13. WHO, *Abortion Care Guideline* (Geneva: WHO, 2022).

14. Sandi Pruitt and Patricia Dolan Mullen, "Contraception or Abortion? Inaccurate Descriptions of Emergency Contraception in Newspaper Articles, 1992–2002," *Contraception* 71, no. 1 (2005): 14–21.

15. WHO, *Abortion Care Guideline*.

16. Tracy Weitz et al., "'Medical' and 'Surgical' Abortion: Rethinking the Modifiers," *Contraception* 69, no. 1 (2004): 77–78.

17. There are older methods of "surgical" abortion such as dilation and curettage, in which a provider dilates the cervix and scrapes the uterus with a sharp object to clear it, but this method is considered obsolete and no longer recommended by WHO.

18. Lucía Berro Pizzarossa and Rishita Nandagiri, "Self-Managed Abortion: A Constellation of Actors, a Cacophony of Laws?," *Sexual and Reproductive Health Matters* 29, no. 1 (2021): 23.

19. Models adapted from Jordan Parsons and Elizabeth Chloe Romanis, *Early Medical Abortion, Equality of Access, and the Telemedical Imperative* (Oxford: Oxford University Press, 2021), 107.

20. See, e.g., Paul Raekstad and Sofa Gradin, *Prefigurative Politics: Building Tomorrow Today* (Bristol: Polity Press, 2020).

21. Author interview with Polish activist and educator, working on abortion access and stigma, 2019 (PL519B).

22. Verónica Undurraga, "Criminalisation under Scrutiny: How Constitutional Courts Are Changing Their Narrative by Using Public Health Evidence in Abortion Cases," *Sexual and Reproductive Health Matters* 27, no. 1 (2019): 41–51.

23. Mariana Prandini Assis, "Liberating Abortion Pills in Legally Restricted Settings: Activism as Public Criminology," in *Routledge Handbook of Public Criminologies*, ed. Kathryn Henne and Rita Shah (London: Routledge, 2020), 120–30; Elyse Ona Singer, "Realizing Abortion Rights at the Margins of Legality in Mexico," *Medical Anthropology* 38, no. 2 (2018): 167–81.

24. Fabiola Orihuela-Cortés and Ma Luisa Marván, "Estigma hacia el aborto y sus consecuencias: Acciones para reducirlo," *Revista Digital Universitaria* 22, no. 4 (2021): 1–12.

25. Mónica Tarducci, "Escenas claves de la lucha por el derecho al aborto en Argentina," *Salud Colectiva* 14 (2018): 425–32.

26. Marina Sitrin, *Everyday Revolutions: Horizontalism and Autonomy in Argentina* (London: Zed Books, 2012); Máiréad Enright and Emilie Cloatre, "Transformative

Illegality: How Condoms 'Became Legal' in Ireland, 1991–1993," *Feminist Legal Studies* 26, no. 3 (2018): 261–84.

27. Michelle Oberman, *Her Body, Our Laws: On the Front Lines of the Abortion War, from El Salvador to Oklahoma* (Boston, MA: Beacon Press, 2018).

28. Mala Htun, *Sex and the State: Abortion, Divorce, and the Family under Latin American Dictatorships and Democracies* (Cambridge: Cambridge University Press, 2003).

29. Enright and Cloatre, "Transformative Illegality," 279.

30. Carol Smart, *Feminism and the Power of Law* (London: Routledge, 2002).

31. Sally Sheldon, *Beyond Control: Medical Power and Abortion Law* (London: Pluto Press, 1997).

32. See, e.g., Ben Kasstan and Maya Unnithan, "Arbitrating Abortion: Sex-Selection and Care Work among Abortion Providers in England," *Medical Anthropology* 39, no. 6 (2020): 491–505.

33. Jennifer Nelson, *More Than Medicine: A History of the Feminist Women's Health Movement* (New York: New York University Press, 2015).

34. Loretta Ross and Rickie Solinger, *Reproductive Justice: An Introduction* (Berkeley: University of California Press, 2017).

35. Zakiya Luna and Kristin Luker, "Reproductive Justice," *Annual Review of Law and Social Science* 9 (2013): 338.

36. Máiréad Enright, Kathryn McNeilly, and Fiona de Londras, "Abortion Activism, Legal Change, and Taking Feminist Law Work Seriously," *Northern Ireland Legal Quarterly* 71 (2020): 359–85.

37. Sheila Jasanoff, *Science at the Bar: Law, Science, and Technology in America* (Cambridge, MA: Harvard University Press, 1997).

38. Chikako Takeshita, *The Global Biopolitics of the IUD: How Science Constructs Contraceptive Users and Women's Bodies* (Cambridge, MA: MIT Press, 2012), 18.

39. Sally Sheldon, "The Medical Framework and Early Medical Abortion in the U.K.: How Can a State Control Swallowing?," in *Abortion Law in Transnational Perspective: Cases and Controversies*, ed. Rebecca Cook, Joanna Erdman and Bernard Dickens (Philadelphia: University of Pennsylvania Press, 2014), 193.

40. Jelinska and Yanow, "Putting Pills into Women's Hands," 87.

41. Margaret MacDonald, "Misoprostol: The Social Life of a Life-Saving Drug in Global Maternal Health," *Science, Technology, & Human Values* 46, no. 2 (2021): 376–401.

42. Silvia de Zordo, "The Biomedicalisation of Illegal Abortion: The Double Life of Misoprostol in Brazil," *História, Ciências, Saúde-Manguinhos* 23, no. 1 (2016): 30.

43. Julia McReynolds-Pérez, "No Doctors Required: Lay Activist Expertise and Pharmaceutical Abortion in Argentina," *Signs* 42, no. 2 (2017): 349–75.

44. Jelinska and Yanow, "Putting Pills into Women's Hands," 87; de Zordo, "The Biomedicalisation of Illegal Abortion."

45. Siri Suh, *Dying to Count: Post-Abortion Care and Global Reproductive Health Politics in Senegal* (New Brunswick, NJ: Rutgers University Press, 2021).

46. MacDonald, "Misoprostol."

47. Andrew Weeks, Christian Fiala, and Peter Safar, "Misoprostol and the Debate over Off-Label Drug Use," *BJOG: An International Journal of Obstetrics & Gynaecology* 112, no. 3 (2005): 269–72.

48. Adele Clarke and Theresa Montini, "The Many Faces of Ru486: Tales of Situated Knowledges and Technological Contestations," *Science, Technology, & Human Values* 18, no. 1 (1993): 42–78.

49. Greer Donley, "Medication Abortion Exceptionalism," *Cornell Law Review* 107 (2021): 627–704.

50. Nina Zamberlin, Mariana Romero, and Silvina Ramos, "Latin American Women's Experiences with Medical Abortion in Settings Where Abortion Is Legally Restricted," *Reproductive Health* 9, no. 1 (2012): 3.

51. Raquel Drovetta, "Safe Abortion Information Hotlines: An Effective Strategy for Increasing Women's Access to Safe Abortions in Latin America," *Reproductive Health Matters* 23, no. 45 (2015): 47–57.

52. Singer, "Realizing Abortion Rights at the Margins."

53. McReynolds-Pérez, "No Doctors Required," 357–59.

54. Pizzarossa and Nandagiri, "Self-Managed Abortion."

55. Donna Haraway, "The Virtual Speculum in the New World Order," *Feminist Review* 55, no. 1 (1997): 22–72.

56. Dorothy Roberts, *Killing the Black Body: Race, Reproduction, and the Meaning of Liberty* (New York: Vintage, 2014); Besty Hartmann, *Reproductive Rights and Wrongs: The Global Politics of Population Control* (Boston, MA: South End Press, 1995); Michelle Murphy, *Seizing the Means of Reproduction: Entanglements of Feminism, Health, and Technoscience* (Durham, NC: Duke University Press, 2012); Takeshita, *The Global Biopolitics of the IUD*.

57. Jennifer Nelson, *Women of Color and the Reproductive Rights Movement* (New York: New York University Press, 2003); Nelson, *More Than Medicine*.

58. Heather Munro Prescott, *The Morning After: A History of Emergency Contraception in the United States* (New Brunswick, NJ: Rutgers University Press, 2011).

59. Jennifer Denbow, *Governed Through Choice: Autonomy, Technology, and the Politics of Reproduction* (New York: New York University Press, 2015); Clarke and Montini, "The Many Faces of Ru486," 59–63.

60. Haraway, "The Virtual Speculum," 39.

61. See, e.g., David Cohen and Carole Joffe, *Obstacle Course: The Everyday Struggle to Get an Abortion in America* (Oakland: University of California Press, 2020). By contrast, scholarship on Latin America, where surgical abortion is unavailable and abortion travel is rare, has focused on medication abortion through support networks and hotlines for misoprostol-only abortion.

62. Carlo Inverardi-Ferri, "Towards a Cultural Political Economy of the Illicit," *Progress in Human Geography* 45, no. 6 (2021): 1646–67.

63. Nicky Gregson and Mike Crang, "Illicit Economies: Customary Illegality, Moral Economies and Circulation," *Transactions of the Institute of British Geographers* 42, no. 2 (2017): 206–19.

64. Alexandra Hall and Georgios Antonopoulos, *Fake Meds Online: The Internet and the Transnational Market in Illicit Pharmaceuticals* (New York: Springer, 2016).

65. Mathieu Quet, "Values in Motion: Anti-Counterfeiting Measures and the Securitization of Pharmaceutical Flows," *Journal of Cultural Economy* 10, no. 2 (2017): 150–62; Julia Hornberger, "From Drug Safety to Drug Security: A Contemporary Shift in the Policing of Health," *Medical Anthropology Quarterly* 32, no. 3 (2018): 365–83.

66. Natalie Rhodes and Remco van de Pas, "Mapping Buyer's Clubs: What Role Do They Play in Achieving Equitable Access to Medicines?," *Global Public Health* 17, no. 9 (2022): 1842–53.

67. Steven Epstein, *Impure Science: AIDS, Activism, and the Politics of Knowledge* (Berkeley: University of California Press, 1996); Sarah Schulman, *Let the Record Show: A Political History of Act Up New York, 1987–1993* (New York: Farrar, Straus and Giroux, 2021).

68. Mathieu Quet, "Pharmaceutical Capitalism and Its Logistics: Access to Hepatitis C Treatment," *Theory, Culture & Society* 35, no. 2 (2018): 76.

69. Quet, "Pharmaceutical Capitalism," 79.

70. Gail Kligman, *The Politics of Duplicity: Controlling Reproduction in Ceausescu's Romania* (Berkeley: University of California Press, 1998).

71. Irene Maffi, "The Production of Ignorance about Medication Abortion in Tunisia: Between State Policies, Medical Opposition, Patriarchal Logics and Islamic Revival," *Reproductive Biomedicine & Society Online* 14 (2022): 111–20; Sally Sheldon, "Empowerment and Privacy? Home Use of Abortion Pills in the Republic of Ireland," *Signs* 43, no. 4 (2018 2018): 823–49.

72. Cordelia Freeman and Sandra Rodriguez, "Not Knowing, Silence and Concealment: Strategic Ignorance in Abortion Practices in Latin America" (Paper presented at the Abortion + SRH Seminar Series, London School of Economics, March 9, 2022).

73. Barbara Sutton, "Zonas de clandestinidad y 'nuda vida': Mujeres, cuerpo y aborto," *Revista Estudos Feministas* 25 (2017): 889–902.

74. Silvia de Zordo and Joanna Mishtal, "Physicians and Abortion: Provision, Political Participation and Conflicts on the Ground—the Cases of Brazil and Poland," *Women's Health Issues* 21, no. 3 (2011): S32–S36; Suh, *Dying to Count*; de Zordo, "The Biomedicalization of Illegal Abortion."

75. Natalie Kimball, *An Open Secret: The History of Unwanted Pregnancy and Abortion in Modern Bolivia* (New Brunswick, NJ: Rutgers University Press, 2020).

76. Linsey McGoey, *The Unknowers: How Strategic Ignorance Rules the World* (London: Bloomsbury, 2019).

77. Anuradha Kumar, Leila Hessini, and Ellen Mitchell, "Conceptualising Abortion Stigma," *Culture, Health & Sexuality* 11, no. 6 (2009): 625–39.

78. Robert Proctor, "Agnotology: A Missing Term to Describe the Cultural Production of Ignorance (and Its Study)," in *Agnotology: The Making and Unmaking of Ignorance*, ed. Robert Proctor and Londa Schiebinger (Stanford, CA: Stanford University Press, 2008), 1–33.

79. Michael Taussig, *Defacement: Public Secrecy and the Labor of the Negative* (Stanford, CA: Stanford University Press, 1999), 50.

80. The exception to this is a set of covert interviews carried out with abortion pill providers in Poland, in which my research assistant made phone calls posing as an abortion seeker.

81. For a discussion of some of the ethical issues, see Jesper Andreasson and Thomas Johansson, "Online Doping: The New Self-Help Culture of Ethnopharmacology," *Sport in Society* 19, no. 7 (2016): 957–72.

82. Author interview with a founder of Women Help Women, 2018 (T1118).

83. Author interview with a volunteer on the Women on Web help desk, 2019 (T819A); Author interview with a doctor who works as a medical supervisor for Women on Web, 2019 (T719B); Author interview with an activist who leads a transnational pill network, 2019 (USA819); Interview T1118.

84. See, e.g., McReynolds Perez, "No Doctors Required"; Drovetta, "Safe Abortion Information Hotlines"; Singer, "Medication Abortion at the Margins"; de Zordo, "The Biomedicalisation of Illegal Abortion"; Assis, "Liberating Abortion Pills."

CHAPTER I. HOW INDIAN ABORTION PILLS TRAVEL THE GLOBE

1. See, e.g., Hall and Antonopoulos, *Fake Meds Online*.

2. Gregson and Crang, "Illicit Economies," 213.

3. Beatrice Couzinet et al., "Termination of Early Pregnancy by the Progesterone Antagonist Ru 486 (Mifepristone)," *New England Journal of Medicine* 315, no. 25 (1986): 1565–70.

4. Peter Hall, "What Has Been Achieved, What Have Been the Constraints and What Are the Future Priorities for Pharmaceutical Product-Related R&D Relevant to the Reproductive Health Needs of Developing Countries?" (World Health Organisation Commission on Intellectual Property Rights, Innovation and Public Health, Geneva, 2005).

5. Étienne-Émile Baulieu and Mort Rosenblum, *The "Abortion Pill": Ru-486, a Woman's Choice* (New York: Simon and Schuster, 1991).

6. Clarke and Montini, "The Many Faces of Ru486," 57.

7. Guttmacher Institute, *Abortion Worldwide*, 25.

8. Gynuity Health Projects, "Mifepristone Approvals" (New York, 2017), https://gynuity.org/assets/resources/biblio_ref_lst_mife_en.pdf, last updated October 2021.

9. PharmaLetter, "Indian Mifepristone Production," *ThePharmaLetter*, December 7, 1992, https://www.thepharmaletter.com/article/indian-mifepristone-production.

10. Kaushik Sunder Rajan, *Pharmocracy: Value, Politics, and Knowledge in Global Biomedicine* (Durham, NC: Duke University Press, 2017).

11. Kalpana Tyagi, "Mergers between Generics: How Competition Commission of India Promotes Innovation and Access through Merger Control," *Global Antitrust Review*, no. 11 (2018): 33–59; Shamim Mondal and Viswanath Pingali, "Competition and Intellectual Property Policies in the Indian Pharmaceutical Sector," *Vikalpa* 42, no. 2 (2017): 61–79.

12. Sudip Chaudhuri, "The Pharmaceutical Industry in India after TRIPS," in *The New Political Economy of Pharmaceuticals: Production, Innovation and Trips in the Global South*, ed. Hans Lofgren and Owen Williams (London: Palgrave Macmillan, 2003), 111–25.

13. Rajan, *Pharmocracy*, 193–98.

14. Both products were reverse-engineered at the Indian Institute of Chemical Technology under A. V. Rama Rao.

15. Timothy Powell-Jackson et al., "Delivering Medical Abortion at Scale: A Study of the Retail Market for Medical Abortion in Madhya Pradesh, India," *PLOS ONE* 10, no. 3 (2015): e0120637; Tania Boler et al., *Medical Abortion in India: A Model for the Rest of the World* (London: Marie Stopes International, 2009).

16. Laura Frye et al., "A Cross-Sectional Analysis of Mifepristone, Misoprostol, and Combination Mifepristone-Misoprostol Package Inserts Obtained in 20 Countries," *Contraception* 101, no. 5 (2020): 315–20.

17. Susheela Singh et al., *Abortion and Unintended Pregnancy in Six Indian States: Findings and Implications for Policies and Programs* (New York: Guttmacher Institute, 2018); Powell-Jackson et al., "Delivering Medical Abortion at Scale."

18. The Medical Termination of Pregnancy Act of 1971 allowed abortion up to twenty weeks of pregnancy for a range of medical and socioeconomic reasons, certified by a doctor. Its rules have since been amended to increase the gestational age limit and remove some restrictions.

19. Dipika Jain, "Time to Rethink Criminalisation of Abortion? Towards a Gender Justice Approach," *National University of Juridical Sciences Law Review* 12 (2019): 21.

20. Chandrasekar et al., *Availability of Medical Abortion Drugs*.

21. Aradhana Srivastava et al., "Pathways to Seeking Medication Abortion Care: A Qualitative Research in Uttar Pradesh, India," *PLOS ONE* 14, no. 5 (2019): e0216738; Boler et al., *Medical Abortion in India*; Powell-Jackson et al., "Delivering Medical Abortion at Scale."

22. V. S. Chandrashekar, D. Choudhuri, and A. Vajpeyi, *Availability of Medical Abortion Drugs in the Markets of Six Indian States* (New Delhi: Foundation for Reproductive Health Services India, 2020).

23. Ann Moore, Alyssa Browne, and Suzanne Bell, "Capturing Medical Methods of Abortion Sales Data in India" (Population Association of America, 2018).

24. Rishita Nandagiri, "'Like a Mother-Daughter Relationship': Community Health Intermediaries' Knowledge of and Attitudes to Abortion in Karnataka, India," *Social Science & Medicine* 239 (2019): 112525.

25. Kalpana Wilson, "In the Name of Reproductive Rights: Race, Neoliberalism and the Embodied Violence of Population Policies," *New Formations* 91 (2017): 50–68.

26. Ryo Yokoe et al., "Unsafe Abortion and Abortion-Related Death among 1.8 million Women in India," *BMJ Global Health* 4, no. 3 (2019): e001491.

27. Chandrasekar et al., *Availability of Medical Abortion Drugs.*

28. Author interview with an abortion and contraception activist based in the southern state of Tamil Nadu, 2022 (IN822).

29. Interview IN822.

30. Jeremy Greene, *Generic: The Unbranding of Modern Medicine* (Baltimore: Johns Hopkins University Press, 2014), 225.

31. Rory Horner and James Murphy, "South-North and South-South Production Networks: Diverging Socio-Spatial Practices of Indian Pharmaceutical Firms," *Global Networks* 18, no. 2 (2018): 326–51; Rajan, *Pharmocracy.*

32. Tyagi, "Mergers between Generics," 33.

33. Rory Horner, "Pharmaceuticals and the Global South: A Healthy Challenge for Development Theory?," *Geography Compass* 10, no. 9 (2016): 363–77; Rory Horner, "Strategic Decoupling, Recoupling and Global Production Networks: India's Pharmaceutical Industry," *Journal of Economic Geography* 14, no. 6 (2014): 1117–40.

34. Greene, *Generic,* 254–55; Horner and Murphy, "South-North and North-South."

35. Horner, "Strategic Decoupling."

36. Nupur Chowdhury et al., *Administrative Structure and Functions of Drug Regulatory Authorities in India* (New Delhi: Indian Council for Research on International Economic Relations, 2015).

37. Jerin Jose Cherian et al., "India's Road to Independence in Manufacturing Active Pharmaceutical Ingredients: Focus on Essential Medicines," *Economies* 9, no. 2 (2021): 1–18.

38. Hall, "What Has Been Achieved."

39. Research assistant interview with managing partner of an Indian firm that manufactures MTP kits for the domestic market, based in Punjab state, 2021 (IN621B).

40. Research assistant interview with employee of an Indian firm that manufactures MTP kits for the domestic market, based in Maharashtra state, 2021 (IN621C).

41. Research assistant interview with operations head of an Indian firm that manufactures MTP kits for the domestic market, based in Punjab state, 2021 (IN621A).

42. Chloe Murtagh et al., "Exploring the Feasibility of Obtaining Mifepristone and Misoprostol from the Internet," *Contraception* 97, no. 4 (2018): 287–91.

43. Murtagh et al., "Exploring the Feasibility of Obtaining Mifepristone."

44. Hall and Antonopoulos, *Fake Meds Online,* 16.

45. Nils Gilman, Jesse Goldhammer, and Steven Weber, *Deviant Globalization: Black Market Economy in the 21st Century* (London: A&C Black, 2011); Saskia Sassen, "Towards a Sociology of Information Technology," *Current Sociology* 50, no. 3 (2002): 365–88; Gregson and Crang, "Illicit Economies."

46. Deborah Cowen, *The Deadly Life of Logistics: Mapping Violence in Global Trade* (Minneapolis: University of Minnesota Press, 2014).

47. Hall and Antonopoulos, *Fake Meds Online,* 83–87.

48. Gregson and Crang, "Illicit Economies," 212.

49. Their practices have also been publicized in US courts, after Rebecca Gomperts sued the US Department of Health and Human Services for seizing pill shipments entering the US and for blocking access to third-party payment platforms.

50. Juliette Jowit and Aparna Pallavi, "From Nagpur to Northern Ireland: Pill Pipeline Helping Women Get Round Abortion Laws," *The Guardian*, January 26, 2016, https://www.theguardian.com/world/2016/jan/06/nagpur-to-northern-ireland-pill-pipeline-helping-women-get-round-abortion-ban.

51. Snehlata Shrivastav, "'When the Pill Reaches Women on Time, I Am Happy,'" *Times of India*, March 16, 2016, https://timesofindia.indiatimes.com/city/nagpur/when-the-pill-reaches-women-on-time-i-am-happy/articleshow/51376696.cms.

52. Author interview with the president of US-based international marketer and manufacturer of sexual and reproductive health supplies, 2021 (USA621).

53. Sarah Hodges, "The Case of the 'Spurious Drugs Kingpin': Shifting Pills in Chennai, India," *Critical Public Health* 29, no. 4 (2019): 473–83.

54. Andrea Di Nicola et al., "Fakecare: Developing Expertise against the Online Trade of Fake Medicines by Producing and Disseminating Knowledge, Counterstrategies and Tools across the EU" (eCrime Research Reports, Trento, Italy, 2015).

55. Veena Das and Ranendra Das, "Urban Health and Pharmaceutical Consumption in Delhi, India," *Journal of Biosocial Science* 38, no. 1 (2006): 69–82.

56. Rosalind Miller et al., "When Technology Precedes Regulation: The Challenges and Opportunities of E-Pharmacy in Low-Income and Middle-Income Countries," *BMJ Global Health* 6, no. 5 (2021): e005405.

57. Vicky Pathare, "MTP Kits at Home," *Pune Mirror*, May 6, 2021, https://punemirror.com/pune/cover-story/mtp-kits-at-home/cid5084614.htm.

58. Research assistant interview with enforcement official of the Food and Drug Control Administration of Maharashtra state, 2021 (IN821A).

59. Hodges, "The Case of the 'Spurious Drugs Kingpin.'"

60. Quet, "Values in Motion," 157.

61. Nishpriha Thakur, "Sub-Standard or Sub-Legal? India's International Pharmaceutical Traders and the Problem of Fake Drugs," *Medical Anthropology Theory* (forthcoming 2023); Emilia Sanabria, *Plastic Bodies: Sex Hormones and Menstrual Suppression in Brazil* (Durham, NC: Duke University Press, 2016).

62. Research assistant interview with enforcement official of the Food and Drug Control Administration of Maharashtra state, 2021 (IN821B).

63. See, e.g., Kanchan Srivastava, "Abortion Kits' Demand Spiked Amid Pandemic Fuelling Illegal Sale & Black Marketing, Amazon Gets FDA Notice," *The Dialogue*, June 23, 2021, https://thedialogue.co.in/article/tRP6NqKmNukFnd4j8fo3/abortion-kits-demand-spiked-amid-pandemic-fuelling-illegal-sale-black-marketing-amazon-gets-fda-notice; Rupsa Chakraborty, "Rampant Illegal Sale of Abortion Pills across Maharashtra," *Hindustan Times*, August 21, 2021, https://www.hindustantimes.com/cities/mumbai-news/rampant-illegal-sale-of-abortion-pills-across-maharashtra-101629570130655.html; Pathare, "MTP Kits at Home."

64. Hornberger, "From Drug Safety," 373.

65. Navtej Purewal, "Sex Selective Abortion, Neoliberal Patriarchy and Structural Violence in India," *Feminist Review* 119, no. 1 (2018): 20–38.

66. Times News Network, "Gujarat: 8 Held for Illegal E-Sales of Pregnancy Termination Kits," *Times of India*, June 13, 2021, https://timesofindia.indiatimes.com /city/ahmedabad/8-held-for-illegal-e-sales-of-pregnancy-termination-kits/article-show/83470052.cms.

67. Press Trust of India, "Over 24,000 Abortion Kits Worth ₹1.5 Crore Seized in Gujarat; 8 Arrested," NDTV, June 14, 2021, https://www.ndtv.com/india-news /over-24-000-abortion-kits-worth-rs-1-5-crore-seized-in-gujarat-8-arrested-2463114.

68. FDA, Warning Letter: Rablon Marcs-Cms 111111, Maryland, USA, August 3, 2019.

69. I made many efforts to contact Rablon's owners and employees for interviews, but they were unwilling to participate.

70. I collected data on 114 online pharmacy websites. I carried out a detailed analysis of the sites that were primarily dedicated to selling abortion pills or that sold abortion pills among other products (n = 29).

71. Hall and Antonopoulos, *Fake Meds Online*, 28–43.

72. Murtagh et al., "Exploring the Feasibility of Obtaining Mifepristone."

73. Hall and Antonopoulos, *Fake Meds Online*, 28–43.

74. Di Nicola et al., "Fakecare," 48.

75. I did not order or test the products from this site. However, following Murtagh et al.'s study, it is important to note that the brands advertised on illicit pharmacy websites regularly differ from the brands of the products actually sent to buyers. See Murtagh et al., "Exploring the Feasibility of Obtaining Mifepristone."

76. International Planned Parenthood Federation, "Medical Abortion Commodities Database" (London, 2021), https://www.medab.org/.

77. Murtagh et al., "Exploring the Feasibility of Obtaining Mifepristone," 289.

CHAPTER 2. ABORTION PILLS IN US CLINICS AND LAWS

1. Gayle Rubin, "The Traffic in Women: Notes on the 'Political Economy' of Sex," in *Toward an Anthropology of Women*, ed. Rayna Reiter (New York: Monthly Review Press, 1975), 160.

2. Rosalind Petchesky, *Abortion and Woman's Choice: The State, Sexuality, and Reproductive Freedom* (New York: Longman, 1984), 291–92.

3. Mary Ziegler, "Sexing Harris: The Law and Politics of the Movement to Defund Planned Parenthood," *Buffalo Law Review* 60 (2012): 701–48.

4. Ross and Solinger, *Reproductive Justice*.

5. Robin West, "From Choice to Reproductive Justice: De-Constitutionalizing Abortion Rights," *Yale Law Journal* 118 (2008): 1415.

6. Mary Ziegler, "After Life: Governmental Interests and the New Antiabortion Incrementalism," *University of Miami Law Review* 73, no. 1 (2018): 78–138.

7. Reva Siegel, "The Right's Reasons: Constitutional Conflict and the Spread of Woman-Protective Antiabortion Argument," *Duke Law Journal* 57 (2008): 1641–92.

8. Paul Saurette and Kelly Gordon, *The Changing Voice of the Anti-Abortion Movement: The Rise of "Pro-Woman" Rhetoric in Canada and the United States* (Toronto: University of Toronto Press, 2016).

9. Carol Sanger, *About Abortion: Terminating Pregnancy in Twenty-First-Century America* (Cambridge, MA: Harvard University Press, 2017), 33.

10. Luna and Luker, "Reproductive Justice," 338.

11. Ross and Solinger, *Reproductive Justice*; West, "From Choice," 1394; Dorothy Roberts, "Reproductive Justice, Not Just Rights," *Dissent* 62, no. 4 (2015): 79–82.

12. Dobbs v. Jackson Women's Health Organization, 597 U.S. _____ (2022), 44 and 25.

13. Dobbs v. Jackson Women's Health Organization, 65.

14. Melissa Haussman, *Reproductive Rights and the State: Getting the Birth Control, Ru-486, and Morning-After Pills and the Gardasil Vaccine to the U.S. Market* (Santa Barbara, CA: ABC-CLIO, 2013), 111–13.

15. Carole Joffe and Tracy Weitz, "Normalizing the Exceptional: Incorporating the 'Abortion Pill' into Mainstream Medicine," *Social Science & Medicine* 56, no. 12 (2003): 2353–66; Clarke and Montini, "The Many Faces of Ru486."

16. Jennifer Jackman, "Anatomy of a Feminist Victory," *Women & Politics* 24, no. 3 (2002): 81–99; Carole Joffe, "Abortion and Medicine: A Sociopolitical History," in *Management of Unintended and Abnormal Pregnancy*, ed. Maureen Paul et al. (Hoboken, NJ: John Wiley, 2009).

17. Mary Ziegler, *Abortion and the Law in America: Roe v. Wade to the Present* (Cambridge: Cambridge University Press, 2020), 160.

18. Sydney Calkin, "Towards a Political Geography of Abortion," *Political Geography* 69 (2019): 22–29.

19. Linda Greenhouse and Reva Siegel, "*Casey* and the Clinic Closings: When Protecting Health Obstructs Choice," *Yale Law Journal* 125 (2016 2016): 1428.

20. Wendy Simonds et al., "Abortion, Revised: Participants in the U.S. Clinical Trials Evaluate Mifepristone," *Social Science & Medicine* 46, no. 10 (1998): 1313–23.

21. Jackman, "Anatomy," 85.

22. Clarke and Montini, "The Many Faces of Ru486," 58.

23. Mary Ziegler, *After Roe: The Lost History of the Abortion Debate* (Cambridge, MA: Harvard University Press, 2015).

24. Haussman, *Reproductive Rights*, 100–105.

25. Mary Ziegler, "The Jurisprudence of Uncertainty: Knowledge, Science, and Abortion," *Wisconsin Law Review* (2018): 317–68.

26. Epstein, *Impure Science*, 6.

27. Ziegler, *After Roe*, 179–80; Ziegler, "The Jurisprudence of Uncertainty," 348–52.

28. Csilla Muhl, "Ru-486: Legal and Policy Issues Confronting the Food and Drug Administration," *Journal of Legal Medicine* 14, no. 2 (1993): 319–47.

29. Haussman, *Reproductive Rights*, 106; Jackman, "Anatomy," 89.

30. Haussman, *Reproductive Rights*, 108–11.

31. Eli Adashi et al., "The Next Two Decades of Mifepristone at FDA: History as Destiny," *Contraception* 109 (2022): 1–7.

32. Clarke and Montini, "The Many Faces of Ru486," 53–55.

33. Munro Prescott, *The Morning After*, 80–81.

34. Nelson, *More Than Medicine*.

35. Joffe and Weitz, "Normalizing the Exceptional," 2355; Haussman, *Reproductive Rights*, 110.

36. CBS News, "Abortion Pill Maker Revealed," October 13, 2000, https://www.cbsnews.com/news/abortion-pill-maker-revealed/.

37. The patent holder of misoprostol, Searle, lobbied to prevent any American companies from making mifepristone before the misoprostol patent ran out in 2000. See Haussman, *Reproductive Rights*, 99–103.

38. Donley, "Early Abortion," 22–25.

39. Joffe and Weitz, "Normalizing the Exceptional."

40. Adashi et al., "The Next Two Decades of Mifepristone," 3.

41. Megan Donovan, "Self-Managed Medication Abortion: Expanding the Available Options for US Abortion Care," *Guttmacher Policy Review* 21 (2018): 41–47; Rachel Jones et al., "Press Release: Medication Abortion Now Accounts for More Than Half of All US Abortions," Guttmacher Institute, February 24, 2022, https://www.guttmacher.org/print/article/2022/02/medication-abortion-now-accounts-more-half-all-us-abortions

42. Ziegler, *Abortion and the Law*, 188.

43. Ziegler, *Abortion and the Law*, 191.

44. Sydney Calkin, "Legal Geographies of Medication Abortion in the USA," *Transactions of the Institute of British Geographers* 47, no. 2 (2022): 378–92.

45. Anna Franzonello, "Confronting Chemical Abortions: The Abortion Industry's Newest Threat to Women's Health," in *Defending Life 2012: Building a Culture of Life, Deconstructing the Abortion Industry*, ed. Americans United for Life (Washington, DC: Americans United for Life, 2012), 58.

46. Ziegler, *Abortion and the Law*; Ziegler, "After Life."

47. Christopher Wittich, Christopher Burkle, and William Lanier, "Ten Common Questions (and Their Answers) about Off-Label Drug Use," *Mayo Clinic Proceedings* 87 (2012): 983.

48. Heather Boonstra, "Medication Abortion Restrictions Burden Women and Providers—and Threaten U.S. Trend toward Very Early Abortion," *Guttmacher Policy Review* 16, no. 1 (2013): 18–23.

49. Daniel Grossman et al., "Effectiveness and Acceptability of Medical Abortion Provided through Telemedicine," *Obstetrics & Gynecology* 118, no. 2 (2011): 296–303.

50. Elizabeth Raymond, Erica Chong, and Paul Hyland, "Increasing Access to Abortion with Telemedicine," *JAMA Internal Medicine* 176, no. 5 (2016): 585–86.

51. Cheryl Sullenger, "Special Report: 'Telemed Abortions' Endanger Women and Drive Up Insurance Costs," *Operation Rescue*, March 29, 2010, https://www .operationrescue.org/archives/special-report-telemed-abortions-endanger-women-and-drive-up-insurance-costs/.

52. Kristin Garrett and Joshua Jansa, "Interest Group Influence in Policy Diffusion Networks," *State Politics & Policy Quarterly* 15, no. 3 (2015): 402.

53. Americans United for Life, *Defending Life 2012*, 64.

54. Americans United for Life, *Defending Life 2016: A State-by-State Legal Guide to Abortion, Bioethics, and the End of Life* (Washington, DC: Americans United for Life, 2016), 258.

55. Mary Tschann et al., "Changes to Medication Abortion Clinical Practices in Response to the Covid-19 Pandemic," *Contraception* 104, no. 1 (2021): 77–81; Ushma Upadhyay, Rosalyn Schroeder, and Sarah Roberts, "Adoption of No-Test and Tele-health Medication Abortion Care among Independent Abortion Providers in Response to Covid-19," *Contraception* 10, no. 2 (2020): 100049.

56. Texas Senate Bill 4 (2021), "relating to abortion . . .," https://capitol.texas.gov /tlodocs/872/billtext/html/SB00004F.HTM.

57. Mandatory counseling "may not be provided by audio or video recording and must be provided at least 24 hours before the abortion is to be performed" (Texas Rev. Code Title 2 § 171.001).

58. An up-to-date list is available through the Guttmacher policy tracker: https:// www.guttmacher.org/state-policy/explore/medication-abortion.

59. Grossman et al., "Effectiveness and Acceptability of Medical Abortion."

60. Caroline Mala Corbin, "Abortion Distortions," *Washington & Lee Law Review* 71 (2014): 1175–1210.

61. Indiana Code IC 16–34–2-1, Sec.1. (a).

62. Idaho Telehealth Access Act 54–5602 (1–5).

63. Idaho Telehealth Access Act 54–5607 (3).

64. Elizabeth Nash, "Ohio as a Window into Recent US Trends on Abortion Access and Restrictions," *American Journal of Public Health* 110, no. 8 (2020): 1115–16.

65. Nash, "Ohio as a Window," 1115–16.

66. Nash, "Ohio as a Window," 1115.

67. Data compiled by the author from Ohio Department of Health, *Induced Abortions in Ohio* annual reports, 2004–20, available at odh.ohio.gov.

68. Ohio Senate Bill 304 "Regards abortion-inducing drugs" as introduced on March 1, 2022, https://legiscan.com/OH/bill/SB304/2021.

69. "Heartbeat" laws like Ohio's ban abortion after fetal cardiac activity can be detected. This can be as early as five weeks, depending on the available technology.

70. ACLU of Ohio, "Legal Landscape of Abortion in Ohio," as of October 18, 2022, https://www.acluohio.org/en/legal-landscape-abortion-ohio.

71. Cohen et al., "The New Abortion Battleground," 11.

72. Mikaela Smith et al., "Abortion Travel within the United States: An Observational Study of Cross-State Movement to Obtain Abortion Care in 2017," *The Lancet Regional Health–Americas* 10 (2022): 100214.

73. Sabrina Tavernise, "New Illinois Abortion Clinic Anticipates Post-Roe World," *New York Times*, October 22, 2019, https://www.nytimes.com/2019/10/22/us/missouri-illinois-planned-parenthood.html.

74. Tessa Weinberg, "With Few In-State Abortions, Missouri Lawmakers Look toward a Post-Roe v. Wade Future," *Missouri Independent*, April 8, 2022, https://missouriindependent.com/2022/04/08/with-few-in-state-abortions-missouri-lawmakers-look-toward-a-post-roe-v-wade-future/.

75. Services like Abortion on Demand, Pills by Post, Carafem, MyAbortionNetwork, among others, offer no-touch telemedicine abortion up to eleven weeks through a model of digital consultation with clinician and medication abortion sent by mail.

76. There is legal uncertainty here, so different no-touch abortion providers interpret the law in different ways. Some do not treat patients who are not physically present in their state, while others treat anyone who gives a postal delivery address where pills can be legally supplied.

77. Cohen et al., "The New Abortion Battleground," 17; and see, e.g., Abortion on Demand, "Logistics: Do I Need to Live in the State Selected?," https://abortionondemand.org/faq/.

78. Example taken from Plan C's public information for pill seekers: https://www.plancpills.org/.

79. Abigail R. A. Aiken and Ushma Upadhyay, "The Future of Medication Abortion in a Post-Roe World," *BMJ* 377 (2022): o1393.

80. Carly Thomsen et al., "US Anti-Abortion Ideology on the Move: Mobile Crisis Pregnancy Centers as Unruly, Unmappable, and Ungovernable," *Political Geography* 92 (2022): 5.

81. Cohen et al., "The New Abortion Battleground."

82. Michele Statz and Lisa Pruitt, "To Recognize the Tyranny of Distance: A Spatial Reading of Whole Woman's Health v. Hellerstedt," *Environment and Planning A: Economy and Space* 51, no. 5 (2019): 1106–27.

83. Beverly Winikoff and Carolyn Westhoff, "Fifteen Years: Looking Back and Looking Forward," *Contraception* 92, no. 3 (2015): 178.

84. Whether a state can prosecute someone for providing (or seeking) an abortion out of state, and whether states could shield their abortion providers from such suits, is unclear and will no doubt be the subject of lawsuits for years to come. For a full discussion of the legal issues, see Cohen et al., "The New Abortion Battleground."

CHAPTER 3. HOW TO SELF-MANAGE ABORTION IN AMERICA

1. Rickie Solinger, *Beggars and Choosers: How the Politics of Choice Shapes Adoption, Abortion, and Welfare in the United States* (New York: Macmillan, 2001), 37.

2. Reagan, *When Abortion Was a Crime*, 70–76.

3. Reagan, *When Abortion Was a Crime*, 208.

4. Reagan, *When Abortion Was a Crime*, 138–39.

5. Solinger, *Beggars and Choosers*, 54–55.

6. Reagan, *When Abortion Was a Crime*, 137.

7. Kristin Luker, *Abortion and the Politics of Motherhood* (Berkeley: University of California Press, 1985), 55–57; Reagan, *When Abortion Was a Crime*, 204–5.

8. Murphy, *Seizing the Means*, 2.

9. Nelson, *More Than Medicine*, 13.

10. Wendy Kline, *Bodies of Knowledge: Sexuality, Reproduction, and Women's Health in the Second Wave* (Chicago: University of Chicago Press, 2010), 71–73; Reagan, *When Abortion Was a Crime*; Nelson, *More Than Medicine*.

11. Drovetta, "Safe Abortion Information," 49.

12. Murphy, *Seizing the Means*, 25–26, 155–59.

13. Murphy, *Seizing the Means*, 150.

14. Murphy, *Seizing the Means*, 65.

15. Murphy, *Seizing the Means*, 35.

16. Murphy, *Seizing the Means*, 62.

17. Petchesky, *Abortion and Woman's Choice*, 128.

18. Wendy Simonds, *Abortion at Work: Ideology and Practice in a Feminist Clinic* (New Brunswick, NJ: Rutgers University Press, 1996).

19. Murphy, *Seizing the Means*, 63–64; Ziegler, *After Roe*; Simonds, *Abortion at Work*.

20. See, e.g., Abigail R. A. Aiken et al., "Motivations and Experiences of People Seeking Medication Abortion Online in the United States," *Perspectives on Sexual and Reproductive Health* 50, no. 4 (2018): 157–63.

21. Nathalie Kapp et al., "Developing a Forward-Looking Agenda and Methodologies for Research of Self-Use of Medical Abortion," *Contraception* 97, no. 2 (2018): 184–88.

22. Pizzarossa and Nandagiri, "Self-Managed Abortion."

23. Abigail R. A. Aiken et al., "Knowledge, Interest, and Motivations Surrounding Self-Managed Medication Abortion among Patients at Three Texas Clinics," *American Journal of Obstetrics and Gynecology* 223, no. 2 (2020): 238.e1–238.e10; Rachel Jones, "How Commonly Do US Abortion Patients Report Attempts to Self-Induce?," *American Journal of Obstetrics and Gynecology* 204, no. 1 (2011): 23; Daniel Grossman et al., "Knowledge, Opinion and Experience Related to Abortion Self-Induction in Texas," *Contraception* 4, no. 92 (2015): 360–61.

24. Rachel Jones, Elizabeth Witwer, and Jenna Jerman, *Abortion Incidence and Service Availability in the United States, 2017* (New York: Guttmacher Institute, 2019), 8; Jones, "How Commonly"; Aiken et al., "Knowledge, Interest"; Grossman et al., "Knowledge, Opinion."

25. Ushma Upadhyay, Alice Cartwright, and Daniel Grossman, "Barriers to Abortion Care and Incidence of Attempted Self-Managed Abortion among Individuals Searching Google for Abortion Care: A National Prospective Study," *Contraception* 106 (2022): 49–56.

26. Jenna Jerman, Tsuyoshi Onda, and Rachel Jones, "What Are People Looking for When They Google 'Self-Abortion'?," *Contraception* 97, no. 6 (2018): 510–14; Cynthia Conti-Cook, "Surveilling the Digital Abortion Diary," *University of Baltimore Law Review* 50 (2020): 1–50; Pizzarossa and Nanagiri, "Self-Managed Abortion."

27. Seth Stephens-Davidowitz, *Everybody Lies: What the Internet Can Tell Us about Who We Really Are* (London: Bloomsbury, 2018).

28. Elizabeth Nash and Joerg Dreweke, "The US Abortion Rate Continues to Drop: Once Again, State Abortion Restrictions Are Not the Main Driver," *Guttmacher Policy Review* 22 (2019): 41–45.

29. Diana Greene Foster, "Dramatic Decreases in US Abortion Rates: Public Health Achievement or Failure?," *American Journal of Public Health* 107, no. 12 (2017): 1861.

30. Foster, "Dramatic Decreases", 1861–62.

31. Kapp et al., "Developing a Forward-Looking Agenda."

32. Caitlin Myers, Rachel Jones, and Ushma Upadhyay, "Predicted Changes in Abortion Access and Incidence in a Post-Roe World," *Contraception* 100, no. 5 (2019): 367–73.

33. Diana Greene Foster, *The Turnaway Study: Ten Years, a Thousand Women, and the Consequences of Having—or Being Denied—an Abortion* (New York: Simon and Schuster, 2020).

34. Sheldon, "Empowerment and Privacy."

35. Freeman and Rodriguez, "Not Knowing."

36. Author interview with operator of an online abortion pill business, 2020 (US1020).

37. Interview US1020.

38. Author interview with US health activist and campaigner working on abortion pill pathways, 2018 (US1018); Author interview with US health activist and campaigner working on abortion pill pathways, 2018 (US1118); Interview USA819.

39. Interviews US1020, US1118, and T819B; see also Lizzie Presser, "Whatever's Your Darkest Question, You Can Ask Me," *California Sunday Magazine*, March 28, 2018, https://story.californiasunday.com/abortion-providers/.

40. I have taken steps to disguise the names and locations of all commenters. I have also reworded the texts slightly so that they are not searchable.

41. John Riddle, *Eve's Herbs: A History of Contraception and Abortion in the West* (Cambridge, MA: Harvard University Press, 1997).

42. McReynolds-Pérez, "No Doctors Required."

43. Author interview with US activist working on DIY medical technologies, including misoprostol, 2019 (US719).

44. Author interview with American living in a southeastern state who bought abortion pills online and used them to self-manage an abortion, 2020 (US520B).

45. Much of the conversation on self-managed abortion has moved to Reddit and Quora in recent years.

46. Aiken et al., "Demand for Self-Managed"; Aiken et al., "Knowledge, Interest"; Dana Johnson et al., "The Economic Context of Pursuing Online Medication Abortion in the United States," *SSM–Qualitative Research in Health* 1 (2021): 100003.

47. Jill Adams and Melissa Mikesell, "And Damned If They Don't: Prototype Theories to End Punitive Policies against Pregnant People Living in Poverty," *Georgetown Journal of Gender & Law* 18 (2017): 324.

48. Interview US1018.

49. Marie Bass, "Toward Coalition: The Reproductive Health Technologies Project," in *Abortion Wars: A Half Century of Struggle, 1950–2000*, ed. Rickie Solinger (Berkeley: University of California Press, 1998); Munro Prescott, *The Morning After*, 80–84.

50. Interviews US1018, US1118, and USA819.

51. See, e.g., comments by the Planned Parenthood of South Texas in Christina Cauterucci, "Why Did Planned Parenthood Halt Abortions in Oklahoma Before the Ban Went into Effect?," *Slate*, May 30, 2022, https://slate.com/news-and-politics/2022/05/planned-parenthood-oklahoma-texas-abortion-bans.html.

52. Author interview with US public health researcher and advocate for medication abortion provision, 2020 (US1220A); Interview US1018.

53. Interview US1118.

54. Olga Khazan, "Women in the U.S. Can Now Get Safe Abortions by Mail," *The Atlantic*, October 18, 2018, https://www.theatlantic.com/health/archive/2018/10/women-on-web-safe-abortion-mail/573322/.

55. Bazelon, "The Dawn of the Post-clinic Abortion."

56. Center for Drug Evaluation and Research, Food and Drug Administration, Warning Letter: Aidaccess.org MARCS-CMS 575658, Issued March 8, 2019; Gomperts vs. Azar et al., United States District Court for the District of Idaho, Case No. 1:19-cv-00345-DCN.

57. Cohen, Donley and Rebouche, "The New Abortion Battleground," 26–27.

58. Abigail R. A. Aiken et al., "Requests for Self-Managed Medication Abortion Provided Using Online Telemedicine in 30 US States before and after the Dobbs v Jackson Women's Health Organization Decision," *JAMA* 328, no. 17 (2022): 1768–70.

59. Elliott Foote, "Prescription Drug Importation: An Expanded FDA Personal Use Exemption and Qualified Regulators for Foreign-Produced Pharmaceuticals," *Loyola Consumer Law Review* 27 (2014): 369–98.

60. Thomas Bollyky and Aaron Kesselheim, "Reputation and Authority: The FDA and the Fight over US Prescription Drug Importation," *Vanderbilt Law Review* 73 (2020): 1343.

61. Peter Reichertz and Melinda Friend, "Hiding behind Agency Discretion: The Food and Drug Administration's Personal Use Drug Importation Policy," *Cornell Journal of Law & Public Policy* 9 (1999): 493–522.

62. Bollyky and Kesselheim, "Reputation and Authority."

63. Liz Hamel et al., "Public Opinion on Prescription Drugs and Their Prices," Kaiser Family Foundation, October 20, 2022, https://www.kff.org/health-costs/poll-finding/public-opinion-on-prescription-drugs-and-their-prices/.

64. Ashley Kirzinger et al., "Kaiser Health Tracking Poll: November 2016," Kaiser Family Foundation, December 1, 2016, https://www.kff.org/health-costs/poll-finding /kaiser-health-tracking-poll-november-2016/.

65. United States Senate, "Combating the Opioid Crisis: Exploiting Vulnerabilities in International Mail," Staff report for the Permanent Subcommittee on Investigations: Committee on Homeland Security and Governmental Affairs (2018), 23; Senate Permanent Subcommittee on Investigations of the Senate Committee on Homeland Security and Governmental Affairs, "Stopping the Shipment of Synthetic Opioids: Oversight of U.S. Strategy to Combat Illicit Drugs," Hearing, 115th Cong. (May 25, 2017), https:// www.c-span.org/video/?429049–1/senate-panel-stopping-flow-synthetic-drugs-us.

66. Jeff Karberg, "Progress in the Challenge to Regulate Online Pharmacies," *Journal of Law & Health* 23 (2010): 113–42.

67. Tammy Whitcomb, Acting Inspector General of the U.S. Postal Service, speaking at the Senate committee hearing "Stopping Flow of Synthetic Drugs" (May 27, 2017), https://www.c-span.org/video/?429049–1/senate-panel-stopping-flow-synthetic-drugs-us.

68. US Food and Drug Administration (USFDA), "U.S. Food and Drug Administration and the International Mail Facilities," updated April 2019, available at https:// www.fda.gov/media/111980/download.

69. Bryan Liang and Tim Mackey, "Online Availability and Safety of Drugs in Shortage: A Descriptive Study of Internet Vendor Characteristics," *Journal of Medical Internet Research* 14, no. 1 (2012): 11; Aaron Wong, "Money, Meet Mouth: The Era of Regulation and Prescription Drug Importation/Reimportation," *Health Law & Policy Brief* 4 (2010): 52.

70. USFDA, "U.S. Food and Drug Administration and the International Mail Facilities."

71. Lana Ivanitskaya et al., "Dirt Cheap and without Prescription: How Susceptible Are Young US Consumers to Purchasing Drugs from Rogue Internet Pharmacies?," *Journal of Medical Internet Research* 12, no. 2 (2010): e1520; Foote, "Prescription Drug"; Karberg, "Progress."

72. Rachel Roth, *Making Women Pay: The Hidden Costs of Fetal Rights* (Ithaca, NY: Cornell University Press, 2000).

73. Roberts, *Killing the Black Body*, 172.

74. See, e.g., Jonah Waterhouse, "The Creepy Ways Gilead in 'The Handmaid's Tale' Resembles Trump's America," *Elle Magazine*, June 29, 2018, https://www.elle .com.au/culture/handmaids-tale-gilead-america-17941.

75. Sophie Lewis, *Full Surrogacy Now: Feminism against Family* (London: Verso Books, 2021), 10.

76. Adams and Mikesell, "Damned If They Don't," 324.

77. Author interview with lawyer and advocate against criminalization of pregnant and abortion-seeking people, 2020 (US1220B).

78. Michele Goodwin, *Policing the Womb: Invisible Women and the Criminalization of Motherhood* (Cambridge: Cambridge University Press, 2020), 30.

79. Farah Diaz-Tello, Melissa Mikesell, and Jill E. Adams, *Roe's Unfinished Promise: Decriminalizing Abortion Once and for All* (Berkeley: University of California and the SIA Legal Team, 2018), 21.

80. Diaz-Tello et al., *Roe's Unfinished Promise*, 17–19.

81. Lynn Paltrow and Jeanne Flavin, "Arrests of and Forced Interventions on Pregnant Women in the United States, 1973–2005: Implications for Women's Legal Status and Public Health," *Journal of Health Politics, Policy and Law* 38, no. 2 (2013): 299–343.

82. Paltrow and Flavin, "Arrests of and Forced Interventions," 309–11.

83. Paltrow and Flavin, "Arrests of and Forced Interventions," 327.

84. Roberts, *Killing the Black Body*, 179.

85. Oberman, *Her Body*, 134.

86. If/When/How Lawyering for Reproductive Justice, "Brief of Experts, Researchers, and Advocates Opposing the Criminalization of People Who Have Abortions as Amici Curiae in Support Of Respondents," filed in *Dobbs vs. Jackson Women's Health Organization*, No. 19–1392, 2021.

87. Cohen et al., "The New Abortion Battleground," 30–31.

88. Missouri SB 603 "enacts provisions extending the laws of Missouri relating to abortion to certain conduct occurring outside the state" (2021).

89. Whitney Arey et al., "A Preview of the Dangerous Future of Abortion Bans—Texas Senate Bill 8," *New England Journal of Medicine* 387, no. 5 (2022): 388–90.

90. Missouri HB 2012 "modifies provisions relating to health care," Amendment 4488H03.01H (2022).

91. Missouri HB 1987 "modifies provisions relating to abortion" (2022).

92. Cohen et al., "The New Abortion Battleground."

CHAPTER 4. THE GEOGRAPHY OF CLANDESTINE
ABORTION IN POLAND

1. Lena Lennerhed, "Sherri Finkbine Flew to Sweden: Abortion and Disability in the Early 1960s," in *Abortion across Borders: Transnational Travel and Access to Abortion Services*, ed. Christabelle Sethna and Gayle Davis (Baltimore: Johns Hopkins University Press, 2019), 41–42.

2. Ewelina Ciaputa, "Abortion and the Catholic Church in Poland," in Sethna and Davis, *Abortion across Borders*, 289.

3. Barbara Einhorn, *Cinderella Goes to Market: Citizenship, Gender and Women's Movements in East Central Europe* (London: Verso, 1993), 75.

4. Ciaputa, "Abortion," 289; Einhorn, *Cinderella Goes to Market*, 86–88.

5. Susan Gal and Gail Kligman, *The Politics of Gender after Socialism: A Comparative-Historical Essay* (Princeton, NJ: Princeton University Press, 2000), 5.

6. Anna Grzymała-Busse, *Nations under God: How Churches Use Moral Authority to Influence Policy* (Princeton, NJ: Princeton University Press, 2015).

7. Atina Krajewska, "Rupture and Continuity: Abortion, the Medical Profession, and the Transitional State—a Polish Case Study," *Feminist Legal Studies* 29, no. 3 (2021): 340–41.

8. Sydney Calkin and Monika Ewa Kaminska, "Persistence and Change in Morality Policy: The Role of the Catholic Church in the Politics of Abortion in Ireland and Poland," *Feminist Review* 124, no. 1 (2020): 86–102.

9. Joanna Mishtal, *The Politics of Morality: The Church, the State, and Reproductive Rights in Postsocialist Poland* (Athens: Ohio University Press, 2015), 41–47.

10. Mishtal, *The Politics of Morality*, 47–9.

11. Grzymała-Busse, *Nations under God*, 158–59.

12. Agnieszka Król and Paula Pustułka, "Women on Strike: Mobilizing against Reproductive Injustice in Poland," *International Feminist Journal of Politics* 20, no. 3 (2018): 370.

13. Gail Kligman and Susan Gal, *Reproducing Gender: Politics, Publics, and Everyday Life after Socialism* (Princeton, NJ: Princeton University Press, 2000); Gal and Kligman, *The Politics of Gender*.

14. Magdalena Grabowska, "Bringing the Second World In: Conservative Revolution(s), Socialist Legacies, and Transnational Silences in the Trajectories of Polish Feminism," *Signs* 37, no. 2 (2012): 385–411.

15. Dorota Szelewa, "The Second Wave of Anti-Feminism? Post-Crisis Maternalist Policies and the Attack on the Concept of Gender in Poland," *Gender rovné příležitosti výzkum* 15, no. 2 (2014): 33–47.

16. Dorota Szelewa, "Killing 'Unborn Children'? The Catholic Church and Abortion Law in Poland since 1989," *Social & Legal Studies* 25, no. 6 (2016): 742.

17. United Nations Population Fund (UNFPA), "Report: Women's Health in Reproductive Age 15–49 Years, Poland 2006" (Polish Office of the United Nations Development Programme, Warsaw), 99–100.

18. Act on Family Planning, Human Embryo Protection, and Conditions for the Lawful Termination of Pregnancy of 1993; English translation available from the Center for Reproductive Rights, https://www.reproductiverights.org/sites/crr.civicactions.net/files/documents/Polish%20abortion%20act—English%20translation.pdf.

19. UNFPA, "Report: Women's Health in Reproductive Age," 99–100.

20. Mishtal, *The Politics of Morality*, 143.

21. Joanna Mishtal, "Neoliberal Reforms and Privatisation of Reproductive Health Services in Post-Socialist Poland," *Reproductive Health Matters* 18, no. 36 (2010): 56–66.

22. Agata Chełstowska, "Stigmatisation and Commercialisation of Abortion Services in Poland: Turning Sin into Gold," *Reproductive Health Matters* 19, no. 37 (2011): 102–3.

23. Mishtal, "Neoliberal Reforms," 61; Krajewska, "Rupture and Continuity," 337.

24. Ciaputa, "Abortion," 288–90.

25. Atina Krajewska, "Revisiting Polish Abortion Law: Doctors and Institutions in a Restrictive Regime," *Social & Legal Studies* (2021): 8.

26. Mishtal, *The Politics of Morality*, 143–50.

27. Author interview with Polish scholar and activist writing and campaigning on reproductive rights, 2019 (PL519C).

28. Author interview with activist and campaigner leading a local branch of a national women's rights group in a large Polish city, 2019 (PL618A); Mishtal, *The Politics of Morality*.

29. Mishtal, "Neoliberal Reforms," 58.

30. Krajewska, "Rupture and Continuity," 341–42.

31. Chełstowska, "Stigmatisation," 100.

32. De Zordo and Mishtal, "Physicians and Abortion," S33; Mishtal, "Neoliberal Reforms," 61.

33. Author interview with Polish activist and lawyer, working on abortion access, 2019 (PL519A); Author interview with Polish politician and campaigner who is a prominent advocate of abortion rights, 2020 (PL220B); Interview PL519B.

34. Chełstowska, "Stigmatisation," 103–4; Krajewska, "Revisiting Polish Abortion Law."

35. Joanna Mishtal, "Matters of 'Conscience': The Politics of Reproductive Healthcare in Poland," *Medical Anthropology Quarterly* 23, no. 2 (2009): 174–80.

36. WHO, *Abortion Care Guideline*, 63.

37. Bartosz Płotka, and Cristina-Iulia Ghenu, "The Implications of Abortion Underground's Institutionalization for the Management Studies," *Revista de Management Comparat International* 18, no. 5 (2017): 485.

38. Ciaputa, "Abortion," 295–96.

39. Anne-Marie Kramer, "The Polish Parliament and the Making of Politics through Abortion: Nation, Gender and Democracy in the 1996 Liberalization Amendment Debate," *International Feminist Journal of Politics* 11, no. 1 (2009): 91.

40. Gal and Kligman, *The Politics of Gender*, 22.

41. David Ost, *The Defeat of Solidarity: Anger and Politics in Postcommunist Europe* (Ithaca, NY: Cornell University Press, 2005).

42. Anna Gwiazda, "The Substantive Representation of Women in Poland," *Politics & Gender* 15, no. 2 (2019): 262–84.

43. Agnieszka Graff, "'Gender Ideology': Weak Concepts, Powerful Politics," *Religion and Gender* 6, no. 2 (2016): 268–72.

44. Weronika Grzebalska and Andrea Pető, "The Gendered Modus Operandi of the Illiberal Transformation in Hungary and Poland," *Women's Studies International Forum* 68, (2018): 164–72.

45. Elżbieta Korolczuk and Agnieszka Graff, "Gender as 'Ebola from Brussels': The Anticolonial Frame and the Rise of Illiberal Populism," *Signs* 43, no. 4 (2018): 797–821.

46. Alicja Curanović, "The International Activity of Ordo Iuris: The Central European Actor and the Global Christian Right," *Religions* 12, no. 12 (2021): 8.

47. Wojciech Sadurski, *Poland's Constitutional Breakdown* (Oxford: Oxford University Press, 2019), 169–73; Graff, "Gender Ideology," 271.

48. Dunja Mijatović, "Commissioner for Human Rights of the Council of Europe: Report Following Her Visit to Poland from 11 to 15 March 2019" (Council of Europe, Commissioner for Human Rights, Strasbourg, 2019).

49. Atina Krajewska, "The History of the Medical Profession in Poland and Its Impact on the on the Development of Abortion Law," Paper presented at workshop "The Impact of the Medical Profession on Abortion Laws in Transitional and Post-Conflict Societies," University of Birmingham, April 4, 2019.

50. Król and Pustułka, "Women on Strike," 375.

51. Elżbieta Korolczuk, "Explaining Mass Protests against Abortion Ban in Poland: The Power of Connective Action," *Zoon Politikon*, no. 7 (2016): 91–113.

52. Public Opinion Research Center Foundation, quoted in Calkin and Kaminska, "Persistence and Change," 97; Mijatović, "Commissioner for Human Rights," 20.

53. Radosław Nawojski, Magdalena Pluta, and Katarzyna Zielińska, "The Black Protests: A Struggle for (Re)Definition of Intimate Citizenship," *Praktyka Teoretyczna* 30, no. 4 (2018): 51–74.

54. Author interview with Polish campaigner working on feminism and church-state separation, 2019 (PL618B).

55. Interview PL220B.

56. Sadurski, *Poland's Constitutional Breakdown*, 61–70.

57. Aleksandra Gliszczyńska-Grabias and Wojciech Sadurski, "The Judgment That Wasn't (but Which Nearly Brought Poland to a Standstill): 'Judgment' of the Polish Constitutional Tribunal of 22 October 2020, K1/20," *European Constitutional Law Review* 17, no. 1 (2021): 138.

58. Human Rights Watch, "Letter: Concerns Regarding the Rule of Law and Human Rights in Poland," Human Rights Watch Press Release, December 18, 2020, https://www.hrw.org/news/2020/12/18/letter-concerns-regarding-rule-law-and-human-rights-poland.

59. Compiled from government data, primarily the annual reports on the implementation of the 1993 law.

60. Interview PL519C.

61. Proctor, "Agnotology," 16.

62. Linsey McGoey, "Strategic Unknowns: Towards a Sociology of Ignorance," *Economy and Society* 41, no. 1 (2012): 1–16.

63. Sheldon, "Empowerment and Privacy."

64. Of the reported 11,271 abortions between 2008 and 2020, 10,801 (95.8%) were granted on grounds of fetal anomaly, 455 (4.04%) on grounds of threat to health or life, and 15 (0.13%) on the grounds of rape.

65. Of these 107 abortions, 75 were granted on the grounds of fetal anomaly before the Constitutional Tribunal's ruling entered into force at the end of January 2021.

Wictor Ferfecki, "A Huge Drop in the Number of Abortions in Poland," *Rzeczpospolita*, July 30, 2022, https://www.rp.pl/spoleczenstwo/art36787631-ogromny-spadek-liczby-aborcji-w-polsce.

66. Kornelia Zaręba et al., "The Influence of Abortion Law on the Frequency of Pregnancy Terminations—a Retrospective Comparative Study," *International Journal of Environmental Research and Public Health* 18, no. 8 (2021): 4099.

67. Wanda Nowicka, "The Anti-Abortion Act in Poland—the Legal and Actual State," in *Reproductive Rights in Poland: The Effects of the Anti-Abortion Law*, ed. Wanda Nowicka (Warsaw: Federation for Women and Family Planning, 2008), 17–44.

68. Mishtal, "Neoliberal Reforms."

69. Kornelia Zaręba et al., "Abortion in Countries with Restrictive Abortion Laws—Possible Directions and Solutions from the Perspective of Poland," *Healthcare* 9, no. 11 (2021): 1594.

70. McGoey, *The Unknowers*, 12–3.

71. Chełstowska, "Stigmatisation."

72. Author interview with staff member in Polish NGO working on sexual and reproductive rights, 2019 (PL519E).

73. Author interview with Polish lawyer and staffer with a reproductive rights NGO, 2019 (PL819C); Interview PL519E.

74. Interview PL819C.

75. Interview PL819C.

76. Author interview with Polish activist living in Sweden, leading an organization to help Polish abortion seekers travel abroad, 2020 (PL220C).

77. Krystyna Kacpura et al., "Twenty Years of Anti-Abortion Law in Poland" (Federation for Women and Family Planning, Warsaw, 2013), 13–14.

78. Mijatović, "Commissioner for Human Rights," 20.

79. Agata Chełstowska et al., "'Good morning, I want to terminate my pregnancy . . .': About Procedures of Access to Legal Abortion in Polish Hospitals." Monitoring Report (Federation for Women and Family Planning, Warsaw, 2016).

80. Magdalena Grabowska, "Cultural War or Business as Usual? Recent Instances and the Historical Origins of the Backlash against Women's Rights and Sexual Rights in Poland," in *Anti-Gender Movements on the Rise? Strategising for Gender Equality in Central and Eastern Europe*, ed. Heinrich Böll Stiftung (Berlin: Heinrich Böll Stiftung, 2015), 54–64.

81. Chełstowska, "Stigmatisation."

82. Interview PL519E.

83. United Nations Human Rights Council, "Report of the Special Rapporteur on the right of everyone to the enjoyment of the highest attainable standard of physical and mental health, Anand Grover. Addendum: Mission to Poland" (United Nations HRC, Geneva, May 20, 2010), https://documents-dds-ny.un.org/doc/UNDOC /GEN/G10/134/03/PDF/G1013403.pdf.

84. Kacpura et al., *Twenty Years of Anti-Abortion Law*, 23; United Nations Office of the High Commissioner, "Press Release: Poland Has Slammed Door Shut on Legal and Safe Abortions—UN Experts" (United Nations, New York, October 27, 2020), https://www.ohchr.org/en/press-releases/2020/10/poland-has-slammed-door-shut-legal-and-safe-abortions-un-experts.

85. Kacpura et al., *Twenty Years of Anti-Abortion Law*, 23.

86. Interview PL519E.

87. Nowicka, "The Anti-Abortion Act."

88. Mishtal, *The Politics of Morality*, 150–54; Ciaputa, "Abortion," 296–97.

89. Interview PL519A.

90. Interview PL519E.

91. Kacpura et al., *Twenty Years of Anti-Abortion Law*, 21.

92. Margit Endler et al., "Safety and Acceptability of Medical Abortion through Telemedicine after 9 Weeks of Gestation: A Population-Based Cohort Study," *BJOG: An International Journal of Obstetrics & Gynecology* 126, no. 5 (2019): 609–18.

93. Abortion Support Network, "Abortion Without Borders Helps More Than 17,000 with Abortion in Six Months after Polish Constitutional Court Ruling," Abortion Support Network, April 22, 2021, https://www.asn.org.uk/press-release-abortion-without-borders-helps-more-than-17000-with-abortion-in-six-months-after-polish-constitutional-court-ruling/.

94. Krajewska, "Revisiting Polish Abortion Law," 8; Ciaputa, "Abortion," 295; Nowicka, "The Anti-Abortion Act," 31.

95. Council of Ministers, Government of Poland, "Report on the Implementation of the 1993 Act on Family Planning, Human Embryo Protection, and Conditions for the Lawful Termination of Pregnancy" (Warsaw, 2019), 118.

96. Freedom of Information request filed with the Polish Ministry of Health (ZPR.0164.11.2021.AB) in August 2021. According to the ministry, its data "do not include the number of illegal terminations of pregnancy for objective reasons, i.e. due to their illegal nature. The data concerning 'the number of Polish women who annually terminate their pregnancy by travelling outside Poland' are not collected either." Original on file with author.

97. Mijatović, "Commissioner for Human Rights," 18.

98. Mijatović, "Commissioner for Human Rights," 20.

99. Antoni Zięba, "Underground Abortion in Poland" (Polish Association of Defenders of Human Life, Krakow, 2006), 1.

100. Zięba, "Underground Abortion in Poland," 4.

101. Jacek Lepiarz, "In Poland, Opposition Lawmakers Criticize 'Pregnancy Register,'" DW.com, June 11, 2022, https://p.dw.com/p/4CZT8.

102. Weronika Strzyżyńska, "Protests Flare across Poland after Death of Young Mother Denied an Abortion," *The Guardian*, January 28, 2022, https://www.theguardian.com/global-development/2022/jan/27/protests-flare-across-poland-after-death-of-young-mother-denied-an-abortion.

103. See, e.g., "Poland Clarifies Abortion Law after Protests over Mother's Death," *BBC News*, November 8, 2021, https://www.bbc.co.uk/news/world-europe-59206683.

CHAPTER 5. ABORTION PILLS IN THE POLISH ABORTION UNDERGROUND

1. Criminal Code of the Republic of Poland 1997 (English version), OSCE Legislation Online, Article 152 §2, https://legislationline.org/sites/default/files/documents/6a/Poland_CC_1997_en.pdf.

2. Quoted in Marta Glanc, "Wydrzynska Trial: Representative of Ordo Iuris in the Room, Limited Number of Seats for Media," *ONET.PL*, April 8, 2022, https://kobieta.onet.pl/wiadomosci/justyna-wydrzynska-proces-na-sali-ordo-iuris/cbrnnqz. In a subsequent court hearing, prosecutors showed clips of Wydrzynska's comments to the media as evidence that she was unrepentant.

3. Abortion Support Network, "Press Release: Abortion Without Borders Helps More Than 34,000 People in Poland Access Abortions," Abortion Support Network, October 21, 2021, https://www.asn.org.uk/abortion-without-borders-helps-more-than-34000-people-in-poland-access-abortions/.

4. Criminal Code of the Republic of Poland, Article 152–153.

5. The restrictions passed in the 1993 law closely mirrored the changes in the Medical Code of Ethics that forbade doctors from providing abortion except for life-saving abortions or where the pregnancy was the result of rape. See Krajewska, "Rupture and Continuity."

6. Krajewska, "Revisiting Polish Abortion Law," 419.

7. Gynuity Health Projects, "Mifepristone Approvals."

8. Someone who tries to self-manage an abortion after 22 weeks can be charged with inducing their own labor and violating article 149 of the Polish Penal Code, which applies to the murder of the child in childbirth.

9. Interview PL519A.

10. Author interview with Polish doctor and activist working with Doctors for Women, 2019 (PL719A); Joanna Caytas, "Women's Reproductive Rights as a Political Price of Post-Communist Transformation in Poland," *Amsterdam Law Forum* 5 (2013): 64–89.

11. Interview PL519A; Author interview with the director of a pan-European abortion travel support group, 2019 (T519A).

12. Foundation for Equality and Emancipation, "Allies or Opponents: Medical Doctors in the Debate on Women's Right to Abortion in Poland" (Warsaw, 2018); de Zordo and Mishtal, "Physicians and Abortion."

13. Foundation for Equality and Emancipation, "Allies or Opponents."

14. Chełstowska, "Stigmatisation."

15. Research assistant interview with Polish woman who formerly worked as a translator for Polish patients in an Austrian abortion clinic, 2020 (PL220D).

16. Author interview with Dutch activist working in a group that helps Polish abortion seekers come to the Netherlands, 2020 (PL220A).

17. We obtained approval from the Queen Mary Ethics of Research Committee to conduct covert interviews over the phone (QMERC2019/68).

18. When Zosia made this call, there was no requirement for doctors to upload pregnancy information into a national database (imposed in 2022). Such a database will make it much harder for Polish women to avoid surveillance and monitoring of their pregnancies.

19. Nowicka, "The Anti-Abortion Act"; Foundation for Equality and Emancipation, "Allies or Opponents"; Interview PL519A.

20. Chełstowska, "Stigmatisation," 103–4.

21. Research assistant interview with Polish woman working as translator and advocate for Polish patients in an Austrian abortion clinic, 2020 (PL320).

22. Author interview with Austrian abortion provider and researcher, 2020 (T120); Interviews PL220A and PL320.

23. Foundation for Equality and Emancipation, "Allies or Opponents," 33–34.

24. Krajewska, "Revisiting Polish Abortion Law."

25. De Zordo and Mishtal, "Physicians and Abortion," 535; Krajewska, "Rupture and Continuity."

26. Federation for Women and Family Planning, "Press Release: Poland Limits Access to Emergency Contraception," June 27, 2017, https://en.federa.org.pl/poland-limits-access-to-emergency-contraception/.

27. Interview PL719A.

28. Interview with Polish doctor and activist, 2019 (PL1119B).

29. See, e.g., "Poland's Lawmakers Reject Bill Seeking to Outlaw Abortion," Associated Press, December 2, 2021, https://apnews.com/article/abortion-health-europe-poland-70271b60f99172d88da03cbb93cc1924.

30. Interview PL519B.

31. Interview PL519A.

32. Grzegorz Sroczyński, "Broniarczyk: We Helped with Two Thousand Abortions. And No One Is Chasing Us," Next Gazeta, November 9, 2020, https://next.gazeta.pl/next/7,151003,26489517,broniarczyk-pomoglysmy-przy-dwoch-tysiacach-aborcji-i-nikt.html.

33. Karolina Domagalska, "Pharmacological Abortion Is a Taboo Subject in Poland. 'We Are for Women Who Make Decisions. It's Their Decision,'" Wysokie Obcasy / Gazeta Wyborcza, February 15, 2018, https://www.wysokieobcasy.pl/wysokie-obcasy/7,163229,23013188,aborcyjny-dream-team-aborcja-farmakologiczna-to-rewolucja.html.

34. For instance, pigulkiaborcyjne.info, a site operated by the Organizacja Pro–Prawo do Życia (Pro–Right to Life Organization).

35. Interviews PL819C, PL519A, and PL519B.

36. Anton Ambroziak, "Shipments with Emergency Contraception and Pharmacological Abortion Kits Are Lost. Poczta Polska Is Responding to the Allegations," OKO.press, November 23, 2017, https://oko.press/poczta-polska-gubia-przesylki-

antykoncepcja-awaryjna-zestawami-aborcji-farmakologicznej-poczta-polska-odpowiada-zarzuty/; Interview PL819C.

37. Interview PL519A.

38. Federation for Women and Family Planning, "Press Release: Sample Letters in Case of Non-Delivery," November 24, 2017, hhttps://federa.org.pl/wzory-pism-przypadku-niedostarczenia-paczki/.

39. Interview PL719B.

40. Author interview with Polish activist living abroad, working with a support group that helps Polish abortion seekers to travel, 2019 (PL819B).

41. Author interview with an activist working in a transnational European network that facilitates abortion pills and travel, 2019 (T2019A).

42. Author interview with a doctor working with a transnational European pill network, 2019 (T2019B).

43. Interview T2019A.

44. Interview T2019A.

45. Mishtal, *The Politics of Morality*.

46. Interviews PL519C and PL618A; Author interview with Polish activist based in London, working in a transnational solidarity group, 2019 (PL519D).

47. The clinic's Polish language site warns, "In Poland, for a long time, we have known 3 websites which, under the name of our clinic, advertise pharmacological abortion. . . . We are prohibited by law from selling drugs online. Any person or website claiming to be able to receive or have received medication through our clinic is not acting in good faith. So be careful!" Retrieved from https://www.vrelinghuis.nl/pl/, last checked May 18, 2022.

48. WHO, *Abortion Care Guideline*.

49. During 2020, I collected data from the website of five Polish pill vendors. As of 2021, three of these five sites no longer existed. I do not name the two sites that are still operating. The three sites thath have been taken offline were called 9 Tygodni (9 Weeks), Girl in Need, and Wszystko o Aborcji (Everything about Abortion). During 2020–21, I made repeated requests for interviews of all five of the vendors listed here, but none agreed to participate.

50. Interview PL220A.

51. Interview PL519A.

52. Inga Koralewska and Katarzyna Zielińska, "'Defending the Unborn,' 'Protecting Women' and 'Preserving Culture and Nation': Anti-Abortion Discourse in the Polish Right-Wing Press," *Culture, Health & Sexuality* (2021): 1–15.

53. Interviews PL220D and PL320; Author interview with German activist leading an abortion fund and travel support group for Polish abortion seekers, 2019 (PL719B).

54. Interview PL519B.

55. Elizabeth Raymond et al., "Efficacy of Misoprostol Alone for First-Trimester Medical Abortion: A Systematic Review," *Obstetrics and Gynecology* 133, no. 1 (2019): 137.

56. Interview PL618A.

57. Polish Council of Ministers, "Report on the Implementation of the Law of 1993 on Family Planning and Termination of Pregnancy," 2006–21 editions, available at http://orka.sejm.gov.pl/.

58. Krajewska, "Revisiting Polish Abortion Law," 413.

59. Mijatović, "Commissioner for Human Rights," 20.

60. Interview PL819C.

61. Krajewska, "Revisiting Polish Abortion Law," 421–22. This figure includes all cases registered under articles 148, 149, 152, 153, 154, 157a, 157, and 160. Together, they encompass abortion, offenses against a pregnant woman and/or a fetus, including manslaughter, neonaticide, abortion with consent, abortion without consent, injury to the "conceived child," and exposure of the pregnant woman to health risks.

62. Krajewska, "Revisiting Polish Abortion Law," 422–23.

63. Interview PL819C.

64. Mijatovic, "Commissioner of Human Rights," 20.

65. Polish Council of Ministers, "Report on the Implementation of the Law of 1993."

66. Krajewska, "Revisiting Polish Abortion Law," 423.

67. Mishtal, *The Politics of Morality*.

68. Jerzy Ferenz, *Analiza Dotycząca Przestępstwa Pomocy W Aborcji* [Analysis of the crime of aiding and abetting an abortion] (Warsaw: Ordo Iuris Institute for Legal Culture, 2017), https://ordoiuris.pl/ochrona-zycia/analiza-dotyczaca-przestepstwa-pomocy-w-aborcji.

69. Mijatovic, "Commissioner of Human Rights," 20.

70. Interview PL519E.

71. Curanović, "The International Activity."

72. Curanović, "The International Activity," 9–10.

73. Ordo Iuris, "Press Release: The Trial of an Abortion Activist Has Begun. Ordo Iuris Joins the Proceedings," Ordo Iuris Institute for Legal Culture, April 9, 2022, https://ordoiuris.pl/ochrona-zycia/ruszyl-proces-dzialaczki-aborcyjnej-ordo-iuris-dolacza-do-postepowania.

74. WHO, "Global Abortion Policies Database: Ukraine," accessed July 4, 2022, https://abortion-policies.srhr.org/country/ukraine/.

75. Leszek Wójtowicz, "She Went to Ukraine to Get An Abortion. The Girl's Mother And Friend Are Convicted," *Dziennik Wschodni*, February 15, 2012, https://www.dziennikwschodni.pl/zamosc/pojechala-na-ukraine-zrobic-aborcje-matka-i-znajomy-dziewczyny-skazani,n,1000145015.html.

76. Ciaputa, "Abortion," 279.

77. United Nations High Commissioner on Refugees, "Operational Data Portal: Ukraine Refugee Situation," accessed July 1, 2022, https://data.unhcr.org/en/situations/ukraine.

78. Claudia Ciobanu, "Ukrainian War Rape Victims Abandoned by Polish State," *Balkan Insight*, July 12, 2022, https://balkaninsight.com/2022/07/12/ukrainian-war-rape-victims-abandoned-by-polish-state/.

79. United Nations Human Rights Council, "Statement: UN Human Rights Council Independent Expert Group on the Issue of Discrimination against Women in Law and in Practice," December 13, 2018, https://www.ohchr.org/en/statements/2018/12/un-human-rights-council-independent-expert-group-issue-discrimination-against.

80. Weronika Strzyżyńska, "'Declare it to a doctor, and it's over': Ukrainian Women Face Harsh Reality of Poland's Abortion Laws," *The Guardian*, May 10, 2022, https://www.theguardian.com/global-development/2022/may/10/ukrainian-women-face-harsh-reality-poland-abortion-laws.

81. Łukasz Kuczera, "Kaja Godek with a New Anti-Abortion Initiative. Jail for Having a Leaflet on Abortion?," *WP Wiadomości*, March 24, 2022, https://wiadomosci.wp.pl/kaja-godek-z-nowa-antyaborcyjna-inicjatywa-wiezienie-za-posiadanie-ulotki-o-przerwaniu-ciazy-6750825762257856a.

82. Aleksandra Lewandowska, "Legal Abortion for Ukrainian Women Victims of Wartime Rape? Ordo Iuris Says 'No,'" *WP Kobieta*, May 13, 2022, https://kobieta.wp.pl/legalna-aborcja-dla-ukrainek-ktore-staly-sie-ofiarami-gwaltow-wojennych-ordo-iuris-mowi-nie-6768399274621856a; Ordo Iuris, "Press Release: Ordo Iuris Monitors Compliance with the Law in Polish Hospitals," Ordo Iuris Institute for Legal Culture, May 17, 2022, https://ordoiuris.pl/ochrona-zycia/ordo-iuris-monitoruje-przestrzeganie-prawa-w-polskich-szpitalach.

CHAPTER 6. IRISH ABORTIONS BY PLANE OR PILL

1. Theresa Reidy, "The 2018 Referendum: Over before It Began!," in *After Repeal: Rethinking Abortion Politics*, ed. Kath Browne and Sydney Calkin (London: Zed Books, 2020), 21–35.

2. RTÉ Behaviour and Attitudes Exit Poll, "Thirty-Sixth Amendment to the Constitution Exit Poll," RTÉ, May 25, 2018, https://www.rte.ie/documents/news/2018/05/rte-exit-poll-final-11pm.pdf.

3. Although the official name for the country is Ireland, I use "Irish Republic" and "Republic of Ireland" throughout to help distinguish between the island of Ireland and the two countries on it.

4. Irish Constitution, art. 40.3.3, as amended in 1983.

5. Cara Delay, "Pills, Potions, and Purgatives: Women and Abortion Methods in Ireland, 1900–1950," *Women's History Review* 28, no. 3 (2019): 480.

6. Lindsey Earner-Byrne, "The Boat to England: An Analysis of the Official Reactions to the Emigration of Single Expectant Irishwomen to Britain, 1922–1972," *Irish Economic and Social History* 30, no. 1 (2003): 52–70.

7. Ann Rossiter, *Ireland's Hidden Diaspora: The "Abortion Trail" and the Making of a London-Irish Underground 1980–2000* (London: IASC Publishing, 2009).

8. Ruth Fletcher, "Post-Colonial Fragments: Representations of Abortion in Irish Law and Politics," *Journal of Law and Society* 28, no. 4 (2002): 568–79; Emily O'Reilly, *Masterminds of the Right* (Cork: Attic Press, 1992).

9. Lisa Smyth, *Abortion and Nation: The Politics of Reproduction in Contemporary Ireland* (London: Routledge, 2005), 63.

10. Ruth Fletcher, "Pro-Life Absolutes, Feminist Challenges: The Fundamentalist Narrative of Irish Abortion Law 1986–1992," *Osgoode Hall Law Journal* 36 (1998): 28.

11. Linda Connolly and Tina O'Toole, *Documenting Irish Feminisms: The Second Wave* (Bognor Regis, UK: Woodfield Press, 2005), 71; Sandra McAvoy, "The Catholic Church and Fertility Control in Ireland: The Making of a Dystopian Regime," in *The Abortion Papers Ireland: Volume 2*, ed. Aideen Quilty, Sinead Kennedy, and Catherine Conlon (Cork: Cork University Press, 2015), 47–62.

12. Author interview with Irish activist who participated in the Anti-Amendment Campaign in 1983 and campaigned for repeal in 2018, 2018 (ROI518B).

13. Luke Field, "The Abortion Referendum of 2018 and a Timeline of Abortion Politics in Ireland to Date," *Irish Political Studies* 33, no. 4 (2018): 610.

14. Fiona de Londras and Máiréad Enright, *Repealing the 8th: Reforming Irish Abortion Law* (Bristol: Policy Press, 2018).

15. Irish Constitution, art. 40.3.3, as amended in 1992.

16. Smyth, *Abortion and Nation*, 112.

17. Kate Gleeson, "A woman's work is . . . unfinished business: Justice for the Disappeared Magdalen Women of Modern Ireland," *Feminist Legal Studies* 25, no. 3 (2017): 291–312.

18. Clara Fischer, "Abortion and Reproduction in Ireland: Shame, Nation-Building and the Affective Politics of Place," *Feminist Review* 122, no. 1 (2019): 37–38.

19. Eithne Luibhéid, *Pregnant on Arrival: Making the Illegal Immigrant* (Minneapolis: University of Minnesota Press, 2013), 37.

20. Ruth Fletcher, "Reproducing Irishness: Race, Gender, and Abortion Law," *Canadian Journal of Women and the Law* 17, no. 2 (2005): 365–404; Fletcher, "Post-Colonial Fragments."

21. Smyth, *Abortion and Nation*, 46.

22. Poster reprinted in Kath Browne and Catherine Nash, "In Ireland We 'Love Both'? Heteroactivism in Ireland's Anti-Repeal Ephemera," *Feminist Review* 124, no. 1 (2020): 59.

23. Quoted in Jean Engela, "Irish Center for Bio-Ethical Reform Report," CBR Communiqué, March 2019, https://www.abortionno.org/wp-content/uploads/2019/11/CBR-Communique-March-2019.pdf.

24. Sydney Calkin, "Healthcare Not Airfare! Art, Abortion and Political Agency in Ireland," *Gender, Place & Culture* 26, no. 3 (2019): 344–45.

25. Delay, "Pills, Potions, and Purgatives."

26. Abortion travelers to England almost exclusively attend independent abortion clinics there because they provide one-day abortion services.

27. Data compiled from the UK Department of Health annual report on abortion, "Abortion Statistics for England and Wales," available at https://www.gov.uk/government/statistics/.

28. Ruth Fletcher, "Negotiating Strangeness on the Abortion Trail," in *Revaluing Care in Theory, Law and Policy: Cycles and Connections*, ed. Rosie Harding, Ruth Fletcher, and Chris Beasley (London: Routledge, 2016), 17.

29. Rossiter, *Ireland's Hidden Diaspora*.

30. Deirdre Duffy, "From Feminist Anarchy to Decolonisation: Understanding Abortion Health Activism before and after the Repeal of the 8th Amendment," *Feminist Review* 124, no. 1 (2020): 69–85.

31. Author interview with director of a pan-European abortion travel support group, 2017 (T317).

32. Ruth Fletcher, "Peripheral Governance: Administering Transnational Health-Care Flows," *International Journal of Law in Context* 9 (2013): 172.

33. Fletcher, "Peripheral Governance," 177.

34. Fletcher, "Peripheral Governance," 172.

35. De Londras and Enright, *Repealing the 8th*, 4.

36. Allison Clifford, "Abortion in International Waters Off the Coast of Ireland: Avoiding a Collision between Irish Moral Sovereignty and the European Community," *Pace International Law Review* 14 (2002): 387.

37. Carrie Lambert-Beatty, "Twelve Miles: Boundaries of the New Art/Activism," *Signs* 33, no. 2 (2008): 320–22.

38. Rebecca Gomperts, "Women on Waves: Where Next for the Abortion Boat?," *Reproductive Health Matters* 10, no. 19 (2002): 181.

39. Gomperts, "Women on Waves," 181–82.

40. Author interview with a leader in Women on Web/Women on Waves, 2018 (T718A).

41. Alan MacSimoin, "How Free Can You Be If You Can't Even Control Your Own Body?," *Red & Black Revolution*, no. 14 (2008): 21.

42. Sydney Calkin, "Towards a Political Geography of Abortion," *Political Geography* 69 (2019): 22–29.

43. Sally Sheldon, "How Can a State Control Swallowing? The Home Use of Abortion Pills in Ireland," *Reproductive Health Matters* 24, no. 48 (2016): 91.

44. Author interview with Irish pro-choice activist and campaigner who worked on medication abortion provision from the mid-2000s, 2018 (ROI718A).

45. Author interview with Derry-based activist and campaigner in Alliance for Choice, 2018 (NI818A).

46. Interview ROI718A.

47. Tamara Hervey and Sally Sheldon, "Abortion by Telemedicine in the European Union," *International Journal of Gynaecology & Obstetrics* 145, no. 1 (2019): 125–28.

48. Travel to the Netherlands fell off almost entirely: in 2006, 461 residents of Ireland obtained abortions in Dutch clinics, while in 2016 that number had dropped to only twenty-two. See, e.g., (Netherlands) Health Care and Youth Inspectorate, "Jaarrapportage 2018 Van De Wet Afbreking Zwangerschap / Annual Report 2018 of the Termination of Pregnancy Act," 2018.

49. Irish Family Planning Association, "Abortion in Ireland: Statistics," IPFA.ie, accessed 1 February 2018.

50. Amnesty International, "She Is Not a Criminal: The Impact of Ireland's Abortion Law" (London, 2015); Gynuity Health Projects, "Mifepristone Approvals."

51. Interviews ROI718A and T718A.

52. Sheldon, "Empowerment and Privacy."

53. Offences Against the Person Act, 1861, §58–59.

54. Protection of Life During Pregnancy Act, 2013, §22.

55. Abigail R. A. Aiken et al. "Self-Reported Outcomes and Adverse Events after Medical Abortion through Online Telemedicine: Population Based Study in the Republic of Ireland and Northern Ireland," *BMJ: British Medical Journal* 357 (2017); Abigail R. A. Aiken, Rebecca Gomperts, and James Trussell, "Experiences and Characteristics of Women Seeking and Completing At-Home Medical Termination of Pregnancy through Online Telemedicine in Ireland and Northern Ireland: A Population-Based Analysis," *BJOG: An International Journal of Obstetrics & Gynaecology* 124, no. 8 (2017): 1208–15.

56. Author interview with activist involved in pill provision and lobbying for reforms, 2020 (NI220); Interview ROI718A.

57. Amnesty International, "She Is Not a Criminal," 95.

58. Interview T718A.

59. Interview T718A; and see, e.g., Aiken et al., "Self-Reported Outcomes and Adverse Events"; Aiken et al. "Experiences and Characteristics of Women."

60. Interview USA819; Interview T1118.

61. Women Help Women, "In Solidarity with Repeal the 8th! Referendum in Ireland on May 25th!," April 10, 2018, https://womenhelp.org/en/page/900/in-solidarity-with-repeal-the-8th-referendum-in-ireland-on-may-25th.

62. Women on Web studies do not differentiate between requests that originate in the Republic of Ireland and in Northern Ireland, so the data here include unknown numbers of Northern Irish abortion seekers.

63. Health Products Regulatory Authority, "The Dangers of Buying Prescription Medicines Online" (Dublin, n.d.).

64. For more detail on customs seizures of abortion pills compared to other products, see Sydney Calkin, "Transnational Abortion Pill Flows and the Political Geography of Abortion in Ireland," *Territory, Politics, Governance* 9, no. 2 (2021): 175–76.

65. Sheldon, "Empowerment and Privacy," 840.

66. Interview NI818A.

67. Sheldon, "Empowerment and Privacy," 840.

68. Jowit and Pallavi, "From Nagpur"; Bazelon, "The Dawn."

69. Sheldon, "Empowerment and Privacy," 840.

70. Amnesty International, "She Is Not a Criminal," 95.

71. Carol Ryan, "Abortion by Post," *Irish Times*, March 15, 2011, https://www.irishtimes.com/news/health/abortion-by-post-1.573017; Grainne Ní Aodha, "Here's

the Number of Abortion Pills Seized in Ireland in the Past 10 Years," *TheJournal.ie*, April 3, 2018, https://www.thejournal.ie/abortion-pill-use-in-ireland-3892752-Apr2018/. The data appear in two forms: "consignments" seized indicates the number of packages, while the raw number of pills received counts all pills seized across the consignments.

72. Blanaid Murphy, "Deadly Haul of 'Online Drugs' Seized in Five Locations around Ireland," *Irish Mirror*, September 6, 2016.

73. Interview ROI718A.

74. Information compiled by the author from the Irish Health Products Regulatory Authority, the UK Department of Health annual reports, Dutch Department of Health annual reports, Women Help Women data, and Women on Web data published in Aiken et al. "Self-Reported Outcomes and Adverse Events"; Aiken et al., "Experiences and Characteristics of Women."

75. Catherine Nash, Lorraine Dennis, and Brian Graham, "Putting the Border in Place: Customs Regulation in the Making of the Irish Border, 1921–1945," *Journal of Historical Geography* 36, no. 4 (2010): 421–31.

76. Gordon Anthony, *Brexit and the Irish Border: Legal and Political Questions* (London and Dublin: British Academy and Royal Irish Academy, 2017), 3–4.

77. Jonathan Tonge, "The Impact of Withdrawal from the European Union upon Northern Ireland," *Political Quarterly* 87, no. 3 (2016): 342.

78. Sheldon, "Empowerment and Privacy," 840.

79. UK Medicines and Healthcare Products Regulatory Agency communication, on file with author.

80. Interview NI818A.

81. Interview NI220.

82. Amnesty International, "She Is Not a Criminal," 95.

83. Author interview with an activist working in ROSA, 2018 (ROI1118A).

84. Interview NI220.

85. Interviews ROI1118A and NI220.

86. Author interview with Irish activist affiliated with ROSA, based in west of Ireland, 2019 (ROI819); Interview T719B.

87. Author interview with activist in the west of Ireland involved in pro-choice campaigning and pill networks, 2021 (ROI421); Interview ROI819.

88. Sheldon, "Empowerment and Privacy," 839–41.

89. Enright and Cloatre, "Transformative Illegality," 279.

90. Enright and Cloatre, "Transformative Illegality," 282–83.

91. This agency was also called the Crisis Pregnancy Programme at a different point in time, but for the sake of clarity I refer to it only as the Crisis Pregnancy Agency.

92. Fletcher, "Peripheral Governance," 167.

93. Health Service Executive, "Number of Women Giving Irish Addresses at UK Abortion Clinics Decreases for Ninth Year in a Row," news release, May 24, 2011; Health Service Executive, "Number of Women Giving Irish Addresses at UK Abortion Clinics Decreases for Tenth Year in a Row According to Department of Health UK,"

news release, May 2012; Health Service Executive, "Number of Women Giving Irish Addresses at UK Abortion Clinics Decreases," news release, July 11, 2013.

94. Health Service Executive, "Number of Women Giving Irish Addresses at Abortion Clinics in 2014," news release, June 9, 2015.

95. Health Service Executive, "UK Records Show Decrease in Women Giving Irish Addresses at Abortion Clinics," news release, May 17, 2016.

96. Health Service Executive, "Over 50% Decrease in the Number of Women Giving Irish Addresses at Abortion Clinics in England and Wales," news release, May 13, 2017.

97. Sheldon, "Empowerment and Privacy," 839.

98. Sheldon, "How Can a State Control Swallowing?," 96.

99. Kara Aitken, Paul Patek, and Mark Murphy, "The Opinions and Experiences of Irish Obstetric and Gynaecology Trainee Doctors in Relation to Abortion Services in Ireland," *Journal of Medical Ethics* 43, no. 11 (2017): 778–83.

100. Sheldon, "Empowerment and Privacy," 839.

101. Interview NI818A.

102. Amnesty International, "She Is Not a Criminal," 95.

103. Ryan, "Abortion by Post."

104. Emilie Cloatre and Máiréad Enright, "'On the Perimeter of the Lawful': Enduring Illegality in the Irish Family Planning Movement, 1972–1985," *Journal of Law and Society* 44, no. 4 (2017): 486.

105. Cloatre and Enright, "On the Perimeter," 488.

106. Cloatre and Enright, "On the Perimeter," 497.

107. Sheldon, "Empowerment and Privacy."

CHAPTER 7. ABORTION PILLS AND IRELAND'S 8TH AMENDMENT
REFERENDUM

1. Abigail R. A. Aiken et al., "Experiences of Women in Ireland Who Accessed Abortion by Travelling Abroad or by Using Abortion Medication at Home: A Qualitative Study," *BMJ Sexual & Reproductive Health* 44, no. 3 (2018): 181–86.

2. Fiona de Londras, "Protection of Life During Pregnancy Act 2013," in *Women's Legal Landmarks: Celebrating the History of Women and Law in the UK and Ireland*, ed. Erika Rackley and Rosemary Auchmuty (London: Bloomsbury, 2018), 597.

3. Health Service Executive External Independent Committee, "Investigation of Incident 50278 from Time of Patient's Self Referral to Hospital on the 21st of October 2012 to the Patient's Death on the 28th of October, 2012" (Health Service Executive, Dublin, June 2013), https://www.hse.ie/eng/services/news/nimtreport50278.pdf.

4. Fergal Bowers, "Midwife Confirms She Told Savita Halappanavar Ireland a 'Catholic Country,'" *RTE News*, April 11, 2013, https://www.rte.ie/news/health/2013/0410/380613-savita-halappanavar-inquest/.

5. Quilty, Kennedy, and Conlon, *The Abortion Papers Ireland: Volume 2*; Orla McDonnell and Padraig Murphy, "Mediating Abortion Politics in Ireland: Media Framing of the Death of Savita Halappanavar," *Critical Discourse Studies* 16, no. 1 (2019): 1–20.

6. Claire Murray, "The Protection of Life During Pregnancy Act 2013: Suicide, Dignity and the Irish Discourse on Abortion," *Social & Legal Studies* 25, no. 6 (2016): 667–98.

7. Protection of Life During Pregnancy Act of 2013, sec. 7–9.

8. De Londras, "Protection of Life," 597–99.

9. Oireachtas Éireann, Joint Committee on Health and Children, "Debate: Implementation of Government Decision Following Expert Group Report into Matters Relating to A, B and C v. Ireland" (Oireachtas Éireann, Dublin, January 10, 2013).

10. Protection of Life During Pregnancy Act, 2013, sec. 22.

11. Dáil Éireann, "Protection of Life During Pregnancy Bill 2013: Report Stage" (Oireachtas Éireann, Dublin, July 11, 2013).

12. Oireachtas Éireann, Joint Committee on Health and Children, "Debate."

13. Dáil Éireann, "Protection of Life During Pregnancy Bill 2013: Report Stage."

14. Fletcher, "Pro-Life Absolutes," 27.

15. Solinger, *Beggars and Choosers*, 37.

16. Dáil Éireann, "Protection of Life During Pregnancy Bill 2013: Report Stage"; Oireachtas Éireann, Joint Committee on Health and Children, "Debate: Implementation of Government Decision Following Expert Group Report into Matters Relating to A, B and C v. Ireland" (Oireachtas Eireann, Dublin, January 3, 2013).

17. Field, "The Abortion Referendum," 614.

18. Mary Minihan, "Was Citizens' Assembly Best Way to Deal with Abortion Question?," *Irish Times*, April 29, 2017, https://www.irishtimes.com/news/politics/was-citizens-assembly-best-way-to-deal-with-abortion-question-1.3065226.

19. Citizens' Assembly, "First Report and Recommendations of the Citizens' Assembly: The Eighth Amendment of the Constitution" (Dublin, 2017), 39.

20. Fiona de Londras, "Intersectionality, Repeal, and Reproductive Rights in Ireland," in *Intersectionality and Human Rights*, ed. Peter Dunne and Shreya Atrey (Oxford: Hart Publishing, 2019), 4.

21. De Londras, "Intersectionality, Repeal," 5.

22. Citizens' Assembly, "First Report," 4.

23. Elzbieta Drążkiewicz-Grodzicka and Maire Ní Mhórdha, "Of Trust and Mistrust: The Politics of Repeal," in *After Repeal: Rethinking Abortion Politics*, ed. Kath Browne and Sydney Calkin (London: Zed Books, 2020), 97.

24. Oireachtas Éireann, Joint Committee on the 8th Amendment of the Constitution, "Engagement with Ms Justice Mary Laffoy, Citizens' Assembly" (Dublin, September 9, 2017).

25. Catherine Noone, "Senator Catherine Noone," interview by Hugh Linehan, *Irish Times*, Inside Politics Podcast, December 20, 2017, Audio 33:02, https://www.irishtimes.com/podcasts/inside-politics/.

26. Cianan Brennan, "14 TDs in Dáil Chamber as Bríd Smith Produces Packet of Abortion Pills," *TheJournal.ie*, October 25, 2016, https://www.thejournal.ie/eighth-amendment-debate-3046112-Oct2016/.

27. TD Bríd Smith, quoted in *Dáil Éireann Debates*, Vol. 926, No. 1, October 14, 2016.

28. Interview ROI1118A.

29. Author interview with Irish senator who served on 2013 and 2018 legislative committees on abortion legislation, 2019 (ROI719).

30. Author interview with public health researcher working on self-managed abortion, 2018 (T518).

31. Abigail Aiken, Opening Statement to the Joint Oireachtas Committee on the 8th Amendment to the Constitution, Oireachtas Éireann, October 11, 2017.

32. See, e.g., TD Lisa Chambers (Fianna Fáil), in *Dáil Éireann Debates*, Vol. 963, No. 7, January 18, 2018; TD Mick Barry (People Before Profit), in *Dáil Éireann Debates*, Vol. 966, No. 6, March 9, 2018.

33. Author interview with staff member on the policy team of a large Irish reproductive rights NGO, 2019 (ROI919).

34. Interview T718A.

35. Author interview with Abigail Aiken.

36. Joint Oireachtas Committee on the 8th Amendment, "Report of the Joint Committee on the 8th Amendment of the Constitution" (Oireachtas Éireann, Dublin, 2017), 11.

37. Joint Oireachtas Committee on the 8th Amendment, *Report*, 11.

38. Interview ROI719.

39. Sen. Ronán Mullen (Ind.), quoted in *Seanad Éireann Debates*, Vol. 257, No. 1, March 27, 2018; see also statements by Ronán Mullen, quoted in *Seanad Éireann Debates*, Vol. 255, No. 5, January 17, 2018; and statements by TD Peadar Tóibín (Sinn Fein), quoted in *Dáil Éireann Debates*, Vol. 964, No. 1, January 23, 2018, and Vol. 964, No. 2, January 25, 2018; and Minority Report of TD Peter Fitzpatrick, TD Mattie McGrath, and Sen. Ronan Mullen on the Joint Oireachtas Committee on the 8th Amendment, 17.

40. TD Michael Collins (Ind.), quoted in *Dáil Éireann Debates*, Vol. 964, No. 1, January 23, 2018; and Vol. 964, No. 2, January 25, 2018.

41. Quoted in *Dáil Éireann Debates*, Vol. 966, No. 6, March 9, 2018.

42. Quoted in *Dáil Éireann Debates*, Vol. 963, No. 7, January 18, 2018.

43. Quoted in *Dáil Éireann Debates*, Vol. 963, No. 6, January 17, 2018.

44. Quoted in *Dáil Éireann Debates*, Vol. 257, No. 1, March 27, 2018.

45. Máiréad Enright, "'No. I Won't Go Back': National Time, Trauma and Legacies of Symphysiotomy in Ireland," in *Law and Time*, ed. Sian Beynon-Jones and Emily Grabham (London: Routledge, 2018), 47.

46. Quoted in *Dáil Éireann Debates*, Vol. 966, No. 7, March 20, 2018.

47. See, e.g., Health Minister Simon Harris (Fine Gael), in *Seanad Éireann Debates*, Vol. 257, No. 1, March 27, 2018; Sen. Jerry Buttimer (Fine Gael), in *Seanad Éireann Debates*, Vol. 255, No. 5, January 17, 2018; TD Fergus O'Dowd (Fine Gael), in *Dáil Éireann Debates*, Vol. 966, No. 7, March 20, 2018; Health Minister Simon Harris (Fine Gael) and TD Bill Kelleher (Fine Gael), in *Dáil Éireann Debates*, Vol. 966, No. 6, March 9, 2018; TD Maria Bailey (Fine Gael), in *Dáil Éireann Debates*, Vol. 964, No. 3, January 25, 2018.

48. Takeshita, *The Global Biopolitics*, 18.

49. Quoted in *Dáil Éireann Debates*, Vol. 964, No. 1, January 23, 2018; and Vol. 964, No. 2, January 25, 2018.

50. Quoted in *Dáil Éireann Debates*, Vol. 966, No. 6, March 9, 2018.

51. Quoted in *Dáil Éireann Debates*, Vol. 966, No. 6, March 9, 2018.

52. Aiken et al., "Self-reported Outcomes and Adverse Events," 4.

53. Celeste Condit, *Decoding Abortion Rhetoric: Communicating Social Change* (Champaign: University of Illinois Press, 1994), 23–24.

54. Solinger, *Beggars and Choosers*, 60.

55. Interview ROI919A.

56. Aiken et al., "Experiences and Characteristics of Women," 1209.

57. Author interview with Irish senator and member of the Joint Committee on the 8th Amendment, 2019 (ROI1219).

58. Vincent Browne, "Martin Is Adept at Not Putting a Foot Wrong," *Irish Times*, February 23, 2002, https://www.irishtimes.com/news/martin-is-adept-at-not-putting-a-foot-wrong-1.1051581.

59. TD Micheál Martin (Fianna Fáil), in *Dáil Éireann Debates*, Vol. 963, No. 7, January 18, 2018.

60. Pam Lowe, *Reproductive Health and Maternal Sacrifice: Women, Choice and Responsibility* (New York: Springer, 2016).

61. TD Hildegarde Naughton (Fine Gael), in *Dáil Éireann Debates*, Vol. 963, No. 6, January 17, 2018.

62. TD Alan Farrell (Fine Gael), in *Dáil Éireann Debates*, Vol. 963, No. 7, January 18, 2018.

63. Quoted in *Dáil Éireann Debates*, Vol. 966, No. 7, March 20, 2018.

64. Erica Millar, *Happy Abortions: Our Bodies in the Era of Choice* (London: Zed Books, 2017), 122–24.

65. Smyth, *Abortion and Nation*, 129.

66. Interview ROI718A.

67. Vivienne Clarke and Marie O'Halloran, "Varadkar: Only a Matter of Time before Someone 'Bleeds to Death' If Abortion No Vote," *Irish Times*, May 18, 2018, https://www.irishtimes.com/news/politics/varadkar-only-a-matter-of-time-before-someone-bleeds-to-death-if-abortion-no-vote-1.3500220.

68. Varadkar, quoted in Clarke and O'Halloran, "Varadkar."

69. Ela Drążkiewicz et al., "Repealing Ireland's Eighth Amendment: Abortion Rights and Democracy Today," *Social Anthropology* 28, no. 3 (2020): 582.

70. Philip Ryan, "Repeal Won't Lead to Abortion Free-for-All, Says Varadkar," *Irish Independent*, April 22, 2018, https://www.independent.ie/irish-news/politics/repeal-wont-lead-to-abortion-freeforall-says-varadkar-36830613.html.

71. Author interview with leading figure in Irish campaign for abortion reform who played a public role in Together for Yes, 2017 (ROI317A).

72. Together for Yes, "Learning from the 2018 Together for Yes Campaign," 2019, https://www.togetherforyes.ie/app/uploads/2019/11/2019_TFY_Review.pdf.

73. Field, "The Abortion Referendum," 12.

74. Aideen O'Shaughnessy, "Bodies of Change: Analysing the Embodied and Affective Movement for Abortion Rights in Ireland" (PhD diss., University of Cambridge, 2022), DOI:10.17863/CAM.87018.

75. Interview ROI518B.

76. Máiréad Enright, "'The Enemy of the Good': Reflections on Ireland's New Abortion Legislation," *feminists@law* 8, no. 2 (2018): 8, Ruth Fletcher, "#Repealedthe8th: Translating Travesty, Global Conversation, and the Irish Abortion Referendum," *Feminist Legal Studies*, no. 26 (2018): 233–59.

77. Interview ROI718A.

78. Interview ROI317A.

79. De Londras, "Intersectionality, Repeal," 8–10.

80. Ailbhe Conneely, "Group Says Repeal of Eighth Amendment Required to Regulate Abortion Pill Usage," *RTE*, April 11, 2018, https://www.rte.ie/news/eighth-amendment/2018/0411/953646-together-for-yes/; Michelle Hennessy, "'Please Come Home Mam, I'm in Agony': Parents of Women Who Had Crisis Pregnancies Urge Yes Vote," *TheJournal.ie*, May 23, 2018, https://www.thejournal.ie/abortion-pill-4029566-May2018/.

81. Author interview with activist working with several pro-choice and feminist groups in Belfast, 2018 (NI518A); Interview ROI718A.

82. Reprinted in Clara Fischer, "Feminists Redraw Public and Private Spheres: Abortion, Vulnerability, and the Affective Campaign to Repeal the Eighth Amendment," *Signs* 45, no. 4 (2020): 995.

83. Interview ROI919.

84. Interviews NI220, NI518A, and ROI518B.

85. Together for Yes, "Briefing on the Proposal to Regulate Termination of Pregnancy in Early Pregnancy (12 Weeks): Medical Abortion" (Dublin, 2018), https://www.togetherforyes.ie/medical-abortion/.

86. Reidy, "The 2018 Referendum."

87. RTÉ Behaviour & Attitudes Exit Poll, "Thirty-Sixth Amendment."

88. Health (Regulation of Termination of Pregnancy) Act 2018, sec. 23 (2).

89. Minister Simon Harris (Fine Gael), in *Seanad Éireann Debates*, Vol. 262, No. 3, December 11, 2018.

90. TD Stephen Donnelly (Fianna Fáil), in committee debate on the Health (Regulation of Termination of Pregnancy) Bill 2018, November 6, 2018.

91. Enright, "The Enemy of the Good."

92. Health (Regulation of Termination of Pregnancy) Act 2018, sec. 23 (3).

93. Catherine Shanahan, "Abortion Pill Approved for the First Time," *Irish Examiner*, December 4, 2018, https://www.irishexaminer.com/news/arid-30889664.html.

94. Sydney Calkin and Ella Berny, "Legal and Non-Legal Barriers to Abortion in Ireland and the United Kingdom," *Medicine Access@ Point of Care* 5 (2021): 2–4.

95. Abortion Rights Campaign and Lorraine Grimes, "Too Many Barriers: Experiences of Abortion in Ireland after Repeal Report" (Abortion Rights Campaign,

Dublin, 2021), https://www.abortionrightscampaign.ie/wp-content/uploads/2021/09/Too-Many-Barriers-Report_ARC1.pdf.

96. "Significant Decrease in Number of Abortion Pills Seized This Year," *Irish Pharmacist*, July 29, 2020, https://irishpharmacist.ie/2020/07/29/significant-decrease-in-number-of-abortion-pills-seized-this-year/.

CHAPTER 8. FROM CRIMINALIZATION TO DECRIMINALIZATION IN NORTHERN IRELAND

1. For clarity, in this chapter I use "Ireland" only to refer to the island of Ireland, not the two countries on it. With regard to the latter, I refer to "Republic of Ireland" and "Northern Ireland."

2. Offences Against the Person Act 1861.

3. Katherine Side, "Contract, Charity, and Honorable Entitlement: Social Citizenship and the 1967 Abortion Act in Northern Ireland after the Good Friday Agreement," *Social Politics: International Studies in Gender, State & Society* 13, no. 1 (2006): 89–116.

4. Jennifer Thomson, *Abortion Law and Political Institutions: Explaining Policy Resistance* (New York: Springer, 2018), 68–69.

5. Although residents of the United Kingdom, taxpayers, and contributors to the National Health Service, Northern Irish people were treated as nonresidents for the purposes of abortion and forced to pay out of pocket at English clinics until 2017.

6. UK Department of Health data are not available for 1996, 1998, or 2002. Northern Ireland termination of pregnancy statistics are released by the Department of Health of Northern Ireland but no data is available before 2008.

7. Steve Clements and Roger Ingham, *Improving Knowledge Regarding Abortions Performed on Irish Women in the UK* (Dublin: Health Service Executive, Crisis Pregnancy Agency, 2007), 9.

8. Kate Hayward and Ben Rosher, "Political Attitudes at a Time of Flux," ARK Research Brief (Queens University Belfast, June 2020); Jocelyn Evans and Jonathan Tonge, "Social Class and Party Choice in Northern Ireland's Ethnic Blocs," *West European Politics* 32, no. 5 (2009): 1012–30.

9. Paul Mitchell, "Transcending an Ethnic Party System: The Impacts of Consociational Governance on Electoral Dynamics and the Party System," in *Aspects of the Belfast Agreement*, ed. Rick Wilford (Oxford: Oxford University Press, 2001), 28–29.

10. Jennifer Thomson, "Abortion and Same-Sex Marriage: How Are Non-Sectarian Controversial Issues Discussed in Northern Irish Politics?," *Irish Political Studies* 31, no. 4 (2016): 483–501.

11. Lisa Smyth, "The Cultural Politics of Sexuality and Reproduction in Northern Ireland," *Sociology* 40, no. 4 (2006): 668.

12. MLA Paul Givan, quoted in Official Report (Hansard), Tuesday, March 12, 2013 (Northern Ireland Assembly, Belfast, 2013).

13. Robin Whitaker and Gorotti Horgan, "Abortion Governance in the New Northern Ireland," in *A Fragmented Landscape: Abortion Governance and Protest Log-*

ics in Europe, ed. Silvia de Zordo, Joanna Mishtal, and Lorena Anton (New York: Berghahn Books, 2016); Smyth, "The Cultural Politics of Sexuality."

14. Sally Sheldon et al., "'Too Much, Too Indigestible, Too Fast'? The Decades of Struggle for Abortion Law Reform in Northern Ireland," *Modern Law Review* 83, no. 4 (2020): 761–69.

15. Thomson, "Abortion and Same-Sex Marriage"; Claire Pierson, "One Step Forwards, Two Steps Back: Women's Rights 20 Years after the Good Friday Agreement," *Parliamentary Affairs* 71, no. 2 (2018): 461–81.

16. Thomson, *Abortion Law*, 26; Claire Pierson et al., "After a CEDAW Optional Protocol Inquiry into Abortion Law: A Conversation with Activists for Change in Northern Ireland," *International Feminist Journal of Politics* 24, no. 2 (2022): 321.

17. Enright, McNeilly, and de Londras, "Abortion Activism," 365.

18. Interview NI818A; Jane Dreaper, "Women 'Using Web for Abortions,'" *BBC News*, July 11, 2008, http://news.bbc.co.uk/1/hi/health/7500237.stm.

19. MHRA communication, on file with author.

20. Author interview with Northern Irish lawyer involved in defending people charged with abortion-related crimes, 2021 (NI721).

21. Chi Chi Izundu, "Abortion Pill Online Sales 'Increasing in Britain,'" *BBC News*, February 15, 2017, https://www.bbc.co.uk/news/health-38960437; "BBC Grossly Exaggerated Number of Women Directly Ordering Abortion Pills from Overseas Providers FOI Reveals," *Right to Life News*, July 22, 2019, https://righttolife.org.uk /news/bbc-grossly-exaggerated-number-of-women-directly-ordering-abortion-pills-from-overseas-providers-foi-reveals.

22. Interpol, "Pharmaceutical Crime Operations: Operation Pangea," n.d., https:// www.interpol.int/en/Crimes/Illicit-goods/Pharmaceutical-crime-operations.

23. Interviews NI818A and NI721.

24. Author interview with activist working with several pro-choice and feminist groups in Belfast, 2018 (NI518A); Author interview with activist affiliated with Alliance for Choice, working in rural Northern Ireland, 2018 (NI518B); Interview NI220.

25. Interview NI518A.

26. Alliance for Choice, "Open Letter," March 11, 2013, reprinted in "Mass Civil Disobedience in North Illuminates Role of States In Abortion Discussion," *Workers Social Movement*, March 11, 2013, http://www.wsm.ie/c/mass-civil-disobedience-abortion-northern-ireland.

27. Marie-Lise Drapeau-Bisson, "Beyond Green and Orange: Alliance for Choice—Derry's Mobilisation for the Decriminalisation of Abortion," *Irish Political Studies* 35, no. 1 (2020): 90–114; Pierson, "One Step Forwards, Two Steps Back," 475–76.

28. Emma Campbell of Alliance for Choice, quoted in Enright, McNeilly, and de Londras, "Abortion Activism," 369.

29. Interview NI818A. The text of the letter was reprinted in Sam McBride, "We've Broken the Law—Prosecute Us, over 200 Abortion Activists Challenge Police," *Belfast Newsletter*, June 24, 2015, http://www.newsletter.co.uk/news/regional/we-ve-broken-the-law-prosecute-us-over-200-abortion-activists-challenge-police-1-6813947.

30. Amelia Gentleman, "Northern Irish Women Ask to Be Prosecuted for Taking Abortion Pills," *The Guardian*, May 23, 2016, https://www.theguardian.com/world/2016/may/23/northern-ireland-women-ask-to-be-prosecuted-for-taking-abortion-pills.

31. Interview NI518B.

32. Enright, McNeilly, and de Londras, "Abortion Activism," 370.

33. Interview ROI1118A.

34. The parallels between 1971 and 2014 were inexact: when the 1971 activists went to Belfast to buy condoms and bring them back to Dublin, the condoms were legally purchased in Northern Ireland. When ROSA went to Belfast to collect abortion pills and bring them back to Dublin, abortion pills were illegal in both jurisdictions, and the media compounded this confusion by inaccurately reporting that the activists had obtained the pills at Marie Stopes Belfast.

35. Interview ROI1118A; Máiréad Enright, "Law, Disobedience and 'the Abortion Pill': #Abortionpilltrain," *Human Rights Ireland* (Blog), November 1, 2014; last accessed September 1, 2017.

36. "'Abortion Drone' Delivers Pills to Northern Ireland," *Belfast Telegraph*, June 21, 2016, https://www.belfasttelegraph.co.uk/news/northern-ireland/abortion-drone-delivers-pills-to-northern-ireland-34819010.html; Andy Cuthbertson, "Abortion Robots Confiscated by Police for Distributing Pills at Belfast Protest," *Independent*, June 5, 2018, https://www.independent.co.uk/life-style/gadgets-and-tech/news/abortion-robot-belfast-protest-northern-ireland-pills-deliver-a8377591.html.

37. Author interview with activist and campaigner in Alliance for Choice, 2018 (NI818B); Interview NI721.

38. Interview ROI1118A; Socialist Party, "Defending Rosa & a Combative Socialist Feminist Approach," *Socialist Party* (Blog), June 28, 2018, https://socialistparty.ie/2018/06/defending-rosa-combative-socialist-feminist-approach/.

39. Sheldon, "Empowerment and Privacy," 49.

40. Kline, *Bodies of Knowledge*, 74.

41. Laura Kaplan, *The Story of Jane: The Legendary Underground Feminist Abortion Service* (Chicago: University of Chicago Press, 1997), 198.

42. Danièle Stewart, "The Women's Movement in France," *Signs* 6, no. 2 (1980): 350–54.

43. Author interview with Irish politician who has campaigned on abortion reform and medication abortion, 2018 (ROI1118B); Interview ROI1118A.

44. Sheldon et al., "Too Much, Too Indigestible," 23.

45. Ellen Coyne, "Northern Ireland Abortion Law Used to Arrest Violent Men," *The Times of London*, September 21, 2015, https://www.thetimes.co.uk/article/northern-ireland-abortion-law-used-to-arrest-violent-men-fv2b52gvnlj.

46. BPAS, "JR76 Case Report" (British Pregnancy Advisory Service, London, n.d.), https://www.bpas.org/media/3060/jr76-case-report.pdf; Interview NI721.

47. Sara Ramshaw, "Commentary on Family Planning Association of Northern Ireland v the Minister for Health, Social Services and Public Safety," in *Northern/Irish*

Feminist Judgments, ed. Aoife O'Donoghue, Julie McCandless, and Máiréad Enright (Oxford: Hart Publishing, 2016), 436–37; Henry McDonald, "Pro-Choice Activists Picket Derry Police Station over Mother's Abortion Trial," *The Guardian*, July 15, 2015, https://www.theguardian.com/uk-news/2015/jul/15/pro-abortion-campaigners-picket-derry-police-station-mother-prosecution; BPAS, "JR76 Case Report."

48. Deborah McAleese, "Why We Reported Abortion Pills Girl to Northern Ireland Police," *Belfast Telegraph*, April 26, 2016, https://www.belfasttelegraph.co.uk/news/northern-ireland/why-we-reported-abortion-pills-girl-to-northern-ireland-police-34602857.html.

49. "Woman Who Bought Drugs Online to Terminate Pregnancy Given Suspended Sentence," *BBC News*, April 4, 2016, https://www.bbc.co.uk/news/uk-northern-ireland-35962134.

50. "Man and Woman Cautioned over Abortion Pills," *BBC News*, January 18, 2017, https://www.bbc.co.uk/news/world-europe-38669974.

51. Hervey and Sheldon, "Abortion by Telemedicine," 125–28.

52. Author interview with activist working on pro-choice and feminist campaigns in Belfast, 2018 (NI518C); Interview NI818A.

53. Interview NI818B.

54. Interview NI818B.

55. Interview NI721; Tyler McNally, "A Shot across the Bow," *The Last Round* (Blog), June 17, 2017, https://lastroundblog.wordpress.com/2017/06/17/a-shot-across-the-bow/; Lisa Smyth, "Northern Ireland Abortion Pills Raid Woman Helen Crickard Won't Be Charged," *Belfast Telegraph*, April 18, 2017, https://www.belfasttelegraph.co.uk/news/northern-ireland/northern-ireland-abortion-pills-raid-woman-helen-crickard-wont-be-charged-35630380.html.

56. Interview NI518A.

57. Interview NI518A.

58. Sheldon, "Empowerment and Privacy," 838.

59. House of Commons, Women and Equalities Committee, "Abortion Law in Northern Ireland: Eighth Report of Session 2017–19."

60. "John Larkin Abortion Comments Totally Wrong—Sinn Fein," *BBC News*, October 19, 2012, https://www.bbc.co.uk/news/uk-northern-ireland-20010143.

61. Author interview with activist working in Alliance for Choice, 2018 (NI1018); Interviews NI518B, NI518C, NI818A, and NI818B.

62. Thomson, *Abortion Law*, 182–83.

63. Interview NI721.

64. Catherine O'Rourke, "Advocating Abortion Rights in Northern Ireland: Local and Global Tensions," *Social & Legal Studies* 25, no. 6 (2016): 730–31; Thomson, *Abortion Law*, 780–81.

65. Department of Health, Social Services and Public Safety, "The Limited Circumstances for a Lawful Termination of Pregnancy in Northern Ireland: A Guidance Document for Health and Social Care Professionals on Law and Clinical Practice" [Draft] (Belfast, 2013).

66. Whitaker and Horgan, "Abortion Governance," 254.

67. O'Rourke, "Advocating Abortion Rights," 730.

68. Clare Dyer, "Abortion numbers Halve in Northern Ireland as Doctors Fear Prison," *BMJ: British Medical Journal* 352 (2016): i1135.

69. Niamh Griffin, "Patients, Not Criminals: Northern Ireland Grapples with How to Provide Legal Abortion," *BMJ: British Medical Journal* 367 (2019): l6318; Thomson, *Abortion Law*, 180.

70. Interviews NI518A and NI518B.

71. MacDonald, "Misoprostol."

72. Thomson, *Abortion Law*, 73; Sheldon et al., "Too Much, Too Indigestible," 24.

73. Enright, McNeilly, and de Londras, "Abortion Activism," 373.

74. Sheldon et al., "Too Much, Too Indigestible," 24.

75. Interviews NI1018 and NI818B.

76. Interviews NI518A, NI818B, and NI721.

77. Thomson, *Abortion Law*, 60.

78. See, e.g., Henry McDonald, "Belfast Council Passes Abortion Pills Motion against Prosecutions," *The Guardian*, April 10, 2018, https://www.theguardian.com/world/2018/apr/09/belfast-council-to-debate-abortion-pills-motion-northern-ireland.

79. Thomson, "Abortion and Same Sex Marriage"; Claire Pierson and Jennifer Thomson, "Allies or Opponents? Power-Sharing, Civil Society, and Gender," *Nationalism and Ethnic Politics* 24, no. 1 (2018): 100–115.

80. Thomson, *Abortion Law*, 189.

81. Interview NI721.

82. See, e.g., the press release from the Women's Equality Party, "Press Release: DUP Deal Is Threat to Human Rights," June 26, 2017, https://www.womensequality.org.uk/dup_deal.

83. The request was submitted by the Family Planning Association Northern Ireland, Alliance for Choice, and Northern Ireland Women's European Platform.

84. O'Rourke, "Advocating Abortion Rights."

85. Interview NI818B.

86. Committee on the Elimination of Discrimination against Women (CEDAW), "Report of the Inquiry Concerning the United Kingdom of Great Britain and Northern Ireland under Article 8 of the Optional Protocol to the Convention on the Elimination of All Forms of Discrimination against Women" (United Nations, New York, 2018), 18–19.

87. CEDAW, "Report of the Inquiry," 21–22.

88. O'Rourke, "Advocating Abortion Rights," 724.

89. Enright, McNeilly, and de Londras, "Abortion Activism, Legal Change," 375; Interviews NI518A and NI818B.

90. O'Rourke, "Advocating Abortion Rights," 724.

91. David Torrance, *Devolution in Northern Ireland, 1998–2020* (London: House of Commons, 2020).

92. Sheldon et al., "Too Much, Too Indigestible," 28–32.

93. Interview NI721.

94. UK Parliament, Northern Ireland (Executive Formation) Act 2019, s9.

95. Author interview with Emma Campbell, 2020.

96. Sheldon, *Beyond Control*.

97. Shanti Das, "Women Accused of Illegal Abortions in England and Wales after Miscarriages and Stillbirths," *The Guardian*, July 2, 2022, https://www.theguardian.com/world/2022/jul/02/women-accused-of-abortions-in-england-and-wales-after-miscarriages-and-stillbirths.

98. Pierson et al., "After a CEDAW," 312.

99. Pierson et al., "After a CEDAW," 313.

CHAPTER 9. LOOKING FORWARD

1. Michelle Goodwin and Mary Ziegler, "Whatever Happened to the Exceptions for Rape and Incest?," *The Atlantic*, November 29, 2021, https://www.theatlantic.com/ideas/archive/2021/11/abortion-law-exceptions-rape-and-incest/620812/.

2. See, e.g., Frances Stead Sellers and Fenit Nirappil, "Confusion Post-Roe Spurs Delays, Denials for Some Lifesaving Pregnancy Care," *Washington Post*, July 16, 2022, https://www.washingtonpost.com/health/2022/07/16/abortion-miscarriage-ectopic-pregnancy-care/.

3. Elizabeth Nash and Isabel Guarnieri, "13 States Have Abortion Trigger Bans—Here's What Happens When Roe Is Overturned," Guttmacher Institute, June 6, 2022, www.guttmacher.org/article/2022/06/13-states-have-abortion-trigger-bans-heres-what-happens-when-roe-overturned.

4. Goodwin, *Policing the Womb*, 30–31; Diaz-Tello et al., *Roe's Unfinished Promise*.

5. Quet, "Pharmaceutical Capitalism,"; Gavin Brown and Cesare Di Feliciantonio, "Geographies of PrEP, TasP and Undetectability: Reconceptualising HIV Assemblages to Explore What Else Matters in the Lives of Gay and Bisexual Men," *Dialogues in Human Geography* 12, no. 1 (2022): 100–118.

6. Murtagh et al., "Exploring the Feasibility."

7. Liza Fuentes et al., "Texas Women's Decisions and Experiences Regarding Self-Managed Abortion," *BMC Women's Health* 20, no. 1 (2020): 1–12.

8. Interview NI518.

9. Nisha Verma et al., "Interim Clinical Recommendations: Self-Managed Abortion," Society of Family Planning, 2022, https://doi.org/10.46621/ZRDX9581.

10. Conti-Cook, "Surveilling the Digital Abortion Diary," 1.

11. Interview T1118.

12. Sophie Kasakove, "Woman in Texas Charged with Murder in Connection with 'Self-Induced Abortion,'" *New York Times*, April 11, 2022, https://www.nytimes.com/2022/04/09/us/self-induced-abortion-murder-charge.html/.

13. Pew Research Center, "America's Abortion Quandary," May 6, 2022, https://www.pewresearch.org/religion/2022/05/06/americas-abortion-quandary/

14. Interviews PL519A and PL519B.

15. Enright and Cloatre, "Transformative Illegality," 279.

16. Joanna Erdman, Kinga Jelinska, and Susan Yanow, "Understandings of Self-Managed Abortion as Health Inequity, Harm Reduction and Social Change," *Reproductive Health Matters* 26, no. 54 (2018): 13–19.

17. Parsons and Romanis, *Early Medical Abortion*, 166.

18. Aiken et al., "Knowledge, Interest, and Motivations," 238; Margit Endler et al., "Telemedicine for Medical Abortion: A Systematic Review," *BJOG: An International Journal of Obstetrics & Gynaecology* 126, no. 9 (2019): 1094–1102.

19. María Lafaurie et al., "Women's Perspectives on Medical Abortion in Mexico, Colombia, Ecuador and Peru: A Qualitative Study," *Reproductive Health Matters* 13, no. 26 (2005): 75–83; Simonds et al., "Abortion, Revised."

20. Caroline Moreau et al., "Medical vs. Surgical Abortion: The Importance of Women's Choice," *Contraception* 84, no. 3 (2011): 228.

21. Jelinska and Yanow, "Putting Abortion Pills into Women's Hands," 86–89.

22. Abortion Rights Campaign, "Too Many Barriers."

23. Caroline Moreau et al. "Abortion Regulation in Europe in the Era of COVID-19: A Spectrum of Policy Responses," *BMJ Sexual & Reproductive Health* 47, no. 4 (2021): e14.

24. Calkin and Berny, "Legal and Non-Legal Barriers."

25. BPAS, "Pills by Post: Telemedical Abortion at the British Pregnancy Advisory Service" (London, September 2020), https://www.bpas.org/media/3385/bpas-pills-by-post-service.pdf; Abigail R. A. Aiken et al., "Demand for Self-Managed Online Telemedicine Abortion in Eight European Countries during the COVID-19 Pandemic: A Regression Discontinuity Analysis," *BMJ Sexual & Reproductive Health* 47, no. 4 (2021): 238–45.

26. Endler et al. "Telemedicine for Medical Abortion"; Sarah Baum et al., "'It's Not a Seven-Headed Beast': Abortion Experience among Women That Received Support from Helplines for Medication Abortion in Restrictive Settings," *Health Care for Women International* 41, no. 10 (2020): 1128–46.

27. Mariana Prandini Assis and Sara Larrea, "Why Self-Managed Abortion Is So Much More Than a Provisional Solution for Times of Pandemic," *Sexual and Reproductive Health Matters* 28, no. 1 (2020): 1779633.

28. Melissa Murray, "Race-ing Roe: Reproductive Justice, Racial Justice, and the Battle for Roe v. Wade," *Harvard Law Review* 134 (2020): 2025.

29. Loretta Ross, "What Is Reproductive Justice?," In *Reproductive Justice Briefing Book: A Primer on Reproductive Justice and Social Change*, ed. SisterSong (Atlanta, GA: Pro-Choice Public Education Project and SisterSong Women of Color Reproductive Justice Collective, 2007), 4–5.

30. Rachel Jones and Jenna Jerman, "Population Group Abortion Rates and Lifetime Incidence of Abortion: United States, 2008–2014," *American Journal of Public Health* 107, no. 12 (2017): 1904–9.

31. See, e.g., Alexa Solazzo, "Different and Not Equal: The Uneven Association of Race, Poverty, and Abortion Laws on Abortion Timing," *Social Problems* 66, no. 4 (2019): 519–47.

32. Foster, *The Turnaway Study*.

33. Roberts, "Reproductive Justice," 81.

34. Elizabeth Raymond et al., "TelAbortion: Evaluation of a Direct to Patient Telemedicine Abortion Service in the United States," *Contraception* 100, no. 3 (2019): 173–77.

35. Sarah Raifman et al., "Medication Abortion: Potential for Improved Patient Access through Pharmacies," *Journal of the American Pharmacists Association* 58, no. 4 (2018): 377–81.

36. Donley, "Early Abortion Exceptionalism."

37. Petchesky, *Abortion and Woman's Choice*, 291–92.

BIBLIOGRAPHY

Adams, Jill, and Melissa Mikesell. "And Damned If They Don't: Prototype Theories to End Punitive Policies against Pregnant People Living in Poverty." *Georgetown Journal of Gender & Law* 18 (2017): 283–332.

Adashi, Eli, Rohit Rajan, Daniel O'Mahony, and Glenn Cohen. "The Next Two Decades of Mifepristone at FDA: History as Destiny." *Contraception* 109 (2022): 1–7.

Aiken, Abigail R. A., Kathleen Broussard, Dana M. Johnson, and Elisa Padron. "Motivations and Experiences of People Seeking Medication Abortion Online in the United States." *Perspectives on Sexual and Reproductive Health* 50, no. 4 (2018): 157–63.

Aiken, Abigail R. A., Kathleen Broussard, Dana Johnson, Elisa Padron, Jennifer Starling, and James Scott. "Knowledge, Interest, and Motivations Surrounding Self-Managed Medication Abortion among Patients at Three Texas Clinics." *American Journal of Obstetrics and Gynecology* 223, no. 2 (2020): e1–38.

Aiken, Abigail R. A., Irena Digol, James Trussell, and Rebecca Gomperts. "Self-Reported Outcomes and Adverse Events after Medical Abortion through Online Telemedicine: Population-Based Study in the Republic of Ireland and Northern Ireland." *BMJ: British Medical Journal* 357 (2017): j2011.

Aiken, Abigail R. A., Rebecca Gomperts, and James Trussell. "Experiences and Characteristics of Women Seeking and Completing At-Home Medical Termination of Pregnancy through Online Telemedicine in Ireland and Northern Ireland: A Population-Based Analysis." *BJOG: An International Journal of Obstetrics & Gynaecology* 124, no. 8 (2017): 1208–15.

Aiken, Abigail R. A., Dana M. Johnson, Kathleen Broussard, and Elisa Padron. "Experiences of Women in Ireland Who Accessed Abortion by Travelling Abroad or by Using Abortion Medication at Home: A Qualitative Study." *BMJ Sexual & Reproductive Health* 44, no. 3 (2018): 181–86.

Aiken, Abigail R. A., Evdokia Romanova, Julia Morber, and Rebecca Gomperts. "Safety and Effectiveness of self-Managed Medication Abortion Provided Using Online Telemedicine in the United States: A Population-Based Study." *The Lancet Regional Health—Americas* 10 (2022): 1–8.

Aiken, Abigail R. A., Jennifer Starling, Rebecca Gomperts, James Scott, and Catherine Aiken. "Demand for Self-Managed Online Telemedicine Abortion in Eight European Countries during the COVID-19 Pandemic: A Regression Discontinuity Analysis." *BMJ Sexual & Reproductive Health* 47, no. 4 (2021): 238–45.

Aiken, Abigail R. A., Jennifer Starling, James Scott, and Rebecca Gomperts. "Requests for Self-Managed Medication Abortion Provided Using Online Telemedicine in 30 US States before and after the Dobbs v Jackson Women's Health Organization Decision." *JAMA* 328, no. 17 (2022): 1768–70.

Aiken, Abigail R. A., and Ushma D. Upadhyay. "The Future of Medication Abortion in a Post-Roe World." *BMJ: British Medical Journal* 377 (2022): 1393.

Aitken, Kara, Paul Patek, and Mark Murphy. "The Opinions and Experiences of Irish Obstetric and Gynaecology Trainee Doctors in Relation to Abortion Services in Ireland." *Journal of Medical Ethics* 43, no. 11 (2017): 778–83.

Amnesty International. "She Is Not a Criminal: The Impact of Ireland's Abortion Law." London, 2015.

Andreasson, Jesper, and Thomas Johansson. "Online Doping: The New Self-Help Culture of Ethnopharmacology." *Sport in Society* 19, no. 7 (2016): 957–72.

Anthony, Gordon. "Brexit and the Irish Border: Legal and Political Questions." In "Royal Irish Academy & British Academy Brexit Briefing," 1–9. British Academy and Royal Irish Academy, 2017.

Arey, Whitney, Klaira Lerma, Anitra Beasley, Lorie Harper, Ghazaleh Moayedi, and Kari White. "A Preview of the Dangerous Future of Abortion Bans—Texas Senate Bill 8." *New England Journal of Medicine* 387, no. 5 (2022): 388–90.

Assis, Mariana Prandini. "Liberating Abortion Pills in Legally Restricted Settings: Activism as Public Criminology." In *Routledge Handbook of Public Criminologies*, edited by Kathryn Henne and Rita Shah, 120–30. London: Routledge, 2020.

Assis, Mariana Prandini, and Joanna Erdman. "Abortion Rights beyond the Medico-Legal Paradigm." *Global Public Health* 17, no. 10 (2022): 2235–50.

Assis, Mariana Prandini, and Sara Larrea. "Why Self-Managed Abortion Is So Much More Than a Provisional Solution for Times of Pandemic." *Sexual and Reproductive Health Matters* 28, no. 1 (2020): 37–39.

Bass, Marie. "Toward Coalition: The Reproductive Health Technologies Project." In *Abortion Wars: A Half Century of Struggle, 1950–2000*, edited by Rickie Solinger, 251–68. Berkeley: University of California Press, 1998.

Baulieu, Etienne-Emile, and Mort Rosenblum. *The "Abortion Pill": RU-486: A Woman's Choice*. New York: Simon & Schuster, 1991.

Baum, Sarah, A. Ramirez, S. Larrea, S. Filippa, I. Egwuatu, J. Wydrzynska, M. Piasecka, S. Nmezi, and K. Jelinska. 2020. "'It's Not a Seven-Headed Beast: Abortion Experience among Women That Received Support from Helplines for Medication

Abortion in Restrictive Settings." *Health Care for Women International* 41, no. 10 (2020): 1128–46.

Bearak, Jonathan, Anna Popinchalk, Bela Ganatra, Ann-Beth Moller, Özge Tunçalp, Cynthia Beavin, Lorraine Kwok, and Leontine Alkema. "Unintended Pregnancy and Abortion by Income, Region, and the Legal Status of Abortion: Estimates from a Comprehensive Model for 1990–2019." *The Lancet Global Health* 8, no. 9 (2020): e1152–e1161.

Boler, Tania, Cicely Marston, Nick Corby, and Elizabeth Gardiner. *Medical Abortion in India: A Model for the Rest of the World*. London: Marie Stopes International, 2009.

Bollyky, Thomas, and Aaron Kesselheim. "Reputation and Authority: The FDA and the Fight over US Prescription Drug Importation." *Vanderbilt Law Review* 73 (2020): 1331–1400.

Boonstra, Heather. "Medication Abortion Restrictions Burden Women and Providers—and Threaten U.S. Trend toward Very Early Abortion." *Guttmacher Policy Review* 16, no. 1 (2013): 18–23.

Brown, Gavin, and Cesare Di Feliciantonio. "Geographies of PrEP, TasP and Undetectability: Reconceptualising HIV Assemblages to Explore What Else Matters in the Lives of Gay and Bisexual Men." *Dialogues in Human Geography* 12, no. 1 (2022): 100–118.

Browne, Kath, and Catherine Jean Nash. "In Ireland We 'Love Both'? Heteroactivism in Ireland's Anti-Repeal Ephemera." *Feminist Review* 124, no. 1 (2020): 51–67.

Calkin, Sydney. "Healthcare Not Airfare! Art, Abortion and Political Agency in Ireland." *Gender, Place & Culture* 26, no. 3 (2019): 338–61.

———. "Legal Geographies of Medication Abortion in the USA." *Transactions of the Institute of British Geographers* 47, no. 2 (2022): 378–92.

———. "Towards a Political Geography of Abortion." *Political Geography* 69 (2019): 22–29.

———. "Transnational Abortion Pill Flows and the Political Geography of Abortion in Ireland." *Territory, Politics, Governance* 9, no. 2 (2021): 163–79.

Calkin, Sydney, and Ella Berny. "Legal and Non-Legal Barriers to Abortion in Ireland and the United Kingdom." *Medicine Access@Point of Care* 5 (2021): 1–10.

Calkin, Sydney, and Monika Ewa Kaminska. "Persistence and Change in Morality Policy: The Role of the Catholic Church in the Politics of Abortion in Ireland and Poland." *Feminist Review* 124, no. 1 (2020): 86–102.

Caytas, Joanna. "Women's Reproductive Rights as a Political Price of Post-Communist Transformation in Poland." *Amsterdam Law Forum* 5 (2013): 64–89.

Chandrashekar, V. S., Debanjana Choudhuri, and Ananya Vajpeyi. *Availability of Medical Abortion Drugs in the Markets of Six Indian States*. New Delhi: Foundation for Reproductive Health Services (FRHS) India, 2020.

Chaudhuri, Sudip. "The Pharmaceutical Industry in India after Trips." In *The New Political Economy of Pharmaceuticals: Production, Innovation and Trips in the Global South*, edited by Hans Löfgren and Owen Williams, 111–25. London: Palgrave Macmillan, 2003.

Chełstowska, Agata. "Stigmatisation and Commercialisation of Abortion Services in Poland: Turning Sin into Gold." *Reproductive Health Matters* 19, no. 37 (2011): 98–106.

Cherian, Jerin Jose, Manju Rahi, Navdeep Rinwa, Shubhra Singh, Sanapareddy Eswara Reddy, Yogendra Kumar Gupta, Vishwa Mohan Katoch, et al. "India's Road to Independence in Manufacturing Active Pharmaceutical Ingredients: Focus on Essential Medicines." *Economies* 9, no. 2 (2021): 1–18.

Chowdhury, Nupur, Pallavi Joshi, Arpita Patnaik, and Arpita Saraswathy. *Administrative Structure and Functions of Drug Regulatory Authorities in India.* New Delhi: Indian Council for Research on International Economic Relations, 2015.

Ciaputa, Ewelina. "Abortion and the Catholic Church in Poland." In *Abortion across Borders: Transnational Travel and Access to Abortion Services,* edited by Christabelle Sethna and Gayle Davis, 278–309. Baltimore: Johns Hopkins University Press, 2019.

Clarke, Adele, and Theresa Montini. "The Many Faces of Ru486: Tales of Situated Knowledges and Technological Contestations." *Science, Technology, & Human Values* 18, no. 1 (1993): 42–78.

Clements, Steve, and Roger Ingham. *Improving Knowledge Regarding Abortions Performed on Irish Women in the UK.* Dublin: Health Service Executive, Crisis Pregnancy Agency, 2007.

Clifford, Allison. "Abortion in International Waters Off the Coast of Ireland: Avoiding a Collision between Irish Moral Sovereignty and the European Community." *Pace International Law Review* 14 (2002): 385–434.

Cloatre, Emilie, and Máiréad Enright. "'On the Perimeter of the Lawful': Enduring Illegality in the Irish Family Planning Movement, 1972–1985." *Journal of Law and Society* 44, no. 4 (2017): 471–500.

Cohen, David S., Greer Donley, and Rachel Rebouché. "The New Abortion Battleground." *Columbia Law Review* 123, no. 1 (2023): 1–100.

Cohen, David, and Carole Joffe. *Obstacle Course: The Everyday Struggle to Get an Abortion in America.* Oakland: University of California Press, 2020.

Condit, Celeste. *Decoding Abortion Rhetoric: Communicating Social Change.* Champaign: University of Illinois Press, 1994.

Connolly, Linda, and Tina O'Toole. *Documenting Irish Feminisms: The Second Wave.* Bognor Regis, UK: Woodfield Press, 2005.

Conti-Cook, Cynthia. "Surveilling the Digital Abortion Diary." *University of Baltimore Law Review* 50 (2020): 1–76.

Corbin, Caroline Mala. "Abortion Distortions." *Washington & Lee Law Review* 71 (2014): 1175–1210.

Couzinet, Beatrice, Nelly LeStrat, Andre Ulmann, Etienne Emile Baulieu, and Gilbert Schaison. "Termination of Early Pregnancy by the Progesterone Antagonist Ru 486 (Mifepristone)." *New England Journal of Medicine* 315, no. 25 (1986): 1565–70.

Cowen, Deborah. *The Deadly Life of Logistics: Mapping Violence in Global Trade.* Minneapolis: University of Minnesota Press, 2014.

Curanović, Alicja. "The International Activity of Ordo Iuris: The Central European Actor and the Global Christian Right." *Religions* 12, no. 12 (2021): 1–20.

Das, Veena, and Ranendra Das. "Urban Health and Pharmaceutical Consumption in Delhi, India." *Journal of Biosocial Science* 38, no. 1 (2006): 69–82.

Davies, Norman. *God's Playground: A History of Poland*. Oxford: Oxford University Press, 2005.

Delay, Cara. "Pills, Potions, and Purgatives: Women and Abortion Methods in Ireland, 1900–1950." *Women's History Review* 28, no. 3 (2019): 479–99.

De Londras, Fiona. "Intersectionality, Repeal, and Reproductive Rights in Ireland." In *Intersectionality and Human Rights*, edited by Peter Dunne and Shreya Atrey, 1–24. Oxford: Hart Publishing, 2019.

———. "Protection of Life During Pregnancy Act 2013." In *Women's Legal Landmarks: Celebrating the History of Women and Law in the UK and Ireland*, edited by Erika Rackley and Rosemary Auchmuty, 597–604. London: Bloomsbury, 2018.

De Londras, Fiona, and Máiréad Enright. *Repealing the 8th: Reforming Irish Abortion Law*. Bristol: Policy Press, 2018.

Denbow, Jennifer. *Governed through Choice: Autonomy, Technology, and the Politics of Reproduction*. New York: New York University Press, 2015.

De Zordo, Silvia. "The Biomedicalisation of Illegal Abortion: The Double Life of Misoprostol in Brazil." *História, Ciências, Saúde-Manguinhos* 23, no. 1 (2016): 19–36.

De Zordo, Silvia, and Joanna Mishtal. "Physicians and Abortion: Provision, Political Participation and Conflicts on the Ground—the Cases of Brazil and Poland." *Women's Health Issues* 21, no. 3 (2011): S32–S36.

Diaz-Tello, Farah, Melissa Mikesell, and Jill Adams. *Roe's Unfinished Promise: Decriminalizing Abortion Once and for All*. SIA Legal Team. Available at SSRN 3082643 (2017).

Di Nicola, Andrea, E. Martini, G. Baratto, G. Antonopoulos, D. Boriero, W. Da Col, and Y. Zabyelina. "Fakecare: Developing Expertise against the Online Trade of Fake Medicines by Producing and Disseminating Knowledge, Counterstrategies and Tools across the EU." eCrime Research Reports, Trento, Italy, 2015.

Donley, Greer. "Medication Abortion Exceptionalism." *Cornell Law Review* 107 (2021): 627–704.

Donovan, Megan. "Self-Managed Medication Abortion: Expanding the Available Options for US Abortion Care." *Guttmacher Policy Review* 21 (2018): 41–47.

Drapeau-Bisson, Marie-Lise. "Beyond Green and Orange: Alliance for Choice—Derry's Mobilisation for the Decriminalisation of Abortion." *Irish Political Studies* 35, no. 1 (2020): 90–114.

Drążkiewicz, Ela, Thomas Strong, Nancy Scheper-Hughes, Hugh Turpin, A. Jamie Saris, Joanna Mishtal, Helena Wulff, et al. "Repealing Ireland's Eighth Amendment: Abortion Rights and Democracy Today." *Social Anthropology* 28, no. 3 (2020): 561–84.

Drążkiewicz-Grodzicka, Elzbieta, and Maire Ní Mhórdha. "Of Trust and Mistrust: The Politics of Repeal.'" In *After Repeal: Rethinking Abortion Politics*, edited by Kath Browne and Sydney Calkin, 90–106. London: Zed Books, 2020.

Duffy, Deirdre Niamh. "From Feminist Anarchy to Decolonisation: Understanding Abortion Health Activism before and after the Repeal of the 8th Amendment." *Feminist Review* 124, no. 1 (2020): 69–85.

Dyer, Clare. "Abortion Numbers Halve in Northern Ireland as Doctors Fear Prison." *BMJ: British Medical Journal* 352 (2016): i135.

Earner-Byrne, Lindsey. "The Boat to England: An Analysis of the Official Reactions to the Emigration of Single Expectant Irishwomen to Britain, 1922–1972." *Irish Economic and Social History* 30, no. 1 (2003): 52–70.

Einhorn, Barbara. *Cinderella Goes to Market: Citizenship, Gender and Women's Movements in East Central Europe*. London: Verso, 1993.

Endler, Margit, Leona Beets, Kristina Gemzell Danielsson, and Rebecca Gomperts. "Safety and Acceptability of Medical Abortion through Telemedicine after 9 Weeks of Gestation: A Population-Based Cohort Study." *BJOG: An International Journal of Obstetrics & Gynaecology* 126, no. 5 (2019): 609–18.

Endler, Margit, Antonella Lavelanet, Amanda Cleeve, Bela Ganatra, Rebecca Gomperts, and Kristina Gemzell-Danielsson. "Telemedicine for Medical Abortion: A Systematic Review." *BJOG: An International Journal of Obstetrics & Gynaecology* 126, no. 9 (2019): 1094–1102.

Enright, Máiréad. "The Enemy of the Good': Reflections on Ireland's New Abortion Legislation." *feminists@law* 8, no. 2 (2018): 1–12.

———. "Law, Disobedience and 'the Abortion Pill': #Abortionpilltrain." *Human Rights Ireland* [Blog]. Published November 1, 2014; last accessed September 1, 2017. http://humanrights.ie/law-culture-and-religion/law-disobedience-and-the-abortion-pill-abortionpilltrain/.

———. "'No. I Won't Go Back': National Time, Trauma and Legacies of Symphysiotomy in Ireland." In *Law and Time*, edited by Sian Beynon-Jones and Emily Grabham, 46–74. London: Routledge, 2018.

Enright, Máiréad, and Emilie Cloatre. "Transformative Illegality: How Condoms 'Became Legal' in Ireland, 1991–1993." *Feminist Legal Studies* 26, no. 3 (2018): 261–84.

Enright, Máiréad, Kathryn McNeilly, and Fiona de Londras. "Abortion Activism, Legal Change, and Taking Feminist Law Work Seriously." *Northern Ireland Legal Quarterly* 71 (2020): 359–85.

Epstein, Steven. *Impure Science: AIDS, Activism, and the Politics of Knowledge*. Berkeley: University of California Press, 1996.

Erdman, Joanna, Kinga Jelinska, and Susan Yanow. "Understandings of Self-Managed Abortion as Health Inequity, Harm Reduction and social Change." *Reproductive Health Matters* 26, no. 54 (2018): 13–19.

Evans, Jocelyn, and Jonathan Tonge. "Social Class and Party Choice in Northern Ireland's Ethnic Blocs." *West European Politics* 32, no. 5 (2009): 1012–30.

Field, Luke. "The Abortion Referendum of 2018 and a Timeline of Abortion Politics in Ireland to Date." *Irish Political Studies* 33, no. 4 (2018): 608–28.

Fischer, Clara. "Abortion and Reproduction in Ireland: Shame, Nation-Building and the Affective Politics of Place." *Feminist Review* 122, no. 1 (2019): 32–48.

———. "Feminists Redraw Public and Private Spheres: Abortion, Vulnerability, and the Affective Campaign to Repeal the Eighth Amendment." *Signs* 45, no. 4 (2020): 995–1010.

Fletcher, Ruth. "Negotiating Strangeness on the Abortion Trail." In *Revaluing Care in Theory, Law and Policy: Cycles and Connections*, edited by Rosie Harding, Ruth Fletcher, and Chris Beasley, 14–30. London: Routledge, 2016.

———. "Peripheral Governance: Administering Transnational Health-Care Flows." *International Journal of Law in Context* 9 (2013): 160–91.

———. "Post-Colonial Fragments: Representations of Abortion in Irish Law and Politics." *Journal of Law and Society* 28, no. 4 (2002): 568–79.

———. "Pro-Life Absolutes, Feminist Challenges: The Fundamentalist Narrative of Irish Abortion Law 1986–1992." *Osgoode Hall Law Journal* 36 (1998): 1–62.

———. "#Repealedthe8th: Translating Travesty, Global Conversation, and the Irish Abortion Referendum." *Feminist Legal Studies*, no. 26 (2018): 233–59.

———. "Reproducing Irishness: Race, Gender, and Abortion Law." *Canadian Journal of Women and the Law* 17, no. 2 (2005): 365–404.

Foote, Elliott. "Prescription Drug Importation: An Expanded FDA Personal Use Exemption and Qualified Regulators for Foreign-Produced Pharmaceuticals." *Loyola Consumer Law Review* 27 (2014): 369–98.

Foster, Diana Greene. "Dramatic Decreases in US Abortion Rates: Public Health Achievement or Failure?" *American Journal of Public Health* 107, no. 12 (2017): 1860–62.

———. *The Turnaway Study: Ten Years, a Thousand Women, and the Consequences of Having—or Being Denied—an Abortion.* New York: Simon and Schuster, 2020.

Foundation for Equality and Emancipation. "Allies or Opponents: Medical Doctors in the Debate on Women's Right to Abortion in Poland." Fundacja na Rzecz R wności i Emancypacji STER [Foundation for Equality and Emancipation STER], Warsaw, 2018.

Freeman, Cordelia, and Sandra Rodriguez. "Not Knowing, Silence and Concealment: Strategic Ignorance in Abortion Practices in Latin America." Paper presented at the Abortion + SRH Seminar Series, London School of Economics, 9 March 2022.

Frye, Laura, Catherine Kilfedder, Jennifer Blum, and Beverly Winikoff. "A Cross-Sectional Analysis of Mifepristone, Misoprostol, and Combination Mifepristone-Misoprostol Package Inserts Obtained in 20 Countries." *Contraception* 101, no. 5 (2020): 315–20.

Fuentes, Liza, Sarah Baum, Brianna Keefe-Oates, Kari White, Kristine Hopkins, Joseph Potter, and Daniel Grossman. "Texas Women's Decisions and Experiences Regarding Self-Managed Abortion." *BMC Women's Health* 20, no. 1 (2020): 1–12.

Gal, Susan, and Gail Kligman. *The Politics of Gender after Socialism: A Comparative-Historical Essay.* Princeton, NJ: Princeton University Press, 2000.

Ganatra, Bela, Caitlin Gerdts, Clémentine Rossier, Brooke Ronald Johnson Jr., Özge Tunçalp, Anisa Assifi, Gilda Sedgh, et al. "Global, Regional, and Subregional Classification of Abortions by Safety, 2010–14: Estimates from a Bayesian Hierarchical Model." *The Lancet* 390, no. 10110 (2017): 2372–81.

Garrett, Kristin, and Joshua Jansa. "Interest Group Influence in Policy Diffusion Networks." *State Politics & Policy Quarterly* 15, no. 3 (2015): 387–417.

Gilman, Nils, Jesse Goldhammer, and Steven Weber. *Deviant Globalization: Black Market Economy in the 21st Century.* London: A&C Black, 2011.

Gleeson, Kate. "A woman's work is . . . unfinished business: Justice for the Disappeared Magdalen Women of Modern Ireland." *Feminist Legal Studies* 25, no. 3 (2017): 291–312.

Gliszczyńska-Grabias, Aleksandra, and Wojciech Sadurski. "The Judgment That Wasn't (but Which Nearly Brought Poland to a Standstill): 'Judgment' of the Polish Constitutional Tribunal of 22 October 2020, K1/20." *European Constitutional Law Review* 17, no. 1 (2021): 130–53.

Gomperts, Rebecca. "Women on Waves: Where Next for the Abortion Boat?" *Reproductive Health Matters* 10, no. 19 (2002): 180–83.

Goodwin, Michele. *Policing the Womb: Invisible Women and the Criminalization of Motherhood.* Cambridge: Cambridge University Press, 2020.

Grabowska, Magdalena. "Bringing the Second World In: Conservative Revolution(s), Socialist Legacies, and Transnational Silences in the Trajectories of Polish Feminism." *Signs* 37, no. 2 (2012): 385–411.

———. "Cultural War or Business as Usual? Recent Instances and the Historical Origins of the Backlash against Women's Rights and Sexual Rights in Poland." In *Anti-Gender Movements on the Rise? Strategising for Gender Equality in Central and Eastern Europe,* edited by Heinrich Böll Stiftung, 54–64. Berlin: Heinrich Böll Stiftung, 2015.

Graff, Agnieszka. "'Gender Ideology': Weak Concepts, Powerful Politics." *Religion and Gender* 6, no. 2 (2016): 268–72.

Greene, Jeremy. *Generic: The Unbranding of Modern Medicine.* Baltimore: Johns Hopkins University Press, 2014.

Greenhouse, Linda, and Reva Siegel. "Casey and the Clinic Closings: When Protecting Health Obstructs Choice." *Yale Law Journal* 125 (2016): 1428–80.

Gregson, Nicky, and Mike Crang. "Illicit Economies: Customary Illegality, Moral Economies and Circulation." *Transactions of the Institute of British Geographers* 42, no. 2 (1 June 2017): 206–19.

Griffin, Niamh. "Patients, not Criminals: Northern Ireland Grapples with How to Provide Legal Abortion." *BMJ: British Medical Journal* 367 (2019): l6318.

Grossman, Daniel, Kate Grindlay, Todd Buchacker, Kathleen Lane, and Kelly Blanchard. "Effectiveness and Acceptability of Medical Abortion Provided through Telemedicine." *Obstetrics & Gynecology* 118, no. 2 (2011): 296–303.

Grossman, Daniel, E. Hendrick, Liza Fuentes, Kari White, Kristine Hopkins, Amanda Stevenson, Celia Hubert Lopez, Sara Yeatman, and Joseph Potter. "Knowledge, Opinion and Experience Related to Abortion Self-Induction in Texas." *Contraception* 4, no. 92 (2015): 360–61.

Grzebalska, Weronika, and Andrea Pető. "The Gendered Modus Operandi of the Illiberal Transformation in Hungary and Poland." *Women's Studies International Forum* 68 (2018): 164–72.

Grzymała-Busse, Anna. *Nations under God: How Churches Use Moral Authority to Influence Policy*. Princeton, NJ: Princeton University Press, 2015.

Guttmacher Institute. *Abortion Worldwide 2017: Unequal Progress and Unequal Access*. Washington, DC: Guttmacher Institute, 2018.

Gwiazda, Anna. "The Substantive Representation of Women in Poland." *Politics & Gender* 15, no. 2 (2019): 262–84.

Hall, Alexandra, and Georgios Antonopoulos. *Fake Meds Online: The Internet and the Transnational Market in Illicit Pharmaceuticals*. New York: Springer, 2016.

Hall, Peter. "What Has Been Achieved, What Have Been the Constraints and What Are the Future Priorities for Pharmaceutical Product-Related R&D Relevant to the Reproductive Health Needs of Developing Countries?" WHO Commission on Intellectual Property Rights, Innovation and Public Health, Geneva, 2005.

Haraway, Donna. "The Virtual Speculum in the New World Order." *Feminist Review* 55, no. 1 (1997): 22–72.

Hartmann, Betsy. *Reproductive Rights and Wrongs: The Global Politics of Population Control*. Boston, MA: South End Press, 1995

Haussman, Melissa. *Reproductive Rights and the State: Getting the Birth Control, Ru-486, and Morning-After Pills and the Gardasil Vaccine to the U.S. Market*. Santa Barbara, CA: ABC-CLIO, 2013.

Hervey, Tamara, and Sally Sheldon. "Abortion by Telemedicine in the European Union." *International Journal of Gynaecology & Obstetrics* 145, no. 1 (2019): 125–28.

Hodges, Sarah. "The Case of the 'Spurious Drugs Kingpin': Shifting Pills in Chennai, India." *Critical Public Health* 29, no. 4 (2019): 473–83.

Hornberger, Julia. "From Drug Safety to Drug Security: A Contemporary Shift in the Policing of Health." *Medical Anthropology Quarterly* 32, no. 3 (2018): 365–83.

Horner, Rory. "Pharmaceuticals and the Global South: A Healthy Challenge for Development Theory?" *Geography Compass* 10, no. 9 (2016): 363–77.

———. "Strategic Decoupling, Recoupling and Global Production Networks: India's Pharmaceutical Industry." *Journal of Economic Geography* 14, no. 6 (2014): 1117–40.

Horner, Rory, and James Murphy. "South-North and South-South Production Networks: Diverging Socio-Spatial Practices of Indian Pharmaceutical Firms." *Global Networks* 18, no. 2 (2018): 326–51.

Htun, Mala Nani. *Sex and the State: Abortion, Divorce, and the Family under Latin American Dictatorships and Democracies*. Cambridge: Cambridge University Press, 2003.

Inverardi-Ferri, Carlo. "Towards a Cultural Political Economy of the Illicit." *Progress in Human Geography* 45, no. 6 (2021): 1646–67.

Ivanitskaya, Lana, Jodi Brookins-Fisher, Irene O'Boyle, Danielle Vibbert, Dmitry Erofeev, and Lawrence Fulton. "Dirt Cheap and without Prescription: How Susceptible Are Young US Consumers to Purchasing Drugs from Rogue Internet Pharmacies?" *Journal of Medical Internet Research* 12, no. 2 (2010): e11.

Jackman, Jennifer. "Anatomy of a Feminist Victory." *Women & Politics* 24, no. 3 (2002): 81–99.

Jain, Dipika. "Time to Rethink Criminalisation of Abortion? Towards a Gender Justice Approach." *National University of Juridical Sciences Law Review* 12 (2019): 21–42.

Jasanoff, Sheila. *Science at the Bar: Law, Science, and Technology in America.* Cambridge, MA: Harvard University Press, 1997.

Jelinska, Kinga, and Susan Yanow. "Putting Abortion Pills into Women's Hands: Realizing the Full Potential of Medical Abortion." *Contraception* 97, no. 2 (2018): 86–89.

Jerman, Jenna, Tsuyoshi Onda, and Rachel K. Jones. "What Are People Looking for When They Google 'Self-Abortion'?" *Contraception* 97, no. 6 (2018): 510–14.

Joffe, Carole. "Abortion and Medicine: A Sociopolitical History." In *Management of Unintended and Abnormal Pregnancy*, edited by Maureen Paul, Steve Lichtenberg, Lynn Borgatta, David A. Grimes, Phillip G. Stubblefield, and Mitchell D. Creinin, 1–9. Hoboken, NJ: Wiley, 2009.

Joffe, Carole, and Tracy Weitz. "Normalizing the Exceptional: Incorporating the 'Abortion Pill' into Mainstream Medicine." *Social Science & Medicine* 56, no. 12 (2003): 2353–66.

Johnson, Dana, Melissa Madera, Rebecca Gomperts, and Abigail R. A. Aiken. "The Economic Context of Pursuing Online Medication Abortion in the United States." *SSM—Qualitative Research in Health* 1 (2021): 1–8.

Jones, Rachel. "How Commonly Do US Abortion Patients Report Attempts to Self-Induce?" *American Journal of Obstetrics and Gynecology* 204, no. 1 (2011): 1–23.

Jones, Rachel, and Jenna Jerman. "Population Group Abortion Rates and Lifetime Incidence of Abortion: United States, 2008–2014." *American Journal of Public Health* 107, no. 12 (2017): 1904–9.

Jones, Rachel, Elizabeth Witwer, and Jenna Jerman. *Abortion Incidence and Service Availability in the United States, 2017.* New York: Guttmacher Institute, 2019.

Kacpura, Krystyna, Karolina Wiekiewicz, Bozena Jawien, Anka Grywacz, and Martyna Zimniewska. "Twenty Years of Anti-Abortion Law in Poland." Federation for Women and Family Planning, Warsaw, 2013.

Kaplan, Laura. *The Story of Jane: The Legendary Underground Feminist Abortion Service.* Chicago: University of Chicago Press, 1997.

Kapp, Nathalie, Kelly Blanchard, Ernestina Coast, Bela Ganatra, Jane Harries, Katharine Footman, Ann Moore, et al. "Developing a Forward-Looking Agenda and Methodologies for Research of Self-Use of Medical Abortion." *Contraception* 97, no. 2 (2018): 184–88.

Karberg, Jeff. "Progress in the Challenge to Regulate Online Pharmacies." *Journal of Law & Health* 23 (2010): 113–42.

Kasstan, Ben, and Maya Unnithan. "Arbitrating Abortion: Sex-Selection and Care Work among Abortion Providers in England." *Medical Anthropology* 39, no. 6 (2020): 491–505.

Kimball, Natalie. *An Open Secret: The History of Unwanted Pregnancy and Abortion in Modern Bolivia.* New Brunswick, NJ: Rutgers University Press, 2020.

Kligman, Gail. *The Politics of Duplicity: Controlling Reproduction in Ceausescu's Romania.* Berkeley: University of California Press, 1998.

Kligman, Gail, and Susan Gal. *Reproducing Gender: Politics, Publics, and Everyday Life after Socialism.* Princeton, NJ: Princeton University Press, 2000.

Kline, Wendy. *Bodies of Knowledge: Sexuality, Reproduction, and Women's Health in the Second Wave.* Chicago: University of Chicago Press, 2010.

Koralewska, Inga, and Katarzyna Zielińska. "'Defending the Unborn,' 'Protecting Women' and 'Preserving Culture and Nation': Anti-Abortion Discourse in the Polish Right-Wing Press." *Culture, Health & Sexuality* (2021): 673–87.

Korolczuk, Elżbieta. "Explaining Mass Protests against Abortion Ban in Poland: The Power of Connective Action." *Zoon politikon*, no. 7 (2016): 91–113.

Korolczuk, Elżbieta, and Agnieszka Graff. "Gender as 'Ebola from Brussels': The Anticolonial Frame and the Rise of Illiberal Populism." *Signs* 43, no. 4 (2018): 797–821.

Krajewska, Atina. "The History of the Medical Profession in Poland and Its Impact on the Development of Abortion Law." Paper presented at workshop "Impact of the Medical Profession on Abortion Laws in Transitional and Post-Conflict Societies," University of Birmingham, April 4, 2019.

———. "Revisiting Polish Abortion Law: Doctors and Institutions in a Restrictive Regime." *Social & Legal Studies* 31, no. 3 (2022): 409–38.

———. "Rupture and Continuity: Abortion, the Medical Profession, and the Transitional State—a Polish Case Study." *Feminist Legal Studies* 29, no. 3 (2021): 323–50.

Kramer, Anne-Marie. "The Polish Parliament and the Making of Politics through Abortion: Nation, Gender and Democracy in the 1996 Liberalization Amendment Debate." *International Feminist Journal of Politics* 11, no. 1 (2009): 81–101.

Król, Agnieszka, and Paula Pustułka. "Women on Strike: Mobilizing against Reproductive Injustice in Poland." *International Feminist Journal of Politics* 20, no. 3 (2018): 366–84.

Kumar, Anuradha, Leila Hessini, and Ellen Mitchell. "Conceptualising Abortion Stigma." *Culture, Health & Sexuality* 11, no. 6 (2009): 625–39.

Lafaurie, María Mercedes, Daniel Grossman, Erika Troncoso, Deborah Billings, and Susana Chávez. "Women's Perspectives on Medical Abortion in Mexico, Colombia, Ecuador and Peru: A Qualitative Study." *Reproductive Health Matters* 13, no. 26 (2005): 75–83.

Lambert-Beatty, Carrie. "Twelve Miles: Boundaries of the New Art/Activism." *Signs* 33, no. 2 (2008): 309–27.

Lennerhed, Lena. "Sherri Finkbine Flew to Sweden: Abortion and Disability in the Early 1960s." In *Abortion across Borders: Transnational Travel and Access to Abortion Services*, edited by Christabelle Sethna and Gayle Davis, 25–45. Baltimore: Johns Hopkins University Press, 2019.

Lewis, Sophie. *Full Surrogacy Now: Feminism against Family.* London: Verso Books, 2021.

Liang, Bryan A., and Tim K. Mackey. "Online Availability and Safety of Drugs in Shortage: A Descriptive Study of Internet Vendor Characteristics." *Journal of Medical Internet Research* 14, no. 1 (2012): e1999.

Lowe, Pam. *Reproductive Health and Maternal Sacrifice: Women, Choice and Responsibility*. New York: Springer, 2016.

Luibhéid, Eithne. *Pregnant on Arrival: Making the Illegal Immigrant*. Minneapolis: University of Minnesota Press, 2013.

Luker, Kristin. *Abortion and the Politics of Motherhood*. Berkeley: University of California Press, 1985.

Luna, Zakiya, and Kristin Luker. "Reproductive Justice." *Annual Review of Law and Social Science* 9 (2013): 327–52.

MacDonald, Margaret. "Misoprostol: the Social Life of a Life-Saving Drug in Global Maternal Health." *Science, Technology & Human Values* 46, no. 2 (2021): 376–401.

MacSimoin, Alan. "How Free Can You Be If You Can't Even Control Your Own Body?" *Red & Black Revolution*, no. 14 (2008): 15–22.

Maffi, Irene. "The Production of Ignorance about Medication Abortion in Tunisia: Between State Policies, Medical Opposition, Patriarchal Logics and Islamic Revival." *Reproductive Biomedicine & Society Online* 14 (2022): 111–20.

McAvoy, Sandra. "The Catholic Church and Fertility Control in Ireland: The Making of a Dystopian Regime." In *The Abortion Papers Ireland: Volume 2*, edited by Aideen Quilty, Sinead Kennedy, and Catherine Conlon, 47–62. Cork: Cork University Press, 2015.

McDonnell, Orla, and Padraig Murphy. "Mediating Abortion Politics in Ireland: Media Framing of the Death of Savita Halappanavar." *Critical Discourse Studies* 16, no. 1 (2019): 1–20.

McGoey, Linsey. "Strategic Unknowns: Towards a Sociology of Ignorance." *Economy and Society* 41, no. 1 (2012): 1–16.

———. *The Unknowers: How Strategic Ignorance Rules the World*. London: Bloomsbury, 2019.

McReynolds-Pérez, Julia. "No Doctors Required: Lay Activist Expertise and Pharmaceutical Abortion in Argentina." *Signs* 42, no. 2 (2017): 349–75.

Mijatović, Dunja. "Commissioner for Human Rights of the Council of Europe: Report Following Her Visit to Poland from 11 to 15 March 2019." Council of Europe, Commissioner for Human Rights, Strasbourg, 2019.

Millar, Erica. *Happy Abortions: Our Bodies in the Era of Choice*. London: Zed Books, 2017.

Miller, Rosalind, Francis Wafula, Chima Onoka, Prasanna Saligram, Anita Musiega, Dosila Ogira, Ikedichi Okpani, et al. "When Technology Precedes Regulation: The Challenges and Opportunities of E-Pharmacy in Low-Income and Middle-Income Countries." *BMJ Global Health* 6, no. 5 (2021): e005405.

Mishtal, Joanna. "Matters of 'Conscience': The Politics of Reproductive Healthcare in Poland." *Medical Anthropology Quarterly* 23, no. 2 (2009): 161–83.

———. "Neoliberal Reforms and Privatisation of Reproductive Health Services in Post-Socialist Poland." *Reproductive Health Matters* 18, no. 36 (2010): 56–66.

————. *The Politics of Morality: The Church, the State, and Reproductive Rights in Postsocialist Poland.* Athens: Ohio University Press, 2015.

Mitchell, Paul. "Transcending an Ethnic Party System: The Impacts of Consociational Governance on Electoral Dynamics and the Party System." In *Aspects of the Belfast Agreement,* edited by Rick Wilford, 28–48. Oxford: Oxford University Press, 2001.

Mondal, Shamim S., and Viswanath Pingali. "Competition and Intellectual Property Policies in the Indian Pharmaceutical Sector." *Vikalpa* 42, no. 2 (2017): 61–79.

Moore, Ann, Alyssa Browne, and Suzanne Bell. "Capturing Medical Methods of Abortion Sales Data in India." Paper presented at the Population Association of America, Denver, CO, 2018. Full paper available at paa.confex.com.

Moreau, Caroline, Mridula Shankar, Anna Glasier, Sharon Cameron, and Kristina Gemzell-Danielsson. "Abortion Regulation in Europe in the Era of COVID-19: A Spectrum of Policy Responses." *BMJ Sexual & Reproductive Health* 47, no. 4 (2021): 1–8.

Moreau, Caroline, James Trussell, Julie Desfreres, and Nathalie Bajos. "Medical vs. Surgical Abortion: The Importance of Women's Choice." *Contraception* 84, no. 3 (2011): 224–29.

Moseson, Heidi, Stephanie Herold, Sofia Filippa, Jill Barr-Walker, Sarah Baum, and Caitlin Gerdts. "Self-Managed Abortion: A Systematic Scoping Review." *Best Practice & Research Clinical Obstetrics & Gynaecology* 63 (2020): 87–110.

Muhl, Csilla. "Ru-486: Legal and Policy Issues Confronting the Food and Drug Administration." *Journal of Legal Medicine* 14, no. 2 (1993): 319–47.

Munro Prescott, Heather. *The Morning After: A History of Emergency Contraception in the United States.* New Brunswick, NJ: Rutgers University Press, 2011.

Murphy, Michelle. *Seizing the Means of Reproduction: Entanglements of Feminism, Health, and Technoscience.* Durham, NC: Duke University Press, 2012.

Murray, Claire. "The Protection of Life During Pregnancy Act 2013: Suicide, Dignity and the Irish Discourse on Abortion." *Social & Legal Studies* 25, no. 6 (2016): 667–98.

Murray, Melissa. "Race-ing Roe: Reproductive Justice, Racial Justice, and the Battle for *Roe v. Wade.*" *Harvard Law Review* 134 (2020): 2025–2102.

Murtagh, Chloe, Elisa Wells, Elizabeth G. Raymond, Francine Coeytaux, and Beverly Winikoff. "Exploring the Feasibility of Obtaining Mifepristone and Misoprostol from the Internet." *Contraception* 97, no. 4 (2018): 287–91.

Myers, Caitlin, Rachel Jones, and Ushma Upadhyay. "Predicted Changes in Abortion Access and Incidence in a Post-Roe World." *Contraception* 100, no. 5 (2019): 367–73.

Nandagiri, Rishita. "'Like a Mother-Daughter Relationship': Community Health Intermediaries' Knowledge of and Attitudes to Abortion in Karnataka, India." *Social Science & Medicine* 239 (2019): 112525.

Nash, Catherine, Lorraine Dennis, and Brian Graham. "Putting the Border in Place: Customs Regulation in the Making of the Irish Border, 1921–1945." *Journal of Historical Geography* 36, no. 4 (2010): 421–31.

Nash, Elizabeth. "Ohio as a Window into Recent US Trends on Abortion Access and Restrictions." *American Journal of Public Health* 110, no. 8 (2020): 1115–16.

Nash, Elizabeth, and Joerg Dreweke. "The US Abortion Rate Continues to Drop: Once Again, State Abortion Restrictions Are Not the Main Driver." *Guttmacher Policy Review* 22 (2019): 41–45.

Nawojski, Radosław, Magdalena Pluta, and Katarzyna Zielińska. "The Black Protests: A Struggle for (Re)Definition of Intimate Citizenship." *Praktyka Teoretyczna* 30, no. 4 (2018): 51–74.

Nelson, Jennifer. *More Than Medicine: A History of the Feminist Women's Health Movement.* New York: New York University Press, 2015.

———. *Women of Color and the Reproductive Rights Movement.* New York: New York University Press, 2003.

Nowicka, Wanda. "The Anti-Abortion Act in Poland—the Legal and Actual State." In *Reproductive Rights in Poland: The Effects of the Anti-Abortion Law,* edited by Wanda Nowicka, 17–44. Warsaw: Federation for Women and Family Planning, 2008.

Oberman, Michelle. *Her Body, Our Laws: On the Front Lines of the Abortion War, from El Salvador to Oklahoma.* Boston, MA: Beacon Press, 2018.

O'Reilly, Emily. *Masterminds of the Right.* Cork: Attic Press, 1992.

Orihuela-Cortés, Fabiola, and Ma Luisa Marván. "Estigma hacia el aborto y sus consecuencias: Acciones para reducirlo." *Revista Digital Universitaria* 22, no. 4 (2021): 1–12.

O'Rourke, Catherine. "Advocating Abortion Rights in Northern Ireland: Local and Global Tensions." *Social & Legal Studies* 25, no. 6 (2016): 716–40.

O'Shaughnessy, Aideen. "Bodies of Change: Analysing the Embodied and Affective Movement for Abortion Rights in Ireland." PhD dissertation, University of Cambridge, 2022. https://doi.org/10.17863/CAM.87018.

Ost, David. *The Defeat of Solidarity: Anger and Politics in Postcommunist Europe.* Ithaca, NY: Cornell University Press, 2005

Paltrow, Lynn, and Jeanne Flavin. "Arrests of and Forced Interventions on Pregnant Women in the United States, 1973–2005: Implications for Women's Legal Status and Public Health." *Journal of Health Politics, Policy and Law* 38, no. 2 (2013): 299–343.

Parsons, Jordan, and Elizabeth Chloe Romanis. *Early Medical Abortion, Equality of Access, and the Telemedical Imperative.* Oxford: Oxford University Press, 2021.

Petchesky, Rosalind. *Abortion and Woman's Choice: The State, Sexuality, and Reproductive Freedom.* London: Longman, 1984.

Pierson, Claire. "One Step Forwards, Two Steps Back: Women's Rights 20 Years after the Good Friday Agreement." *Parliamentary Affairs* 71, no. 2 (2018): 461–81.

Pierson, Claire, Fiona Bloomer, Les Allamby, Emma Campbell, Breedagh Hughes, Laura McLaughlin, and Rachel Powell. "After a CEDAW Optional Protocol Inquiry into Abortion Law: A Conversation with Activists for Change in Northern Ireland." *International Feminist Journal of Politics* 24, no. 2 (2022): 312–28.

Pierson, Claire, and Jennifer Thomson. "Allies or Opponents? Power-Sharing, Civil Society, and Gender." *Nationalism and Ethnic Politics* 24, no. 1 (2018): 100–115.

Pizzarossa, Lucía Berro, and Rishita Nandagiri. "Self-Managed Abortion: A Constellation of Actors, a Cacophony of Laws?" *Sexual and Reproductive Health Matters* 29, no. 1 (2021): 23–30.

Płotka, Bartosz, and Cristina-Iulia Ghenu. "The Implications of Abortion Underground's Institutionalization for the Management Studies." *Revista de Management Comparat International* 18, no. 5 (2017): 482–90.

Powell-Jackson, Timothy, Rajib Acharya, Veronique Filippi, and Carine Ronsmans. "Delivering Medical Abortion at Scale: A Study of the Retail Market for Medical Abortion in Madhya Pradesh, India." *PLOS ONE* 10, no. 3 (2015): e0120637.

Proctor, Robert. "Agnotology: A Missing Term to Describe the Cultural Production of Ignorance (and Its Study)." In *Agnotology: The Making and Unmaking of Ignorance*, edited by Robert Proctor and Londa Schiebinger, 1–36. Stanford: Stanford University Press, 2008.

Pruitt, Sandi, and Patricia Dolan Mullen. "Contraception or Abortion? Inaccurate Descriptions of Emergency Contraception in Newspaper Articles, 1992–2002." *Contraception* 71, no. 1 (2005): 14–21.

Purewal, Navtej. "Sex Selective Abortion, Neoliberal Patriarchy and Structural Violence in India." *Feminist Review* 119, no. 1 (2018): 20–38.

Quet, Mathieu. "Pharmaceutical Capitalism and Its Logistics: Access to Hepatitis C Treatment." *Theory, Culture & Society* 35, no. 2 (2018): 67–89.

———. "Values in Motion: Anti-Counterfeiting Measures and the Securitization of Pharmaceutical Flows." *Journal of Cultural Economy* 10, no. 2 (2017): 150–62.

Quilty, Aideen, Sinead Kennedy, and Catherine Conlon, eds. *The Abortion Papers Ireland: Volume 2*. Cork: Cork University Press, 2015.

Raekstad, Paul, and Sofa Saio Gradin. *Prefigurative Politics: Building Tomorrow Today*. Bristol: Polity Press, 2020.

Raifman, Sarah, Megan Orlando, Sally Rafie, and Daniel Grossman. "Medication Abortion: Potential for Improved Patient Access through Pharmacies." *Journal of the American Pharmacists Association* 58, no. 4 (2018): 377–81.

Rajan, Kaushik Sunder. *Pharmocracy: Value, Politics, and Knowledge in Global Biomedicine*. Durham, NC: Duke University Press, 2017.

Ramshaw, Sara. "Commentary on Family Planning Association of Northern Ireland v the Minister for Health, Social Services and Public Safety." In *Northern/Irish Feminist Judgments*, edited by Aoife O'Donoghue, Julie McCandless, and Mairead Enright, 433–54. Oxford: Hart Publishing, 2016.

Raymond, Elizabeth, Erica Chong, and Paul Hyland. "Increasing Access to Abortion with Telemedicine." *JAMA Internal Medicine* 176, no. 5 (2016): 585–86.

Raymond, Elizabeth, Erica Chong, Beverly Winikoff, Ingrida Platais, Meighan Mary, Tatyana Lotarevich, Philicia Castillo, et al. "TelAbortion: Evaluation of a Direct to Patient Telemedicine Abortion Service in the United States." *Contraception* 100, no. 3 (2019): 173–77.

Raymond, Elizabeth, Margo Harrison, and Mark Weaver. "Efficacy of Misoprostol Alone for First-Trimester Medical Abortion: A Systematic Review." *Obstetrics and Gynecology* 133, no. 1 (2019): 137–47.

Reagan, Leslie. *When Abortion Was a Crime: Women, Medicine, and Law in the United States, 1867–1973*. Berkeley: University of California Press, 1997.

Reichertz, Peter, and Melinda Friend. "Hiding behind Agency Discretion: The Food and Drug Administration's Personal Use Drug Importation Policy." *Cornell Journal of Law & Public Policy* 9 (1999): 493–522.

Reidy, Theresa. "The 2018 Referendum: Over before It Began!" In *After Repeal: Rethinking Abortion Politics*, edited by Kath Browne and Sydney Calkin, 21–35. London: Zed Books, 2020.

Rhodes, Natalie, and Remco van de Pas. "Mapping Buyer's Clubs; What Role Do They Play in Achieving Equitable Access to Medicines?" *Global Public Health* 17, no. 9 (2022): 1842–53.

Riddle, John. *Eve's Herbs: A History of Contraception and Abortion in the West*. Cambridge, MA: Harvard University Press, 1997.

Roberts, Dorothy. *Killing the Black Body: Race, Reproduction, and the Meaning of Liberty*. New York: Vintage, 1999.

———. "Reproductive Justice, Not Just Rights." *Dissent* 62, no. 4 (2015): 79–82.

Ross, Loretta. "What Is Reproductive Justice?" In *Reproductive Justice Briefing Book: A Primer on Reproductive Justice and Social Change*, edited by SisterSong, 4–5. Atlanta, GA: Pro-Choice Public Education Project and SisterSong Women of Color Reproductive Justice Collective, 2007.

Ross, Loretta, and Rickie Solinger. *Reproductive Justice: An Introduction*. Oakland: University of California Press, 2017.

Rossiter, Ann. *Ireland's Hidden Diaspora: The "Abortion Trail" and the Making of a London-Irish Underground 1980–2000*. London: IASC Publishing, 2009.

Roth, Rachel. *Making Women Pay: The Hidden Costs of Fetal Rights*. Ithaca, NY: Cornell University Press, 2000.

Rubin, Gayle. "The Traffic in Women: Notes on the 'Political Economy' of Sex." In *Toward an Anthropology of Women*, edited by Rayna Reiter, 157–210. New York: Monthly Review Press, 1975.

Sadurski, Wojciech. *Poland's Constitutional Breakdown*. Oxford: Oxford University Press, 2019.

Sanabria, Emilia. *Plastic Bodies: Sex Hormones and Menstrual Suppression in Brazil*. Durham, NC: Duke University Press, 2016.

Sanger, Carol. *About Abortion: Terminating Pregnancy in Twenty-First Century America*. Cambridge, MA: Harvard University Press, 2017.

Sassen, Saskia. "Towards a Sociology of Information Technology." *Current Sociology* 50, no. 3 (2002): 365–88.

Saurette, Paul, and Kelly Gordon. *The Changing Voice of the Anti-Abortion Movement: The Rise of "Pro-Woman" Rhetoric in Canada and the United States*. Toronto: University of Toronto Press, 2016.

Schulman, Sarah. *Let the Record Show: A Political History of Act Up New York, 1987–1993.* New York: Farrar, Straus and Giroux, 2021.

Sheldon, Sally. *Beyond Control: Medical Power and Abortion Law.* London: Pluto Press, 1997.

———. "Empowerment and Privacy? Home Use of Abortion Pills in the Republic of Ireland." *Signs* 43, no. 4 (2018): 823–49.

———. "How Can a State Control Swallowing? The Home Use of Abortion Pills in Ireland." *Reproductive Health Matters* 24, no. 48 (2016): 90–101.

———. "The Medical Framework and Early Medical Abortion in the U.K.: How Can a State Control Swallowing?" In *Abortion Law in Transnational Perspective: Cases and Controversies,* edited by Rebecca Cook, Joanna Erdman, and Bernard Dickens, 189–209. Philadelphia: University of Pennsylvania Press, 2014.

Sheldon, Sally, Jane O'Neill, Clare Parker, and Gayle Davis. "'Too Much, Too Indigestible, Too Fast'? The Decades of Struggle for Abortion Law Reform in Northern Ireland." *Modern Law Review* 83, no. 4 (2020): 761–96.

Side, Katherine. "Contract, Charity, and Honorable Entitlement: Social Citizenship and the 1967 Abortion Act in Northern Ireland after the Good Friday Agreement." *Social Politics: International Studies in Gender, State & Society* 13, no. 1 (2006): 89–116.

Siegel, Reva. "The Right's Reasons: Constitutional Conflict and the Spread of Woman-Protective Antiabortion Argument." *Duke Law Journal* 57 (2008): 1641–92.

Simonds, Wendy. *Abortion at Work: Ideology and Practice in a Feminist Clinic.* New Brunswick, NJ: Rutgers University Press, 1996.

Simonds, Wendy, Charlotte Ellertson, Kimberly Springer, and Beverly Winikoff. "Abortion, Revised: Participants in the U.S. Clinical Trials Evaluate Mifepristone." *Social Science & Medicine* 46, no. 10 (1998): 1313–23.

Singer, Elyse Ona. "Realizing Abortion Rights at the Margins of Legality in Mexico." *Medical Anthropology* 38, no. 2 (2018): 167–81.

Singh, Susheela, et al. *Abortion and Unintended Pregnancy in Six Indian States: Findings and Implications for Policies and Programs.* New York: Guttmacher Institute, 2018.

Sitrin, Marina. *Everyday Revolutions: Horizontalism and Autonomy in Argentina.* London: Zed Books, 2012.

Smart, Carol. *Feminism and the Power of Law.* London: Routledge, 2002.

Smith, Mikaela, Zoe Muzyczka, Payal Chakraborty, Elaina Johns-Wolfe, Jenny Higgins, Danielle Bessett, and Alison Norris. "Abortion Travel within the United States: An Observational Study of Cross-State Movement to Obtain Abortion Care in 2017." *The Lancet Regional Health—Americas* 10 (2022): 100214.

Smyth, Lisa. *Abortion and Nation: The Politics of Reproduction in Contemporary Ireland.* London: Routledge, 2005.

———. "The Cultural Politics of Sexuality and Reproduction in Northern Ireland." *Sociology* 40, no. 4 (2006): 663–80.

Solazzo, Alexa. "Different and Not Equal: The Uneven Association of Race, Poverty, and Abortion Laws on Abortion Timing." *Social Problems* 66, no. 4 (2019): 519–47.

Solinger, Rickie. *Beggars and Choosers: How the Politics of Choice Shapes Adoption, Abortion, and Welfare in the United States.* New York: Macmillan, 2001.

———. *Pregnancy and Power: A Short History of Reproductive Politics in America.* New York: New York University Press, 2007.

Srivastava, Aradhana, Malvika Saxena, Joanna Percher, and Nadia Diamond-Smith. "Pathways to Seeking Medication Abortion Care: A Qualitative Research in Uttar Pradesh, India." *PLOS ONE* 14, no. 5 (2019): e0216738.

Statz, Michele, and Lisa Pruitt. "To Recognize the Tyranny of Distance: A Spatial Reading of *Whole Woman's Health v. Hellerstedt.*" *Environment and Planning A: Economy and Space* 51, no. 5 (2019): 1106–27.

Stephens-Davidowitz, Seth. *Everybody Lies: What the Internet Can Tell Us about Who We Really Are.* London: Bloomsbury, 2018.

Stewart, Danièle. "The Women's Movement in France." *Signs* 6, no. 2 (1980): 350–54.

Suh, Siri. *Dying to Count: Post-Abortion Care and Global Reproductive Health Politics in Senegal.* New Brunswick, NJ: Rutgers University Press, 2021.

Sutton, Barbara. "Zonas de clandestinidad y 'nuda vida': Mujeres, cuerpo y aborto." *Revista Estudos Feministas* 25 (2017): 889–902.

Szelewa, Dorota. "Killing 'Unborn Children'? The Catholic Church and Abortion Law in Poland since 1989." *Social & Legal Studies* 25, no. 6 (2016): 741–64.

———. "The Second Wave of Anti-Feminism? Post-Crisis Maternalist Policies and the Attack on the Concept of Gender in Poland." *Gender rovné příležitosti výzkum* 15, no. 2 (2014): 33–47.

Takeshita, Chikako. *The Global Biopolitics of the IUD: How Science Constructs Contraceptive Users and Women's Bodies.* Cambridge, MA: MIT Press, 2012.

Tarducci, Mónica. "Escenas claves de la lucha por el derecho al aborto en Argentina." *Salud Colectiva* 14 (2018): 425–32.

Taussig, Michael. *Defacement: Public Secrecy and the Labor of the Negative.* Stanford: Stanford University Press, 1999.

Thakur, Nishpriha. "Sub-Standard or Sub-Legal? India's International Pharmaceutical Traders and the Problem of Fake Drugs." *Medical Anthropology Theory* (forthcoming 2023).

Thomsen, Carly, Zach Levitt, Christopher Gernon, and Penelope Spencer. "US Anti-Abortion Ideology on the Move: Mobile Crisis Pregnancy Centers as Unruly, Unmappable, and Ungovernable." *Political Geography* 92 (2022): 102523.

Thomson, Jennifer. "Abortion and Same-Sex Marriage: How Are Non-Sectarian Controversial Issues Discussed in Northern Irish Politics?" *Irish Political Studies* 31, no. 4 (2016): 483–501.

———. *Abortion Law and Political Institutions: Explaining Policy Resistance.* New York: Springer, 2018.

Tonge, Jonathan. "The Impact of Withdrawal from the European Union upon Northern Ireland." *Political Quarterly* 87, no. 3 (2016): 338–42.

Torrance, David. *Devolution in Northern Ireland, 1998–2020.* London: House of Commons, 2020.

Tschann, Mary, Elizabeth Ly, Sara Hilliard, and Hannah Lange. "Changes to Medication Abortion Clinical Practices in Response to the Covid-19 Pandemic." *Contraception* 104, no. 1 (2021): 77–81.

Tyagi, Kalpana. "Mergers between Generics: How Competition Commission of India Promotes Innovation and Access through Merger Control." *Global Antitrust Review*, no. 11 (2018): 33–59.

Undurraga, Verónica. "Criminalisation under Scrutiny: How Constitutional Courts Are Changing Their Narrative by Using Public Health Evidence in Abortion Cases." *Sexual and Reproductive Health Matters* 27, no. 1 (2019): 41–51.

Upadhyay, Ushma, Alice Cartwright, and Daniel Grossman. "Barriers to Abortion Care and Incidence of Attempted Self-Managed Abortion among Individuals Searching Google for Abortion Care: A National Prospective Study." *Contraception* 106 (2022): 49–56.

Upadhyay, Ushma, Nicole Johns, Sarah Combellick, Julia Kohn, Lisa Keder, and Sarah Roberts. "Comparison of Outcomes before and after Ohio's Law Mandating Use of the FDA-Approved Protocol for Medication Abortion: A Retrospective Cohort Study." *PLOS Medicine* 13, no. 8 (2016): e1002110.

Upadhyay, Ushma, Rosalyn Schroeder, and Sarah Roberts. "Adoption of No-Test and Telehealth Medication Abortion Care among Independent Abortion Providers in Response to Covid-19." *Contraception: X* 2 (2020): 100049.

Verma, Nisha, Vinita Goyal, Daniel Grossman, Jamila Perritt, and Grace Shih. "Interim Clinical Recommendations: Self-Managed Abortion." *Society of Family Planning* (2022). https://doi.org/10.46621/ZRDX9581.

Weeks, Andrew, Christian Fiala, and Peter Safar. "Misoprostol and the Debate over Off-Label Drug Use." *BJOG: An International Journal of Obstetrics & Gynaecology* 112, no. 3 (2005): 269–72.

Weitz, Tracy, C. Foster, D. Ellertson, D. Grossman, and F. Stewart. "'Medical' and 'Surgical' Abortion: Rethinking the Modifiers." *Contraception* 69, no. 1 (2004): 77–78.

West, Robin. "From Choice to Reproductive Justice: De-Constitutionalizing Abortion Rights." *Yale Law Journal* 118 (2008): 1394–1433.

Whitaker, Robin, and Goretti Horgan. "Abortion Governance in the New Northern Ireland." In *A Fragmented Landscape: Abortion Governance and Protest Logics in Europe*, edited by Silvia De Zordo, Joanna Mishtal, and Lorena Anton, 245–65. New York: Berghahn Books, 2016.

Wilson, Kalpana. "In the Name of Reproductive Rights: Race, Neoliberalism and the Embodied Violence of Population Policies." *New Formations* 91 (2017): 50–68.

Winikoff, Beverly, and Carolyn Westhoff. "Fifteen Years: Looking Back and Looking Forward." *Contraception* 92, no. 3 (2015): 177–78.

Wittich, Christopher, Christopher Burkle, and William Lanier. "Ten Common Questions (and Their Answers) about Off-Label Drug Use." *Mayo Clinic Proceedings* 87 (2012): 982–90.

Wong, Aaron James. "Money, Meet Mouth: The Era of Regulation and Prescription Drug Importation/Reimportation." *Health Law & Policy Brief* 4 (2010): 48–61.

World Health Organization (WHO). *Abortion Care Guideline*. Geneva: WHO, 2022.

Yokoe, Ryo, Rachel Rowe, Saswati Sanyal Choudhury, Anjali Rani, Farzana Zahir, and Manisha Nair. "Unsafe Abortion and Abortion-Related Death among 1.8 Million Women in India." *BMJ Global Health* 4, no. 3 (2019): e001491.

Zaręba, Kornelia, Krzysztof Herman, Ewelina Kołb-Sielecka, and Grzegorz Jakiel. "Abortion in Countries with Restrictive Abortion Laws—Possible Directions and Solutions from the Perspective of Poland." *Healthcare* 9, no. 11 (2021): 1594.

Zaręba, Kornelia, Stanisław Wójtowicz, Jolanta Banasiewicz, Krzysztof Herman, and Grzegorz Jakiel. "The Influence of Abortion Law on the Frequency of Pregnancy Terminations: A Retrospective Comparative Study." *International Journal of Environmental Research and Public Health* 18, no. 8 (2021): 4099.

Zięba, Antoni. "Podziemie aborcyjne w Polsce" [Underground abortion in Poland]. Polskiego Stowarzyszenia Obrońców Życia Człowieka [Polish Association of Defenders of Human Life, Krakow], 2006.

Ziegler, Mary. *Abortion and the Law in America: Roe v. Wade to the Present*. Cambridge: Cambridge University Press, 2020.

———. "After Life: Governmental Interests and the New Antiabortion Incrementalism." *University of Miami Law Review* 73, no. 1 (2018): 78–138.

———. *After Roe: The Lost History of the Abortion Debate*. Cambridge, MA: Harvard University Press, 2015.

———. "The Jurisprudence of Uncertainty: Knowledge, Science, and Abortion." *Wisconsin Law Review* (2018): 317–68.

———. "Sexing Harris: The Law and Politics of the Movement to Defund Planned Parenthood." *Buffalo Law Review* 60 (2012): 701–48.

INDEX

Founded in 1893,
UNIVERSITY OF CALIFORNIA PRESS
publishes bold, progressive books and journals
on topics in the arts, humanities, social sciences,
and natural sciences—with a focus on social
justice issues—that inspire thought and action
among readers worldwide.

The UC PRESS FOUNDATION
raises funds to uphold the press's vital role
as an independent, nonprofit publisher, and
receives philanthropic support from a wide
range of individuals and institutions—and from
committed readers like you. To learn more, visit
ucpress.edu/supportus.